Joslin Diabetes Manual

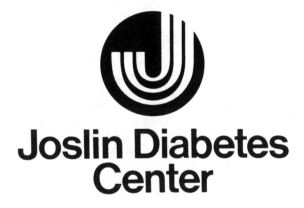

Joslin Diabetes Center

Joslin Diabetes Manual

LEO P. KRALL, M.D.

*Joslin Diabetes Center, New England Deaconess Hospital,
and Harvard Medical School, Boston, Massachusetts.
Past-President, International Diabetes Federation; Chairman of the
Board, Diabetes Research and Education Foundation.*

RICHARD S. BEASER, M.D.

*Joslin Diabetes Center, New England Deaconess Hospital,
and Harvard Medical School, Boston, Massachusetts. Chairman,
Patient Education Committee, Joslin Diabetes Center.*

TWELFTH EDITION

LEA & FEBIGER   1989   PHILADELPHIA, LONDON

Lea & Febiger
200 Chester Field Parkway
Malvern, Pennsylvania   19355-9725
U.S.A.
(215) 251-2230

First Edition, 1918
Second Edition, 1919
Third Edition, 1924
Fourth Edition, 1929
Fifth Edition, 1934
Sixth Edition, 1937
Seventh Edition, 1941
Eighth Edition, 1948
Ninth Edition, 1953
Tenth Edition, 1959
Eleventh Edition, 1978

LIBRARY OF CONGRESS
Library of Congress Cataloging-in-Publication Data

Joslin diabetes manual / by physicians of the Joslin Diabetes Center.
—12th ed. [edited by] Leo P. Krall, Richard S. Beaser.
    p.   cm.
Includes index.
ISBN 0–8121–1120–6
    1. Diabetes.   I. Krall, Leo P.   II. Beaser, Richard S.
III. Joslin Diabetes Center.
[DNLM: 1. Diabetes Mellitus—popular works.   WK 850 J835]
RC660.J58 1988
616.4'62—dc 19
DNLM/DLC
for Library of Congress   88–6852
                                                                     CIP

PRINTED IN THE UNITED STATES OF AMERICA
Print Number 10   9   8   7   6   5   4   3

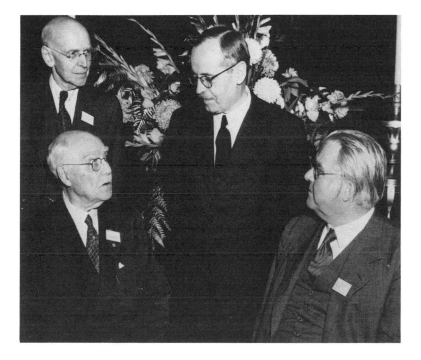

Photograph taken during the celebration of the twenty-fifth anniversary of the discovery of insulin. International Diabetes Clinic, Indianapolis, Indiana, September 23, 1946. Seated, left to right: J. K. Lilly, Sr., chairman of the board, Eli Lilly Co.; H. C. Hagedorn, discoverer of PZI (long-acting protamine zinc) insulin (1936), and, with others, discoverer of intermediate-acting neutral protamine zinc insulin ("Neutral Protamine Hagedorn" or NPH). Standing, left to right: Elliott P. Joslin, M.D., founder of the Joslin Clinic; Professor Bernardo Houssay, who elucidated the relationship of the pituitary gland to diabetes and was co-winner of the Nobel prize for physiology in 1947. (Courtesy of Eli Lilly & Co.)

Prologue

Nearly every book ever written, including books about diabetes, begins with a nonspecific and often confusing chapter. It is variously called the preface, introduction, foreword, or any number of other titles and is most often none of these.

It usually contains a strange collection of items such as a dedication of the book to largely ignored (during the writing and editing) members of the family or to a former professor who has generally long forgotten the authors. There is always profuse thanks to all those who helped in any way in the creation of the medical or literary effort. Family members, however, are usually quite inured to neglect by physicians, former mentors are often skeptical of anything performed by their prodigies, and the section following this one very adequately expresses our gratitude for the enormous input of our many assistants and collaborators.

Because there must be a beginning to everything, however, this could best be described as an overture to the things that follow. It should be what it is—a prologue!

Since the discovery of insulin and especially in the past two decades, the influx of research and clinical advances has made it difficult for anyone with diabetes to understand the game or even who the players are without some form of scorecard. The *Joslin Diabetes Manual*, which was first published 70 years ago, was developed as a guide to help people with diabetes find their way through the jungle of facts and fancies and to impart directions so they might be understood.

The first patient in the Joslin Clinic was seen by the late Dr. Elliott P. Joslin in 1898. Now, more than 160,000 patients later, we have an enormous amount of experience to draw on. This twelfth edition is built on the foundations of the original manual of 1918. The purpose of that first edition was to help people survive. This edition has the same goal, except now there are many more positive things to tell. Indeed, survival is only one goal. Dr. Joslin and his associates did their job well, because the half-millionth copy of the manual was read by someone many years ago. The foundation is the same, but the building is different, taller, more modern. Many of the goals of treatment have changed. In this edition, not only are many topics new, but some were unheard of when past editions were written. To live long is good, but to live more productively and happily is every bit as vital.

Some facts are inescapable. Diabetes began a long time ago. Considering how many factors are involved in its development—heredity, stress, immunologic changes, possibly infections, etc.—it is amazing that so many—possibly 100 million persons in the *known world*—have diabetes. You are not alone!

The Past

Very early medical descriptions of diabetes (1500 B.C.) were reasonably accurate. Arabic and Chinese writings describe the classic symptoms of passing vast amounts of sweet urine through the body. Susruta (400 B.C.) and Charaka (A.D. 6) also were well aware of diabetes. The Greek physician Arteus (ca. A.D. 200) apparently was the first to call it *diabetes* (to flow through; urine). Later the Latin description *mellitus* (sweetened or honey-like) was added.

In the middle of the nineteenth century, a series of discoveries advanced the knowledge of diabetes. For example, in the middle 1860s Langerhans described clusters of cells comprising only a small percentage of all the cells in the pancreas; these were called the islets of Langerhans. In 1889 von Mering and Minkowski found diabetes-like symptoms in dogs whose pancreases had been removed. New discoveries came quickly, and gradually diabetes as a disease was identified. Nothing for treatment was available through, until the beginning of the 1920s—nothing *specific* for treatment, that is. There was treatment that had some measure of success. This was relative starvation. Those with what is now known as type I (insulin-dependent) diabetes had very short careers. In fact, almost half of the people with diabetes who died at the New England Deaconess Hospital at that time, before insulin, succumbed to ketoacidosis and coma. (Now the figure in the better institutions is less that 1%). People with type II (non-insulin-dependent) diabetes often lived for several or more years, if they heroically reduced their weight to live with the small amount of insulin that might be available. In a sense, this was organized starvation, which enabled them to cope until they developed some form of infection (this was

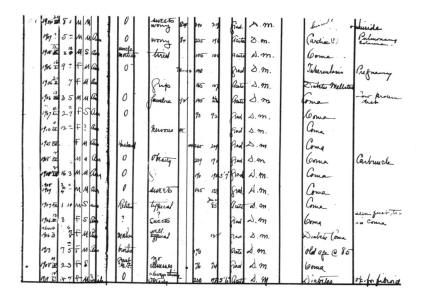

FIG. P–1. Actual notes made by Dr. Elliott P. Joslin concerning the fate of his first 18 patients. Note the cause of death in those preinsulin days was nearly always diabetic coma. A record of all patients was kept during his life and has been ever since.

before antibiotics). If they had insulin resistance, most often they did not survive (Fig. P–1).

Insulin Changes History

Best and Banting made what is considered the first available and useful insulin in 1921, and they history of diabetes changed (Fig. P–2). But this was the result of the efforts of many people working in many places. One of the lesser known pioneers of that time was Dr. Nicholas Paulesco of Bucharest, who reported on the effects of a pancreatic extract he called "pancreine," which apparently depressed blood and urine glucose levels as well as the ketone bodies in dogs whose pancreases had been removed. This probably contained insulin, as did the extracts of others, but the "isletin" of Banting and Best, which led to a Nobel prize, was the most effective and was developed in surroundings (Toronto) that made the manufacture and distribution so possible. Through the summer preceding their earth-shaking discovery they extracted and minced pancreatic

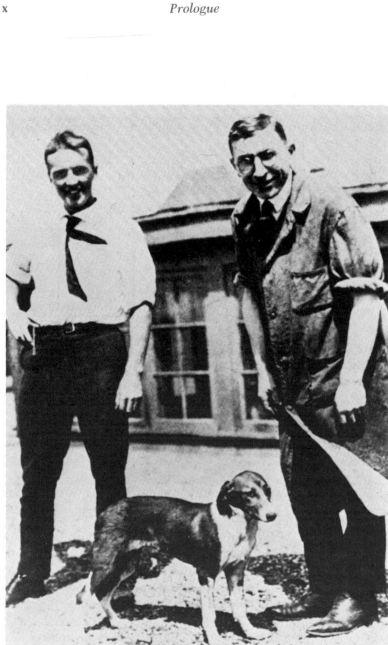

FIG. P–2. Charles Best (left) and Dr. Frederick Banting, with the first dog treated successfully with insulin in 1921. At that time Charles Best was a graduate student, involved with both departments of biology and physiology at the University of Toronto. Dr. Banting was a surgeon. (Courtesy of Charles Best and Eli Lilly Co.).

FIG. P–3. Engraving on the front of the Joslin building with the story of Dr. George Minot. (Original by the late Amelia Peabody.)

tissue from animals and injected this into a dog with diabetes. The results were dramatic. The dog's blood glucose levels fell and insulin had been made possible! In one stroke (the culmination of many, many smaller strokes), life had been substituted for death for the multitudes of people with diabetes, and a whole new era in diabetes treatment began!

It was a year later that insulin was first used in New England. At that time no one had any idea what the proper dose of insulin might be; it was used largely by trial and error. In fact, at the time insulin became available, there were several young men under treatment in Boston. They were gaunt wraiths of humans, barely alive. Insulin saved them, and one of them, Dr. George Minot, later became famous, winning the Nobel prize for his discovery of liver treatment for pernicious anemia (Fig. P–3).

The Interim Period

The initial reaction to insulin was to overestimate its useful effects. It was first considered by many to be a "cure" for diabetes. The euphoria over the discovery of insulin was tempered somewhat when it became evident that the simple intermittent injection of insulin was not enough to alter the basic diabetic state in many individuals. Although blood glucose levels improved and many people were able to lead relatively normal lives, many others still had problems with treatment, and had complications and often died because of inadequate treatment.

About 25 years after use of insulin began, it was found that many people had complications with their eyes, kidneys, nervous systems, and the blood vessels of their limbs. For a period there was a sense of disillusionment and a feeling of betrayal that the miracle medicine was not, after all, the magic hoped for. The fact was that simply giving insulin was not enough. The right amount had to be given at the right time. It took another 25 or 30 years for physicians to realize that tighter control (better stated as an attempt to achieve normal physiology) was necessary.

Into the Future

As the years passed and the number of people with diabetic complications increased, some physicians, including Dr. Elliott P. Joslin, stated that the chances of getting diabetic complications would be reduced if blood glucose levels could be kept as close to normal as possible. While many agreed with him, some did not agree with his aggressive therapeutic approach, which meant a complete change in lifestyle for many.

Even today there are varying viewpoints. More and more physicians, however—especially those expert in diabetes and its complications—believe that the closer the person is to the normal state, the fewer complications will arise. The evidence for this is accumulating year by year. For some complications, such as those associated with pregnancy, nerve damage, or prevention of limb loss, the evidence is quite convincing. For others, the evidence is only suggestive, but ongoing research projects seem to confirm the association between better control and reduction of complications. It is probably safe to say that better treatment can greatly affect those conditions connected with *micro*vascular (smaller blood vessel) complications.

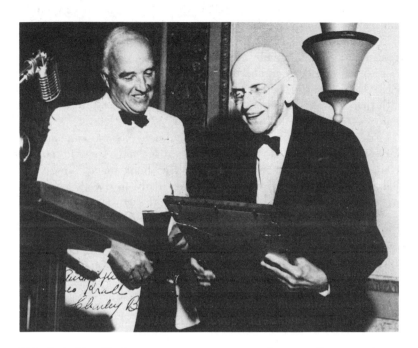

FIG. P–4. Dr. Charles Best presenting an award to Dr. Elliott P. Joslin on the occasion of the latter's 90th birthday in 1959.

Good treatment, however, is more than simply keeping blood glucose levels normal. Ideal treatment means having adequate insulin available at all times. It also means normal blood lipids, electrolytes, proper storage and use of glucose, proper nourishment to all the body cells, and many other factors. Diabetes is more than simply measuring blood sugar levels, but that is still the most accurate way of knowing if sufficient insulin is available.

Can It Be Done?

It would be futile to set normal glucose metabolism as a goal if it were impossible to achieve. It is difficult sometimes, but possible. Research into the normal functioning (physiology) of the body has given us a better understanding of how insulin therapy can more effectively bring glucose levels closer to normal. In addition, technologic advances have provided more and better tools for the treatment of diabetes. While we cannot yet return insulin production and action to natural nondiabetic conditions, we can safely come closer than ever before.

Dr. Elliott P. Joslin (Fig. P–4) focused on diabetes and its treatment when relatively few were doing so. His work included medical care and research, but perhaps his greatest contribution was education of professionals and, even more important, people with diabetes. A plaque on the Joslin auditorium wall says it quite plainly—"Gladly would he teach."

Education is the purpose of this manual. No one can make a person with diabetes do anything. Salvation, such as it is, comes from within. If the facts and ideas in this book make living with diabetes easier, then the efforts of the many involved, past and present, will be worthwhile.

The rest is up to you. This is only the prologue!

Boston, Massachusetts   Leo P. Krall, M.D.
                                          Richard S. Beaser, M.D.

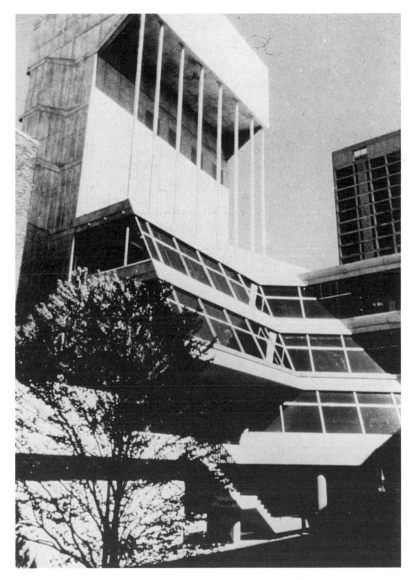

The Joslin Diabetes Center. The clinic moved from what was actually Dr. Joslin's home at 81 Bay State Road, Boston, in 1955. The newest part of the building, the Howard F. Root wing, was completed and dedicated in 1976. This wing houses the basic and clinical research activities, as well as the Joslin Clinic, the Diabetes Treatment Unit, and the administrative offices.

Acknowledgements

Although progress in diabetes has been breathtaking since the previous edition, it is also true that there is nothing *completely* new under the sun. Each generation borrows liberally from the one previous, as can be seen by comparison of the previous eleven editions, which have, in total, reached at least three-quarters of a million people.

Our ability to be authors is possible only because of the research and patient care of our fellow physicians. Therefore this book is not the work of just two authors—it is distilled from the experience of many, past and present. We hope this work will help those who follow.

In preparing the twelfth edition of this manual, we have relied on the experience of the many physicians who have preceded us. Elliott P. Joslin, M.D., Howard F. Root, M.D., and Alexander Marble, M.D., gave us a rich tradition of clinical and research experience. The care of diabetes in mothers and children would be impossible to discuss without the pioneering efforts by Priscilla White, M.D., over her 50 years of clinical practice. Allen P. Joslin, M.D., son of the founder, is known to thousands of patients because of his warm concern. This book also owes much to the clinical experience of the late William B. Hadley, M.D.

The clinic has passed the milestone of 150,000 patients cared for in our Boston facilities, and the enormous gold mine of information provided by the care of these individuals is constantly being studied and restudied in the interest of developing newer and better treatments. It is to these people with diabetes and their relatives and friends who trusted us with their care that this manual is dedicated. The physicians of the Joslin Clinic appreciate all of these fine people who have come and continue to come here over these many years. The physicians past, plus the senior physicians of the clinical and research staff of the Joslin Diabetes Center who have provided care, have all contributed to the preparation of this manual:

Lloyd M. Aiello, M.D.   Robert F. Bradley, M.D.
Donald M. Barnett, M.D.   A. Richard Christlieb, M.D.
William L. Black, M.D.   Ramachandiran Cooppan, M.D.

John D'Elia, M.D.   Eleftheria Maratos-Flier, M.D.
George S. Eisenbarth, M.D.   Lawrence I. Rand, M.D.
B. Dan Ferguson, M.D.   James L. Rosenzweig, M.D.
Om P. Ganda, M.D.   Sabera T. Shah, M.D.
Gisella G. Garan, M.D.   George S. Sharuk, M.D.
Charles A. Graham, M.D.   Donald C. Simonson, M.D.
John W. Hare, M.D.   Robert J. Smith, M.D.
Raymonde D. Herskowitz, M.D.   J. Stuart Soeldner, M.D.
Richard A. Jackson, M.D.   Gordon C. Weir, M.D.
Alan Jacobson, M.D.   Robert Wharton, M.D.
C. Ronald Kahn, M.D.   Mark Williams, M.D.
Antoine Kaldany, M.D.   Joseph I. Wolfsdorf, M.D.
George L. King, M.D.   Gloria Wu, M.D.
Lori Laffel, M.D.   David C. Yoburn, M.D.
John L. Leahy, M.D.   M. Donna Younger, M.D.
Margaret MacLaughlin, M.D.

Of course, these acknowledgments would be incomplete if we did not note the efforts of those who do much of the teaching—the teaching nurses and the dietitians. Through the years, these individuals have established a tradition of excellence that has made the Joslin Diabetes Center stand out as a center for diabetes education. The indivuduals who currently work with us at the Joslin Diabetes Center, or who otherwise contributed significantly through their teaching efforts, include:

TEACHING NURSES
  Brenda Burke, R.N., B.S.N.
  Debra Conboy, R.N., B.S.N.
  Kathryn Connor, R.N., B.S.N.
  Denise Richards Daniels, R.N., B.S.N.
  Jeanne Turley DeFazio, R.N., B.S.N.
  Helen Dennis, R.N., B.S.N.
  Sandra Eaton, R.N., B.S.N.
  Anne Marie Firestone, R.N., B.S.N.
  Suzanne Ghiloni, R.N., B.S.N.
  Deborah Greenwood, R.N., B.S.N.
  Sharon Hucul, R.N., M.P.H., C.D.E.
  Janice Kimmel-Davis, R.N., B.S.N.
  Phyllis Master, R.N., B.S.N.
  Therese McGraw, R.N., B.S.N.
  Linda McKay, R.N., B.S.N.
  Robin Neel, R.N., B.S.N.
  Cynthia Pasquarello, R.N., B.S.N.

Laurinda Poirier, R.N., B.S.N.
Carrie Stewart, R.N., B.S.N.
Anne Vernon, R.N., B.S.N.
Martha S. Wray, R.N., B.S.N.
DIETITIANS
Anna DiCenso, R.D.
Emmy Friedlander, R.D., M.S.
Geoffrey Gallant, R.D.
Joan Hill, R.D.
Susan Holman, R.D., M.S.
Debra Kaplan, R.D., M.S.
Laura Kinzel, R.D., M.S., C.D.E.
Diana Marthinsen, R.D., M.S.
Susan Richards, R.D., M.S.

Chapters 1 and 18 were reviewed by Gordon C. Weir, M.D., medical director of the Joslin Diabetes Center. Chapter 3 was coauthored by Hugo Hollerorth, Ed.D., curriculum developer for the Joslin Diabetes Center. Chapter 4 was coauthored by Laura Kinzel, R.D., M.S., head of the Nutrition Service Department. Debra Kaplan, R.D., M.S., also contributed to this chapter.

Chapter 5, on exercise, was based largely on the writings of Lee Cunninghan, who has provided a great deal of help in developing the Joslin Diabetes Center exercise programs. Anne Marie Firestone, R.N., B.S.N., also contributed to this chapter.

Extensive assistance in the preparation of Chapter 10, on intensive insulin therapy, was provided by Linda McKay, R.N., B.S.N., nurse coordinator of the Joslin Diabetes Center intensive insulin treatment program. Additional input was provided by Steven Edelman, M.D., Fredrick Dunn, M.D., and William L. (Larry) Black, M.D. Additional support came from the Diabetes Control and Complications Trial coordinators, Nancy Mitchell, R.N., and Susan Lemieux, R.N.

Chapter 12, Diabetes in the Young, was coauthored by Joseph I. Wolfsdorf, M.D. Additional assistance was provided by Raymonde D. Herskowitz, M.D., Robert Wharton, M.D., Cynthia Pasquarello, R.N., B.S.N., and Denise Richards Daniels, R.N., B.S.N.

M. Donna Younger, M.D., coauthored Chapter 13, Pregnancy and Diabetes, which owes so much to the fine tradition set by Priscilla White, M.D. Elizabeth Hare, M.S.W., coauthored the section on the psychological aspects of diabetes and pregnancy. John W. Hare, M.D., Suzanne Ghiloni, R.N., B.S.N., and Debra Kaplan, R.D., M.S., also contributed to Chapter 13.

Ramachandiran Cooppan, M.D., assisted in preparing Chapter 14, on diabetes and aging.

Many people contributed to Chapter 16, on the complications of diabetes. Lloyd M. Aiello, M.D., and Jerry Cavallerano, O.D., Ph.D., of the William P. Beetham Eye Unit of the Joslin Diabetes Center provided material for the section on eye care. Fundus sketches were prepared by Sabera T. Shah, M.D. John D'Elia, M.D., chief of the renal section of the Joslin Diabetes Center, provided assistance with the section on kidney complications. A. Richard Christlieb, M.D., assisted with the sections on hypertension. Steven Shama, M.D., helped prepare the section on dermatological complications of diabetes.

Chapter 17 was prepared with assistance from Alan Jacobson, M.D., head of the Joslin Diabetes Center's Mental Health Unit. Additional contributions came from Lloyd M. Aiello, M.D., and John W. Hare, M.D.

We wish to express appreciation to our Adult Nurse Practitioners; Norma Slater, R.N., A.N.P., Elizabeth Blair, R.N., A.N.P., and Patricia Talbot, R.N., A.N.P. Their tireless efforts in patient care and education have been important to us for many years.

We also thank Fredrick L. Dunn, M.D., formerly of the Joslin Diabetes Center and currently codirector of the Diabetes Clinical Service at Duke University Medical Center, and Julie Goodwin, P.A.C., for their review of some of the chapters.

Administrative support was provided through the offices of the administrator of the clinic section, Constance L. Stubbs. Sandra Daise, Nancy Sawyer, Linda Walker, Lisa Finston, and Carol Perry assisted with manuscript preparation. Shiela Meek assisted by taking and preparing many photographs.

Many of the drawings and tables that are new to this edition were prepared by Edith Tagrin and her staff at the Medical Art Department at the Massachusetts General Hospital.

Finally, we thank the Joslin Diabetes Center Patient Education Committee members—Hugo Hollerorth, Ed.D., Sharon Hucul, R.N., M.S., C.D.E., Laura Kinzel, R.D., M.S., C.D.E., and Denise Stevens, R.N., M.S.— who contributed many hours developing content outlines and meticulously reviewing the manuscript.

Boston, Massachusetts   Leo P. Krall, M.D.
                                                 Richard S. Beaser, M.D.

Contents

1. WHAT IS DIABETES? 1

A Definition of Diabetes 2
How the System Normally Works. 3
   The Pancreas 3
   Producing Insulin 6
   Normal Metabolism and Insulin Function 7
   The Fuels We Need 8
      Carbohydrates. 8
      Protein 11
      Fat 12
What Goes Wrong. 13
Types of Diabetes 15
   Type I Diabetes 15
   Type II Diabetes. 17
   Other Types of Diabetes 18
      Increased Risk for Diabetes 18
      Impaired Glucose Tolerance (IGT). 18
      Gestational Diabetes (GDM). 19
      Secondary Diabetes 19
Why People Get Diabetes 19
   Heredity. 19
   Viruses. 21
   Obesity 22
   Aging. 22
   Diet. 22
   Hormones. 23
   Drugs and Medications 23
   Illness 24
   Stress. 24
What Are the Chances of Getting Diabetes? 25
How Do I Know If I Have Diabetes? 26
   Skin Symptoms. 26
   Gynecological Problems. 27
   Impotence 27
   The Nervous System 27

Fatigue. 27
Blurred Vision 27
Detection of Diabetes: Making the Diagnosis 28
Blood Glucose. 29
The Glucose Tolerance Test 29
Urine Glucose. 29
Conclusion 30

2. **TREATING DIABETES MELLITUS** **31**

Goals of Treatment 32
The "Normal" Life 33
The Tools for Treatment 34
Education. 34
Activity. 34
The Place of Diet 34
Oral Medication 35
Insulin. 35

3. **LEARNING FOR LIFE** **38**

Why Educate the Person with Diabetes? 39
More Freedom? 39
Knowledge, Skills, and Attitudes 41
Stages of Learning. 41
Choosing an Educational Program 42
Active Participation 42
Your Own Needs and Problems 43
Attitudes toward Daily Life 44
Other Available Resources 44
Talking to Others with Diabetes. 44
Becoming Less Dependent 45
The Economics of Education 45
Conclusion 45

4. **NUTRITION AND DIABETES** **47**

Body Fuel. 47
Is Diet Obsolete?. 48
Dieting Is Not New 49
A Diabetic Eating Plan 50
Quantity 51
Prescribing Calories 51
Obesity 53
Food Types 55

Fast or Slow Sugars. 55
Glycemic Index. 55
Fiber 56
Carbohydrate 57
Protein. 58
Fat. 58
    Saturated or Un-? 59
    High- and Low-Density Fats. 60
    Reducing Diet Fats and Cholesterol 61
Timing of Eating. 61
The Nutrition Prescription. 61
The Role of the Dietitian. 62
Planning Meals 63
Food Labels 64
Sweeteners 65
    Nutritive Sweeteners. 65
    Non-Nutritive Sweeteners 67
Dietetic Foods. 69
Food Additives 70
The Vitamin Culture 70
    Vitamin C. 74
    The Vitamin E Fad 75
Minerals. 75
    Calcium 76
    Iron 76
    Mineral Excesses. 76
Special Weight-Loss Diets and Other "Specialty" Diets 76
Weight Loss: Group Therapy 77
Pills for Weight Loss 78
Vegetarian Diets 78
Organic Diets 79
Fasting 79
Summary 80

5. EXERCISE WITH DIABETES 81

Why Exercise Helps 81
Exercise without Diabetes 82
Exercise with Diabetes 83
The Exercise Program. 84
    Evaluation before Starting 85
    Prescribing Exercise 85
    The Daily Routine. 87
    Motivation 88
Adjusting Diabetes Treatment to Exercise. 89

Type II Diabetes......................... 89
Type I Diabetes 89
Low-Level Exercise....................... 90
More Vigorous Exercise................... 91
Longer Exercise 91

6. THE ORAL HYPOGLYCEMIC AGENTS.... 94

Looking Back............................... 94
Natural Remedies........................... 95
What Are the Oral Agents?.................. 95
Who Can Use Them?.......................... 95
How Do the Oral Agents Work?............... 97
Available Oral Agents......................100
Possible Undesirable Sulfonylurea Effects..........102
    Low Blood Glucose Reactions................102
    Side Effects...............................103
    Toxicity...................................103
The University Group Diabetes Program
    (UGDP) Report 104
The Good and the Bad of Oral Medications 105
Looking Ahead...............................105
Summary 106

7. INSULIN 107

What Is Insulin?............................109
Characteristics of Insulin..................110
    The Unit..................................110
    Concentration.............................111
    Insulin Type 111
    Insulin Purity 113
    Species...................................114
Insulin Antibodies 115
The Newer Insulins..........................116
Available Insulins..........................116
Emergency Insulins..........................119
Storage.....................................119
Insulins Abroad.............................120
Insulin Syringes............................120
How to Inject a Single Dose of Insulin 122
How to Mix Insulin 126
How to Inject Insulin.......................127
    Avoiding or Removing Bubbles..............128
    Automatic, Button, and Jet Injectors..........128

        Injection Aids for People with Low Vision 130
        Injection Sites 130

8. MONITORING YOUR DIABETES 132

        Why Monitor? 132
        A Brief History of Monitoring 133
        The Glycohemoglobin Measurement 135
        What Does Measuring the Blood Glucose Tell Us? 137
        The Office Blood Glucose Measurement 138
        Self Monitoring of Blood Glucose (SMBG) 139
            Self Blood Testing Materials 139
        Testing Urine for Glucose 146
            Twenty-Four Hour Urine Test 147
            Urine Testing for Acetone 148
        Self Glucose Monitoring Programs 150
            Record Keeping 150
            Frequency of Testing .151
                Level I: Primarily Urine Testing 151
                Level II: Block Testing 152
                Level III: Daily Blood Testing 152
        Conclusions 153

9. CONVENTIONAL TREATMENT OF
    DIABETES WITH INSULIN 154

        Who Needs Insulin? 155
        Starting Insulin 155
        Which Insulin? 156
        Insulin Treatment 156
            Goals 156
            Testing and Monitoring 157
            The Proper Dose 157
            Insulin Adjustment 158
            Adjustment Problems .159
            Know the Peak Activity Time of the
                Insulin You Are Using 159
            Rebound 160

10. INTENSIVE INSULIN THERAPY OF
    TYPE I DIABETES .164

        What Is Intensive Insulin Therapy? 164
        Why Intensive Therapy Makes Sense 165
        Who Needs Intensive Insulin Therapy? 168
        Insulin Dosing Schedules 169

The Dawn Phenomenon. .170
Insulin Infusion Pump 172
Preparing for an Intensive Insulin Program 175
Getting Started 176
Living the Intensive Life .177
　　Algorithm Adjustments 178
　　Adjusting for Hyperglycemia 179
　　Adjusting for Hypoglycemia 181
　　Diet and Weight Gain 182
The Pump. 182
　　The Decision to Use a Pump 183
　　General Pump Care. .183
　　Pump Dose Adjustments 186
　　Sick Days with Pumps. 186
　　Exercise Adjustments with Pumps 187
　　Pump "Vacations" 187
Conclusion 188

11.　TREATING TYPE II DIABETES 189

What Is Type II Diabetes? 189
Treatment of Type II Diabetes. 190
Diet and Weight Loss. 190
Exercise 190
Oral Medication 191
　　Is Diet Still Necessary? 191
Who Might Use the Tablets 191
Combinations of Oral Agents 192
Mixing with Other Medications or Substances 193
Do Oral Tablets Eventually Fail? 193
Insulin Treatment of Type II Diabetes 194

12.　DIABETES IN THE YOUNG 195

You Are Not Alone! 195
Why Do Children Develop Diabetes? 197
Types of Diabetes in Young People 197
Stages of Development of Diabetes. 198
　　Stage I 198
　　Stage II 199
　　Stage III. 199
　　Stage IV 199
Treatment of Diabetes in the Young 200
　　Goals of Treatment 200
　　The Team Approach. .201

Education of the Young .201
Insulin 202
Nutrition 203
The "Free" Diet? 204
Exercise 204
Monitoring Diabetes in Young People 205
Glycosylated Hemoglobin 206
What Every Parent Should Know 207
What the Child Must Know 208
The Emotional Response 209
The Onset of Diabetes 209
The Adolescent 210
Growth and Development 211
Infants with Diabetes 212
The Effect of Menstruation 213
School 213
Leaving the Child with a Babysitter 213
Camps 214
All Our Goals 216

13. PREGNANCY AND DIABETES 218
How Is Pregnancy with Diabetes Different? 220
Gestational Diabetes 221
Effects of Pregnancy on Diabetes 222
Managing Diabetes and Pregnancy 224
Preparing for Pregnancy 225
Managing Your Pregnancy 225
The Course of Pregnancy 226
Monitoring Diabetes during Pregnancy 227
Monitoring Fetal Development 231
Obstetrical Complications 232
Diet 234
Weight 234
The Eating Plan 234
Delivery 235
Breast-Feeding (Nursing) 237
Pregnancy, Diabetes, and Life 237
Conclusion 239

14. DIABETES AND AGING 240
Everybody Is Doing It 240
Effects of Aging on Glucose Tolerance 241
Diabetes Treatment in Mature Individuals 242

Eating. 243
Exercise 243
Pills or Insulin. 243
Monitoring 244
Preventing Complications. 245
Summary 245

15. THE ACUTE COMPLICATIONS OF
    DIABETES. 246

Acute versus Chronic Complications 246
Hypoglycemia (Low Blood Sugar) 247
    The Symptoms of Hypoglycemia. 247
    Severe Reactions. 248
    Reaction Denial. 249
    Rebound: The "Somogyi Effect". 250
    Diagnosing Hypoglycemic Reactions 251
        Pattern Hunting. 251
    Prevention 252
    Treatment. 253
    Glucagon 255
    Are Insulin Reactions Harmful? 256
    Other Causes of Hypoglycemia. 257
The Hyperglycemic "Comas" of Diabetes
(High Blood Sugar) 257
    Ketoacidosis 258
    Hyperosmotic Coma (The Other Coma). 258
    Why These Happen. 259
    Symptoms. 259
    Treatment. 260
    Prevention 261
High and Low 262
Blurred Vision (Presbyopia) 265
Insulin Edema. 266
Diabetes Better, Neuritis Worse? 266
Insulin Allergy. 266
Atrophy and Hypertrophy .267
Insulin Abscess and Infection 267
Insulin Resistance 268
Genital Infections 268

16. THE LONGTERM COMPLICATIONS OF
    DIABETES. 269

The Eyes. 270

Anatomy of the Eye. 270
Subconjunctival Hemorrhage 272
Glaucoma 272
Cataract 273
Diseases of the Retina .274
Treating the Damaged Retina. 275
Photocoagulation by Laser 277
Vitrectomy 279
Eye Examinations for People with Diabetes 280
The Kidneys and Urinary Tract 280
Urinary Tract Infections. 282
Nonfunctioning Bladder (Atony) 282
Kidney Disorders 283
Treating Kidney Disease 283
Neuropathy. 284
Symptoms of Sensory Neuropathies 285
What Causes Neuropathy? 289
Treatment. 289
Cardiovascular Complications. 290
Blood Vessel Changes .291
Infections 291
Feet 292
Skin Care 294
Nail Care 295
Shoes 296
Athlete's Foot 298
Problem Prevention. 299
Skin Problems 300
Is It Caused by My Diabetes? 301
Summary 302

17. LIVING WITH DIABETES 303

Adjusting. 303
Denial 305
Fear 306
Guilt 307
"How Long Will I Live?" 307
Using the Medical System .308
Choosing a Physician 308
How Often to See Your Physician 310
What You Can Do to Help Your Physician. 310
Health Insurance. 310
Life Insurance. 312
The Economics of Diabetes 313

Diabetes and Employment. 313
Educational Opportunities .315
    Career Guidance. 315
Identification Jewelry and Cards 316
Driving Automobiles, Boats, and Other Vehicles 318
Parties and Special Occasions. 318
Alcohol and Diabetes. 319
    How Alcohol Affects Diabetes 319
    Calories from Alcohol .320
Smoking 323
The Drug Culture 324
Usable Medications 326
    Other Problem Medications 326
Surgery and Diabetes 327
Dental Problems 328
Acupuncture 328
Biofeedback, Meditation, and Relaxation Therapy. . . .329
Contact Lenses 330
Ear Piercing 331
Camps for Youngsters with Diabetes. 331
Summertime 331
Sports. 332
Marriage, Childbearing, and Sexual Function 332
    Marriage Counseling 333
    Male Sexual Function .333
    Birth Control 334
    Sexual Activity and Hypoglycemia 335
Traveling with Diabetes. 335
    Before Leaving 335
    Choosing Clothes 336
    Health Record and Identification 337
    Personal Medication 337
    Diabetes during Traveling 338
    Up, Up, and Away! 338
    Time Zones. 339
    Problems en Route 340
    Travel by Ship 340
    On Arriving 342
    "Tourista"—The Curse of the Traveling Class! 342
    Looking for Medical Help 343
    Other Hints 343
For More Information 344

18. A LOOK AHEAD 345

Where We Are Today 346
Research Today, Hopes for Tomorrow 347
    Prevention of Insulin-Dependent Diabetes 347
    Prevention and Treatment of Non-Insulin-
      Dependent Diabetes 348
    Insulin Treatment of Diabetes 349
    Transplanting the Pancreas. 349
    Islet Cell Transplantation 350
    The Artificial Pancreas 350
    Newer Insulins 353
    Treatment and Prevention of Complications 354
    Diabetes Control and Complications Trial (DCCT).354
    Aldose Reductase Inhibitors 355
    Eye Research 355
    Kidney Research 356
    Other Research 356
"Lest We Forget". 357

19. WHAT TO DO UNTIL YOU CAN
    REACH YOUR PHYSICIAN 359

APPENDIXES 367
    1. Food Choice Lists. 368
    2. Cholesterol and Saturated Fat Content of
       Some Foods 389
    3. Oral Hypoglycemic Agents Available Around
       the World by Generic and Trade Names.390
    4. Automatic Insulin Injectors 393
    5. Insulin Pumps 394
    6. White Classification of Diabetes in
       Pregnant Women 395
    7. Resources for the Elderly 396

INDEX 397

1

What Is Diabetes?

The question "What is diabetes?" could just as readily be "Why is diabetes?" because the answer would probably be the same. The interesting thing is that so many factors are required to get diabetes. Despite this there are probably at least 100 million people in the world with diabetes, more than 12 million in the United States alone. It is amazing that so many have become members of this widespread and exclusive group.

There are many reasons for trying to find answers to these questions. Do you have diabetes? Does a child, a parent, a relative, or a friend have it? Are you interested in learning what diabetes means to a person who has it and how diabetes can change the way you or someone you care about lives? These are all good reasons, but the best reason is that knowledge and understanding can help you or someone close to you live better and longer as well as freer from complications. Simple survival is not enough. To live life—to enjoy life—while having diabetes depends on how much you know and what you do about it.

As we shall see, evidence increasingly shows that good care and a sustained effort to achieve blood glucose control that is as close to normal as possible can make the course of the condition smoother and may also prevent complications. Acquiring knowledge leading to better care is not a luxury but a necessity. Although a physician or diabetes educator can offer guidance during office or hospital visits, the person with diabetes must live with it 365 days a year and be prepared to cope constantly with the problems of everyday life.

While a book such as this must be general in nature, it must also be specific enough to provide useful suggestions. Diabetes is a very

1

personal disease, and through self-education, you can acquire the knowledge that applies to you or to the special person with diabetes that you know. Remember, knowledge and understanding are not a *part* of treatment; they *are* the treatment.

A Definition of Diabetes

We need to start with a general explanation of diabetes so we all know what we are talking about. Normally some sugar (glucose) is in the blood at all times. These terms, glucose and sugar, will be used interchangeably, although we almost always mean glucose. The level of glucose is usually between 60 and 120 milligrams percent (mg%), which means that there are 60 to 120 milligrams of glucose in each 100 cubic centimeters (cc) of blood. Milligrams percent is sometimes expressed as milligrams per deciliter (mg/dl). Diabetes mellitus is characterized by a level of glucose in the blood that is above normal much or most of the time.

Glucose is a type of sugar, which is the major fuel for the body. We eat a great deal of glucose each day, as carbohydrates (starches) are made of glucose. When we eat glucose, it gets into the bloodstream and eventually into each of the individual cells (the basic building blocks) of the body to provide them with energy. Glucose cannot just flow into the cells, however. Cells are enclosed in membranes that separate what is inside the cell from what is outside. Somehow, the cell must be told that the glucose waiting outside the cell should be allowed in.

That is what insulin does. Insulin is a substance, called a hormone, that is made in a gland called the pancreas. The pancreas is located deep in the middle of the abdominal cavity, just below and behind the stomach. Insulin is needed to signal to the cells that they should allow the glucose that normally is in the blood to penetrate their outer layer.

If the glucose cannot get into the cells, it "backs up" in the blood. The level of glucose in the blood increases, and a state of diabetes is produced. Such a condition occurs if there is a lack of insulin for whatever reason. Perhaps the pancreas cannot produce enough insulin. Recent research has shown that the condition is really much more complex than that and that there are other reasons glucose does not get into the cells of the body properly. However, we should first discuss how things work *normally*.

How the System Normally Works

Insulin is a hormone, one of the substances that are made in a particular type of cell and that go to other cells to give them certain "information" or to tell them what to do. Insulin tells the cells of the body to allow the sugar in the bloodstream to enter the cells of the body to be used for energy. But to look at the workings in detail, we should start at the beginning. The source of the insulin is the pancreas.

The Pancreas. The pancreas is a gland situated below and behind the stomach (Fig. 1–1). It weighs about half a pound and resembles an elongated cone lying on its side. The broad part, or head, is located next to a curve of the duodenum, the part of the small intestine just beyond the stomach. The pancreas tapers off to the left in the direction of the spleen and left kidney and ends in a portion known as the tail. Within the pancreas, especially at the tail, are very small bits of tissue called islets of Langerhans (Fig. 1–2). These islets contain *beta cells* (first described in 1869), which manufacture, store, and eventually release insulin directly into the bloodstream at the appropriate times.

An *endocrine* gland makes substances (hormones) and releases them directly into the bloodstream, where they can travel to other parts of the body and carry out a specific function. The islet portion of the pancreas, which secretes insulin in this manner, is just such a gland. Other endocrine glands are the thyroid, adrenal, and pituitary glands, each with different hormones that have specific functions.

Each normal pancreas has about 100,000 islets of Langerhans, which are clusters of various types of cells (Fig. 1–2). The most important cell type in these islets is the beta cell. There are usually between 1000 and 2000 beta cells in each islet. These cells make insulin and release it into the blood. These amazing cells are also capable of measuring the blood glucose level within seconds to within a range of 2 mg%. Using this information, they can determine how much insulin is needed, and, within a minute or so, secrete the precise amount of required insulin.

The pancreas has several other important functions. One is to produce enzymes needed for the digestion of various foods in the diet. When foodstuffs made up of starches or proteins are eaten, the pancreas secretes and releases these enzymes, which flow through a duct into the small intestine. The enzymes then split these foodstuffs into simpler substances, which are absorbed into the bloodstream and transported throughout the body for immediate

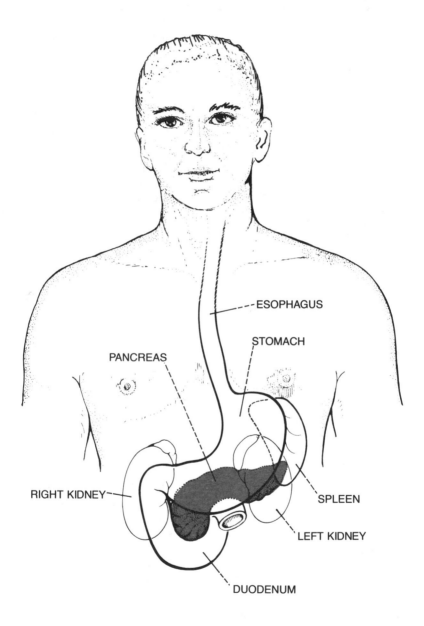

FIG. 1–1. Anatomy of the pancreas. The pancreas is located below and behind the stomach, adjacent to the spleen, kidneys, and duodenum.

ISLET OF LANGERHANS

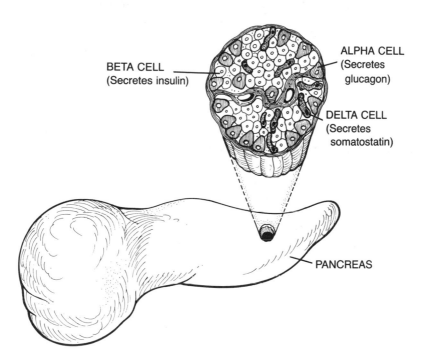

BETA CELL
(Secretes insulin)

ALPHA CELL
(Secretes
glucagon)

DELTA CELL
(Secretes
somatostatin)

PANCREAS

FIG. 1–2. Microscopic anatomy (histology) of the pancreas. The pancreas is made up of many clusters of cells called islets of Langerhans. Within each islet are different types of cells, including the alpha cells, which secrete glucagon, the beta cells, which secrete insulin, and the delta cells, which secrete somatostatin.

use by various tissues or for storage for later needs. The production of digestive enzymes is known as the *exocrine* function of the pancreas gland (the production of substances that get to the site of their action through a duct, rather than by secretion into the bloodstream). In addition to producing insulin, the islets of the pancreas produce other hormones that enter the bloodstream directly. *Alpha cells*, also in the islets, produce and release *glucagon*, which raises the blood sugar level, which is the opposite function of insulin. There is a careful balance between insulin and glucagon which is of primary importance in maintaining the blood glucose level in the normal range. Other substances are produced in the pancreas as well. One important one is *somatostatin*, which is produced in the delta cells of the islets. It probably mediates on behalf of insulin by blocking glucagon and anterior pituitary growth hormone. Gastrin, vasoactive intestinal peptide (VIP), and pancreatic polypeptide (PP), are also produced in the pancreas. There is much current research into the roles of these substances and whether they influence diabetes. It is interesting that the hormones from the pituitary, adrenal, and thyroid glands have an anti-insulin effect (an effect opposite to, or blocking the action of, insulin) so that a normally functioning body has a complete balance between the actions of these various substances.

Producing Insulin. Insulin is a protein made up of a long chain of smaller building blocks called amino acids. The beta cells have the ability to take 86 of these various amino acids and hook them together in a specific order to make a long chain (a protein) known as *proinsulin*. Proinsulin is an early form of insulin.

The proinsulin is placed into small "packages" inside the cell. These are called *secretory granules*. Within these granules, part of the proinsulin chain is cleaved away, leaving insulin itself, which has 51 amino acids, while the cast-off portion of proinsulin has 31 amino acids and is known as C- (or connecting) peptide. (During the cleavage process, 4 amino acids are lost.) Both the insulin and the *C-peptide* are stored in secretory granules, ready for release when the beta cell calls for it. The C-peptide has no known effect, but is released by the beta cells into the circulation. The C-peptide is useful only as a "marker," enabling physicians to determine how much insulin is released.

When the beta cell is signaled by glucose or other foods in the diet, it releases insulin in two stages. During the first stage, which is very rapid, occurring within about 10 minutes, it releases the insulin that was made earlier and is already stored within the secretory granules of the beta cells. A nondiabetic pancreas can store as much as 200 units. The second stage is more complicated. With the increase in the level of glucose in the blood, a signal is sent to the nucleus (or "brain") of the beta cell. In the nucleus is a substance called *DNA* (desoxyribonucleic acid), which is a chain of molecules (nucleic acids) in a specific order which form genes and act as a code to trigger the production of various substances. The DNA coded for insulin production (the insulin gene) gets the signal that the blood glucose level is rising and begins to reproduce its code onto another substance called *messenger RNA* (ribonucleic acid). Just as its name suggests, this messenger RNA transports the code for the production of insulin to the area of the cell that has the capacity to manufacture more insulin, and the further production of this substance begins.

Insulin release into the blood can actually begin even before the blood glucose level becomes elevated. Food entering the digestive tract stimulates the release of insulin from the beta cells. This release depends on the amount and the type of food eaten. Carbohydrates (sugars and starches) are the most effective stimulators. The combined effects of hormones from the digestive tract and the increasing blood sugar level sustains the release and formation of insulin. Protein can also help stimulate insulin secretion.

In people who do not have diabetes, it is almost impossible to raise the blood glucose level no matter what is eaten, because the insulin reserve is plentiful and is secreted in exactly the correct amount. In fact, if a person is given a slow infusion of 5% glucose solution (the standard intravenous glucose solution) in a vein of one arm, the levels of glucose in blood from a vein in the other arm would most often be normal. The person without diabetes can normally manufacture and release as much as 40 to 50 units of insulin daily.

Normal Metabolism and Insulin Function. Like any machine, the body requires materials to make up its structure and replacement materials, like building materials, to replace those that have worn out. In addition, it needs fuel to provide energy for it to function. The fuels that the body uses come from the food we eat, which is made up of carbohydrates (sugars and starches), proteins (amino acids), and fats (fatty acids).

Digestion of the food begins when it arrives in the stomach and is attacked by digestive enzymes. Some of these are also in the mouth and small intestines. The digestive process is like an assembly line. Foods—carbohydrate, protein, and fat—are split apart by enzymes into their basic forms—glucose, amino acid, and fatty acid. Once this process is complete, these basic building blocks of food pass through the wall of the gut and into the bloodstream to be used for energy. Actually, all three provide for energy needs, but they must be further broken down or split apart. This process is known as *metabolism*. It is like the "burning" of fuel to produce energy. The series of chemical reactions in the metabolic pathway which produces energy from glucose is known as the *Krebs cycle*, named after Hans Krebs, the biochemist who first described it. This cycle is probably present in most cells of the body. It is like a furnace for the body—fuel is put in, and energy comes out! This energy fuels our activities such as walking, running, or playing sports, as well as the work of the organs of our body. The waste products of this energy production are carbon dioxide and water. They are disposed of by way of the kidneys and lungs.

Insulin plays a key role in making sure that this machine that is our body runs with a full supply of fuel. Insulin acts like a key that fits into little locks on the surface of the cells known as *receptors*. This unlocking triggers a series of reactions on the surface of the cell and inside the cell (known as "postreceptor events") leading to the opening of a space on the cell surface that allows glucose to enter. Without insulin, the sugar would back up in the blood, unable to get into the cell for use as energy.

The Fuels We Need. The body uses three main fuels, glucose from carbohydrates, amino acids from proteins, and fatty acids from fats. It is important to understand why each of these is needed and how it is used.

CARBOHYDRATES. Carbohydrate is found in most foods that are eaten (fruits, vegetables, pastry, bread, potatoes, etc.) and is frequently called "starch." When these foods are eaten, the carbohydrate is digested (broken apart) into simple sugars and then to basic glucose as it enters the stomach and intestine. Glucose, being smaller than the intricate, branching chains of carbohydrates, can pass through the intestinal wall and enter the blood circulation.

Once in the blood, glucose travels throughout the body. It comes in contact with all cells, including the pancreatic beta cells. These cells make and secrete insulin in response to increased glucose in the blood. This insulin then travels through the bloodstream as noted earlier, and attaches itself to insulin receptors on each cell surface, telling the cells to allow the fuel (glucose) to enter the cells to be used for energy.

Glucose is able to provide energy for immediate needs. As one is eating, however, and shortly afterwards, the energy requirements are fulfilled. The extra energy must be stored for the future. There are two places for this energy to be stored (Fig. 1–3). One is the liver. With insulin's help, extra glucose can be taken up by the liver cells and changed to the storage form called *glycogen*. Glycogen can also be stored in the muscles. Glycogen is important because it is always on call as a source of "quick" energy. Suppose someone with diabetes has taken too much insulin and as a result has a low blood sugar reaction. Even if the person does not eat extra food immediately, the blood glucose level will rise. This is called a "rebound," caused by the release of glycogen from storage in the liver. This release occurs when stimulated by the body's hormonal mechanism made up of *epinephrine* (adrenalin) and *glucagon*. Although all people without and most people with diabetes have this ability to bring blood glucose levels back up to a safe range, people with

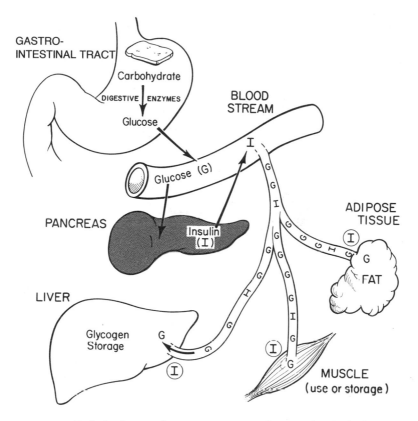

GASTRO-
INTESTINAL TRACT

Carbohydrate

DIGESTIVE ┃ ENZYMES

Glucose

BLOOD
STREAM

I

Glucose (G)

G
G
I

PANCREAS

Insulin
(I)

ADIPOSE
TISSUE

I

G

FAT

LIVER

Glycogen
Storage   G

(I)

(I)

G

MUSCLE
(use or storage)

FIG. 1–3. Carbohydrate is the primary source of energy for the body. The body gets its carbohydrate fuel from sugars and starches. These are digested in the gastrointestinal tract into simple sugars (e.g., glucose), which pass into the bloodstream. Glucose in the bloodstream stimulates the pancreas to secrete insulin. Insulin directs the glucose to muscle for use or storage, to liver for storage as glycogen, or to adipose tissue for storage as fat.

diabetes must treat low blood glucose reactions by eating or drinking substances containing sugar. Don't depend on the usual automatic mechanism always functioning well enough to keep you out of trouble!

Glycogen is also released when muscular exertion requires it for energy. Long-distance runners often eat large quantities of carbohydrate prior to a race to "load" their glycogen stores for the long run.

Unfortunately, while the available glycogen storage space in muscle and liver is limited, there is an almost unlimited storage depot that can hold all of the excess glucose that may be eaten. In

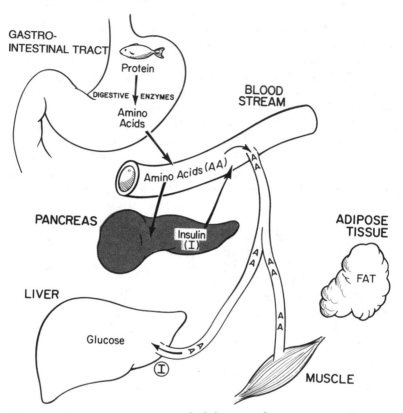

FIG. 1–4. Protein is an important fuel that contributes to many important bodily functions. It comes from meat, seafood, dairy products, and some vegetables such as beans and nuts. Protein is digested in the gastrointestinal tract to its basic building blocks, amino acids. Amino acids pass into the bloodstream, where they can be used for various functions. Protein can stimulate insulin secretion. It can be changed into glucose in the liver.

fact, it can store food energy from any source. It is the *adipose tissue*, or fat cells. Insulin helps promote the change of the excess glucose into fat, which is deposited for long-term storage—for some people, longer than others! As a result, there is a myth that insulin injections make you fat. Insulin doesn't make you fat—excess calories make you fat. Insulin only helps by doing its job! This state of excess fat in the fat cells is called obesity.

The Bible tells about storing food during the fat years to provide for the lean years. People do this, too, but if they don't have the "lean years" and keep storing, their state of being "energy misers" becomes obvious to everyone. The storage places are obvious and are often located in unflattering places!

PROTEIN. Protein is available from the daily diet (e.g., from meat, cheese, and fish). When such foods enter the intestine, enzymes break them down into amino acids, which then enter the circulation (Fig. 1–4). Circulating amino acids can also stimulate the pancreas to secrete insulin. While proteins contribute to various building components of the body such as muscle and bone and to the production of enzymes, they are also "burned" to produce energy in a process similar to the metabolism of glucose. The use of protein as an energy source can occur because amino acids can be changed to glucose in the liver and then used or stored as glycogen. This glucose can also be changed to fat for storage until needed.

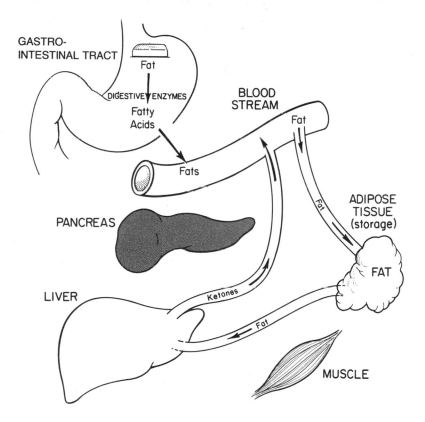

FIG. 1–5. Fat is the third substance the body can use for fuel, although it is not used as rapidly as glucose. Sources of fat include meat, diary products, and vegetable oils. Fats are digested and absorbed as fatty acids, which can be stored in the adipose tissue for later use. When fats are metabolized in the liver for energy, ketones are produced as a by-product.

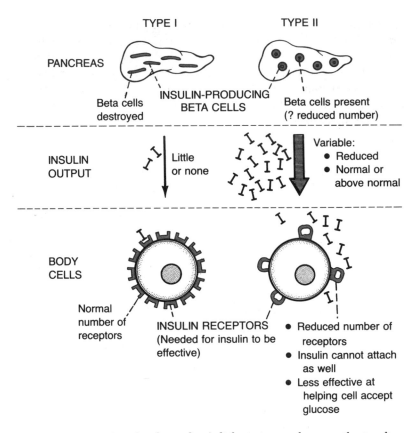

FIG. 1–6. Type I (insulin-dependent) diabetes occurs because the insulin-producing beta cells in the pancreas are destroyed and there is not enough insulin produced. Type II (non-insulin-dependent) diabetes is caused by a relative insulin insufficiency due to insulin resistance—the inability of the insulin to tell the cells to use glucose—plus insufficient insulin to overcome this resistance.

F_AT. The third fuel for the human metabolism is fat, such as is found in oils from corn, peanuts, and olives, as well as fat in meat, fowl, butter, and other dairy products such as milk, cream, and cheese. These foods are digested into fatty acids in the intestine and absorbed into the bloodstream where they are used by the body (Fig. 1–5). Some fats are called "essential fats." The body needs these for metabolism and these must be in the diet. Most fats, however, are either used for energy or stored for later use with the help of insulin. When other fuels are in short supply, such as during prolonged fasting, the level of insulin in the blood falls. The reduced level of circulating insulin promotes the removal of the fat from the storage depots and helps its entry into the circulation. It may then be used by muscle and other organs. However, fat is metabolized ("burned") differently than glucose. When it is metabolized, byproducts may result because fat is not used as efficiently as other fuels. The remaining byproducts are ketones or acetone.

What Goes Wrong

Diabetes occurs when the blood glucose is too high as a result of a deficiency of available, effective insulin. This lack can be *absolute* when the pancreas does not produce enough insulin (or produces none at all) or *relative*, when the pancreas produces a "normal" amount of insulin, but for some reason the body needs more than a normal amount of insulin or the insulin is made ineffective and the pancreas cannot produce enough to compensate (see Fig. 1–6 and the discussion of types of diabetes, below). As a result of these deficiencies, the cells lack fuel, and the body suffers from a lack of energy. People with diabetes complain of weakness and tiredness, and a usually active young child may be tired or listless.

When the cells are starved of their fuel, the body recognizes that not enough food has been eaten and triggers a sense of extreme hunger, called *polyphagia*. The glucose level in the blood rises because it is not used. At the same time, out of desperation, the body turns to stored fuels—glycogen, fat, and protein—to try to meet its energy needs. The level of glucose in the blood continues to rise, as does the blood level of fats. The huge excess of unused glucose circulates through the kidney, which normally rescues useful glucose from the filtered fluid to keep it from being lost in the urine. There is a level of blood glucose, however, known as the *renal threshold*, above which the kidneys cannot keep up with the job of retrieving glucose, and it escapes into the urine. Once this level (usually 160 to 180 mg%) is passed, glucose spills into the urine as from an overflowing dam (Fig. 1–7). As the blood sugar rises, excess glucose appears in the urine. When diabetes is severe, a large proportion of the body's energy needs are lost into the urine in the form of glucose. Enormous amounts, as much as 200 grams (800 calories) daily, can be lost this way.

An interesting historical footnote is appropriate here. In his second edition of the textbook *Treatment of Diabetes* in 1917, long before the discovery of insulin and during World War I, Dr. Elliott P. Joslin wrote, "It is desirable in peace, but a duty in war, for every diabetic patient to keep sugar-free. The food which the untreated

diabetic patient wastes in a week would feed a soldier for a day."
(Indeed, 5600 calories would do it!) This appears a bit far-fetched at
this time, but tells of the desperation of physicians in the preinsulin
days to try to save their patients.

The body knows when the urine is too loaded with sugar and is
too concentrated and tries to dilute it by allowing more and more
fluid to flow through the kidneys. Hence, the person with high
blood glucose levels and *glycosuria* (much urine sugar) experiences
frequent urination of large amounts of fluid, known as *polyuria*
(much urine). With the fluid loss, the body senses increasing
dehydration, and the thirst center is triggered, making the individual drink more fluid. This increased thirst is known as *polydipsia*
(much drinking).

This vicious cycle of glucose and water loss, and the attempts to
correct this loss, lead to the classic symptoms of diabetes. All of
these are due to the body's inability to use glucose properly as the
body fuel. When a person has the type of diabetes with a severe lack
of insulin, this absence allows the fat cells to release fats, which are
converted by the liver into ketones. These *ketones* are acidic. If this
process proceeds rapidly or for a long enough time, blood ketone
levels rise to high levels and becomes *ketoacidosis*, which is indeed
quite dangerous.

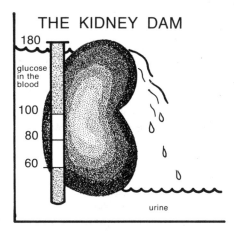

FIG. 1–7. The kidney dam. The figures 60 to 100 mg% of blood represent
the normal fasting level of glucose in the blood. Ordinarily glucose does not
appear in the urine until much higher levels are reached between 160 and
180 mg% of blood or higher). In this respect, the kidney can be considered
a dam. (Adapted from Rossini, A.: The great diabetes machine. *Diabetes
Forecast*, 29:22, 1976.)

Types of Diabetes

Since the previous edition of this book was published, diabetes has been classified into two major types. These have been designated *type I* and *type II*. This use of roman numerals probably dignifies the importance of this classification. This is always the way of designating important events such as Superbowl XX, World War I and World War II, etc. These types of diabetes are, indeed, quite important!

The two types of diabetes occur by two different mechanisms (Table 1–1). Diabetes can be due to a shortage or lack of insulin. This is called type I diabetes, or *insulin-dependent diabetes mellitus (IDDM)*. Insulin injections are a must because the person's own production is reduced or absent.

Type II, *non-insulin dependent diabetes mellitus* (NIDDM), has only a "relative" insulin lack. The body does produce some insulin, sometimes quite a bit, but the need for insulin is so increased that production cannot keep up with this need.

Type I diabetes was formerly called "juvenile diabetes" or "juvenile-onset diabetes," while type II was known as "adult-onset diabetes." Age is not necessarily a factor, however, as both of these occur in various age groups. Some older people can have type I diabetes, and occasionally younger people have type II diabetes. Diabetes is now labeled by the mechanisms that caused the diabetes to occur: "insulin-dependent" (IDDM), due to a lack of insulin, and "non-insulin-dependent" (NIDDM), due to a relative insufficiency of insulin supply.

In some parts of the tropics there is an increasingly common type of diabetes that might be classified as type III. This is called "tropical" or "malnutrition" diabetes. The cause is not completely known, but it is found in areas with very deficient diets.

Type I Diabetes. Type I diabetes, or IDDM, results from decreased insulin production by the pancreas (Fig. 1–6). Persons with this type of diabetes must take supplementary insulin by injections because there is no way to take this insulin orally.

This type of diabetes occurs because the beta cells do not function. These cells are probably destroyed by the body's own defense mechanisms that turn against these cells. Normally, the body's immune system directs antibodies and white blood cells against foreign substances such as viruses and other enemies it wants to destroy. These natural defenses are essential to health. For some reason, however, in persons with type I diabetes these defenses are directed against the islet cells, leading to their

TABLE 1–1. Comparison of Type I and Type II Diabetes

ITEM	TYPE I DIABETES	TYPE II DIABETES
Percentage of all people with diabetes	20%	80%
Other current names	Insulin-dependent diabetes	Non-insulin-dependent diabetes
Former names	Juvenile diabetes, brittle diabetes	Adult-onset diabetes, stable diabetes
Age of discovery	Usually below 40, but not always	Usually over 40, but not always
Condition when discovered	Usually moderately to severely ill	Often not ill at all or having mild symptoms
Cause of diabetes	Reduced or absent insulin production	Insulin resistance and relative or absolute deficiency of insulin
Insulin level	None to small amounts	Slightly decreased to high levels
Weight	Often thin or normal weight, often losing weight at diagnosis	Usually overweight, but 20% are normal weight
Acute complications	Ketoacidosis	Nonketotic hypcrosmolar hyperglycemic coma; not usually prone to ketoacidosis
Usual treatment	Insulin, eating plan, exercise	Diet, exercise. If needed, oral agents, insulin

destruction. This is called an *autoimmune reaction* (an immune reaction against the body's own tissue). Some studies have tried to identify the presence of islet cell antibodies in the blood of persons that are destined to develop diabetes but do not yet have it. Although it is not certain that diabetes will develop, the presence of these antibodies helps predict who might get it. The presence of these antibodies suggests that the person should be especially vigilant for signs or symptoms of diabetes. Ultimately it is hoped that a way can be developed to *stop* the diabetes from occurring before it happens.

Most often the person with type I diabetes is young, and the onset is fairly rapid—perhaps over a few days or weeks. However, some older people can also get type I diabetes. In older people, type I diabetes often has a slower onset. It even may act like type II diabetes for long periods. Ultimately, though, the true insulin requirements become evident, and insulin therapy must be started. Although both types of diabetes can begin with weight loss, the type I individuals tend to be at or below their "ideal" body weight at the start, and may even lose more weight rapidly. They can show ketones in their urine. This suggests a true insulin lack and the burning of fat for energy. On some occasions, the onset of type I diabetes is with coma due to ketoacidosis.

Type II Diabetes. Type II diabetes (NIDDM) is probably caused by resistance to the normal insulin action and a *relative* reduction of insulin secretion (Fig. 1–6). This insulin lack can be caused by a reduced number of insulin-producing beta cells. Insulin resistance occurs when the normal interaction between insulin and the insulin receptors on the cells of the body is less effective, and the glucose is unable to enter the cells.

   People with this type of diabetes often have other family members with the same problem, so there must be an inherited component to this condition. People with type II diabetes are usually *above* their ideal body weight. Obesity plays a role in producing or unmasking this condition. Overeating also contributes to the problem because the body cannot handle large quantities of food consumed. As a result, diet is a primary treatment of this form of diabetes.

   The pancreas of a person with type II diabetes recognizes that the blood glucose level is elevated and as a result calls for more insulin. Although the pancreas secretes insulin—perhaps more than usual—it is not enough to overcome this resistance. Thus type II diabetes is a *relative* insulin deficiency; that is, the insulin produced is insufficient to overcome the insulin resistance.

   If the pancreas could produce enough insulin to overcome insulin resistance, things might remain stable. Unfortunately, though, although production is increased at first, sometimes it cannot be maintained, even with dietary restrictions to reduce the insulin resistance. Fortunately, the oral *sulfonylurea* medications ("oral agents") often help. These medications probably improve the balance between the insulin supply and the amount of insulin needed in two ways. First, it is likely that they make the beta cells more sensitive to glucose so that glucose can stimulate insulin secretion more effectively. Second, they may also reduce insulin resistance. The pills, however, are *not* insulin and are also ineffective without an apropriate diet. Only when the imbalance between insulin production and insulin needs becomes very great will insulin injections be needed in this patient.

People with type II diabetes are usually over age 40. Even this is not an absolute requirement, however, and type II diabetes is sometimes found in younger individuals. Most people with type II diabetes, whether older or younger, are above their ideal body weight. Type II diabetes in children or adolescents is called "maturity-onset diabetes of the young" (MODY). About 85% of all people with diabetes have type II.

Although it is usually easy to determine the type of diabetes, some people show characteristics of both types, and classifying them is difficult. There is no routine test to tell the types. Most decisions for treatment are made based on the severity of the diabetes at a given time. Even if the type of diabetes is not obvious at the onset, care and watchful follow-up by the physician will dictate what treatment is needed.

Other Types of Diabetes. While most people with abnormal glucose levels fall into (or between) one of the two categories, there are other types of abnormalities that should be mentioned. Some of these are not diabetes, but may be way stations on the road to developing it. The National Diabetes Data Group, along with other worldwide diabetes organizations, reclassified these various stages and types.

INCREASED RISK FOR DIABETES. There are two categories that are not diabetes as presently diagnosed but may represent an increased risk of developing diabetes later. People with *previous abnormality of glucose tolerance* (PrevAGT), formerly known as prediabetes, have no current evidence of abnormal glucose metabolism, but have at one time had impaired glucose tolerance or elevated blood sugar. This may have been influenced by stress. People who have had temporary elevations in blood glucose during pregnancy or illness are in this group. People with *potential abnormality of glucose tolerance* (PotAGT), formerly known as potential diabetes or also prediabetes, are those with no evidence of a blood glucose abnormality. However, they are at increased risk to develop diabetes. These include people with islet cell antibodies, or an identical twin or another close relative of someone with type I diabetes.

IMPAIRED GLUCOSE TOLERANCE (IGT). The diagnosis of diabetes is based on specific elevations in blood glucose levels, usually during a *glucose tolerance test* (GTT). However, between the normal levels of glucose and levels that are diagnostic for diabetes is a zone that is neither of the above. These persons are said to have impaired glucose tolerance. They do not usually have the classic symptoms of diabetes and thus may be in a stage of developing diabetes. Although diabetes may eventually develop, many may also remain in this class for many years, and some return to normal. Certainly, however, the potential is there, and this group should make special efforts to maintain normal body weight and to watch for suggestive symptoms.

GESTATIONAL DIABETES MELLITUS (GDM). These women have evidence of abnormal glucose metabolism during pregnancy. They have an increased risk both for diabetes-associated complications during pregnancy and for developing real diabetes after the baby is born. If true diabetes develops, it may be years later or immediately.

SECONDARY DIABETES. This diabetes is due to some process that either reduces the insulin production or increases the insulin resistance. This process might reduce the number of pancreatic beta cells, for example. It could be a pancreatic disease or possible tumors of the pancreas. Certainly, diabetes from the surgical removal of the pancreas would be in this group. Patients with this type of diabetes must be treated in the same way as those with type I diabetes.

___

Why People Get Diabetes

Although we have discussed some of the causes of diabetes, there is still the question, what is it that makes people get diabetes? What triggers the events that cause diabetes to arise from these influences? There are a number of contributing factors.

Heredity. That heredity is involved in causing diabetes has been known for a long time; diabetes seems to occur in certain families. If one identical twin develops diabetes, the other is highly likely to develop diabetes. This occurs in about 90% of identical twins with type II diabetes and about 50% of identical twins with type I diabetes.

When a parent passes an inheritable trait on to an offspring, the parent does so by means of genes, which are like blueprints that direct the offspring to develop that same trait. Genes are found in each and every cell and are a part of chromosomes. These contain

DNA (desoxyriboneucleic acid), the long chain-like molecule that carries the "code" that is the inherited message. All cells in a given individual contain the same chromosomal information or genes, but each cell can use some bits of information that are needed for its particular function. It also ignores information that it does not need. For example, the eyes pay close attention to the information determining eye color, but pay no attention to the information determining the shape of the toes. There is specific information in beta cells which allows them to become beta cells.

Certain characteristics dominate over others when the information received from one parent differs from that received from the other. If both parents have blue eyes, their children should also have blue eyes. However, if one parent has blue eyes, but the other has brown eyes, and if all the children from this mating have brown eyes, the gene for brown eyes was *dominant*. If both parents have brown eyes, each due to a combination of blue and brown that their parents had, some of their offspring could have blue eyes if one blue gene from each parent happened to combine. In such a case, the trait for blue eyes would be said to be *recessive*.

This description of genetics is simplified; in fact, there are often multiple combinations of genes that contribute to a specific inherited trait. No theory of inheritance based on a gene has been compatible with the actual inheritance patterns of either type I or type II diabetes. Children of two diabetic parents have only about a 30% chance of developing diabetes. While studies of identical twins suggest a definite genetic link, it is not absolute. The current theory is that there are many factors that can predispose to diabetes—it is *multifactoral*—and that multiple genes may be involved or even a genetic trait making the individual susceptible to some external factor, such as a virus, which might precipitate the development of diabetes.

One factor that makes study difficult is that we don't always know the details about our ancestors' medical problems. A study in Oxford, Massachusetts, of all people with diagnosed diabetes showed that only 25% knew of relatives with diabetes at the start of the study, but after 15 years, because of an increased awareness of diabetes in the community, nearly 80% of them knew or had heard of some relative who had diabetes, either previously undiagnosed, simply unknown, or developed after the initial interview.

There also seems to be a difference between the frequency of inheriting type I and type II diabetes. People with type II diabetes appear to have many more relatives with diabetes than people with type I. People with type I diabetes often report fewer relatives with diabetes or more distant relatives (such as a distant cousin or aunt) with the disease. Recently research into organ transplantation has lead to *tissue typing*, which is similar to blood typing (A, B, O, AB, etc.) used for blood transfusions. Tissue types are determined by comparison of *antigens*. Antigens are recognizable, unique markers on the surfaces of all cells. These antigens are determined by genes, just as other traits are. The genes that control these antigens have been studied and labeled. This system of genes is known as the human lymphocyte antigen (HLA) system. When these genes produce a specific cell surface marker antigen, the body uses that antigen as a way to identify that cell, just as people on a sports team can be differentiated by their uniforms. If the body's immune system plans to attack itself (autoimmune response), it makes antibodies and white blood cells designed to attack these specific antigens, even though they are supposed to identify the cell as a normal part of the body. This "mistaken identity" can mark the cell for destruction.

Researchers studying type I diabetes have found that two specific HLA system antigens (known as HLA-B8 and HLA-B15) are more common in people with type I diabetes than in the general population. There may be others. Ongoing research is discovering other antigens that may increase the likelihood of type I diabetes. While there is as yet no practical use for this information in predicting diabetes, and HLA types are strictly a research tool, insight into this antigen system gives us new understanding of how people can develop type I diabetes. Unfortunately, no HLA types have yet been discovered for type II diabetes. Other diseases—for example, some thyroid diseases and adrenal failure—have been found to be caused by autoimmune tissue destruction as well. Research into HLA relationships with disease processes continues.

Viruses. The possibility that viruses may help cause diabetes has long been considered. In 1864, a Norwegian scientist reported that a patient developed diabetes following a mumps infection. More recently, a study reported that in Sweden, the onset of diabetes following a mumps epidemic was greater than expected. English scientists have found a relationship in children between diabetes and a strain of viruses known as "coxsackie." Cases of diabetes, along with virus infections, were more frequent during the winter months than summer. In studies of this diabetes/virus association, the British Diabetic Association reported an increased incidence of new cases of type I diabetes at about 4 to 5 years of age and even more at ages 12 to 13. They noted that at these ages the children received heavy exposure to various viruses as they started primary and secondary schools, respectively.

With present theories suggesting that genetic traits predispose individuals to diabetes, it seems logical to look for another factor that starts the process going. Viruses might be just that. This would help explain the situation in which only one twin (with the same genes as his or her sibling) gets diabetes. Only one of the pair might have been exposed to the virus.

Obesity. Although heredity may be responsible for predisposing someone to type II diabetes, obesity may be the "stress" factor that triggers it by promoting insulin resistance. To make things worse, obesity tends to run in families, although environment, such as ethnic life-style or an overweight mother overfeeding her child, is at least as important. The primary therapy of type II diabetes in the obese person is diet. When an obese person loses weight, the blood glucose levels often become normal, although there is still a tendency to elevated blood glucose at times. Obesity is therefore a major factor in the development of type II diabetes.

IN TYPE II DIABETES, IT MIGHT BE SAID THAT HEREDITY MAY LOAD THE CANNON, BUT STRESS OR OBESITY PULLS THE TRIGGER.

Aging. Type II diabetes seems to be more common after age 40. In most people glucose tolerance declines with aging. The relationship between diabetes and age will be discussed further in Chapter 14.

Diet. An interesting relationship exists between food eaten and the onset of diabetes. For instance, the rate of diabetes among Yemenite Jews, who had a low incidence of diabetes while eating a very high protein and low carbohydrate diet, increased when they were exposed to a "Western" diet with refined sugars and a high carbohydrate content. Also, the incidence of diabetes increases with degree of wealth. Do wealthier people eat more, or do they buy food that provides poorer nutrition? In African communities, diabetes is rare except among groups that eat high starch and refined foods. It is interesting that the prevalence of diabetes among Indians living in a relatively poor area is about 1%. Among Indians living in a big industrial city such as Bombay or Calcutta, this changes to 2%. Among Indians who have migrated to South Africa, the United Kingdom, or the United States, however, the rate rises to 4% or more.

It must be emphasized that eating sugar does not cause diabetes. Rather, if someone had the genetic predisposition to develop an intolerance to glucose, eating more glucose might make the individual more obese, which would make the glucose intolerance more evident!

The absence of fiber in the diet has been suggested as a causative factor. High fiber diets seem to decrease the incidence of diabetes.

Hormones. Many hormones are present in humans. For example, the sex hormones determine whether we are male or female. Pituitary hormones send messages to other glands to make their own particular hormones, and the thyroid hormones regulate the body's rate of metabolism. New hormones are being discovered yearly. As we learn more about these hormones, we can better understand how they work and how they can affect various body functions.

Although these hormones are closely regulated, occasionally, changes in amounts can occur. These affect blood glucose metabolism. For example, excess growth hormone from the *pituitary gland* counteracts insulin's effects and produces a diabetic-like state. An excess of cortisol from the *adrenal* does the same thing. Hormone output can fluctuate according to the time of day. An increase of growth hormone probably causes a need for increased amounts of insulin in the early morning hours, just before awakening. This is known as the *dawn phenomenon* and causes difficulty in glucose regulation of a person with type I diabetes. *Glucagon* has the opposite effect of insulin and probably works with insulin to maintain proper blood glucose levels. There also are other hormones, such as *somatostatin*, discussed earlier, that can affect both insulin and glucagon levels and can balance the action of both these hormones. Disease states that involve increased secretion of hormones can also cause diabetes. These include acromegaly (growth hormone excess), Cushing's disease (cortisol excess), and tumors secreting excess glucagon (glucagonomas).

Drugs and Medications. Most medications, while prescribed for a specific reason, can have other effects on various bodily functions in addition to the intended effect for which they were given. Sometimes, one of these side effects can disturb diabetes control. For example, diuretic (fluid-removing) medications may be used to treat high blood pressure. However, this beneficial effect is accompanied by the loss of potassium, which is not good. A lower potassium level can cause an increase in the blood sugar level, especially in those predisposed to diabetes. Changing the medication or just replacing the lost potassium will improve blood sugar levels.

Other medications may affect blood sugars as well. Oral contraceptive agents (birth control pills) may increase blood sugar levels by interfering with insulin availability. Cortisone, which is like cortisol and is a product of the adrenal gland, and similar medications such as prednisone (corticosteroid medications) can also increase the blood sugar, sometimes quite substantially, although these medications are usually used for short periods. Excess amounts of thyroid hormone, due to an overactive thyroid gland or too much replacement medication, increase the rate of metabolism, thereby increasing the amount of insulin required. While most of these medications do not *cause* diabetes, they can make diabetes worse, or unmask diabetes in someone who is a candidate to get it anyway.

Illness. The stress resulting from many illnesses can lead to higher blood glucose levels in some people with diabetes. In anyone predisposed to diabetes it can result in high blood sugar levels where none had been found previously. For persons with no past evidence of diabetes, the blood sugars often return to normal once the stress of the illness subsides. It is also possible that the disease may unmask the diabetes which was present but undiscovered earlier.

People with diabetes, especially if blood sugars have been elevated, are more likely to have infections that take longer to resolve. It was once thought that the elevated blood glucose was a breeding ground for bacteria, promoting infections. This is not really the case, unless sugar is present in the urine. What probably happens is that the phagocytes, white blood cells that fight off infections, work poorly in the presence of elevated blood sugar levels, allowing the infection to get the upper hand.

Stress. Many people think "stress diabetes" is a special form of the disease. Others think there is no way that they can control their diabetes because of the tremendous stress (psychological) that they have undergone. Does stress really play a part in causing or worsening diabetes?

Predisposing factors have already been discussed. Many types of stress, especially physical stress such as illness or injury, may unmask the onset of diabetes in some predisposed to it. It does not cause it unless injury destroys the pancreas itself. Various factors have been identified as potential stresses. Aging may reduce the insulin output. Infection, as previously mentioned, and multiple childbirth have been considered as possible influences on the development of diabetes in those who are likely to succumb anyway.

Nevertheless, diabetes is often discovered when an individual is receiving care for another illness. Type II diabetes often begins slowly and subtly, and it is likely that slightly elevated blood glucose levels were present for some time previously, only to be discovered by blood or urine screening tests performed as part of the care of the other problem.

Occasionally a person finds he has diabetes after some traumatic experience such as an auto accident. In the hospital he is found to have diabetes. Unless the pancreas was badly damaged (most unlikely), what probably happened was that he had diabetes without symptoms, and it was discovered during routine testing. Another person with full-blown diabetes insisted that this was new and blamed it on a severe aggravation a month earlier. His employment records showed that a blood glucose test had been done a half dozen years earlier. The test showed a glucose level of 165 mg% 2 hours after breakfast. Was that diabetes then? Probably not, but it was abnormal and the diabetes may have increased as he grew a bit older and a bit heavier.

Chronic mental stress probably does not cause much of a direct elevation in blood glucose levels, although it is often blamed. More often, chronic stress is a distraction and is often an excuse or reason for not properly caring for the diabetes.

What Are the Chances of Getting Diabetes?

With all of the things that can influence getting diabetes, it seems as if it should be very common. Well, as diseases go, it is one of the more common ones—about 5% of the population has it, with higher levels in select populations. Of course, your chances of getting diabetes are greater if you are related to someone who has it.

For type I diabetes, which appears in less than 1% of the whole population, if you have a sibling (brother or sister) with diabetes, your chances of developing type I diabetes is 5%. If you have a father with diabetes, the chance that you will develop diabetes before the age of 20 is 5 to 10%. If your mother is the one with diabetes, however, the risk is only half of this. The risk is greater if more than one relative has diabetes—if two siblings have type I diabetes, the risk is 10% for the third to develop it. If the relative with type I diabetes is an aunt, uncle, or grandchild, the risk drops to 1 to 2%.

It is important to remember that there are many factors that contribute to type II diabetes, and the inheritance, and the ultimate result of the inheritance in the form of diabetes, differ depending on which traits are actually inherited.

The odds of getting type II diabetes are increased by the presence of any other factors that have just been discussed. Overall, however, the offspring of someone with type II diabetes may have as much as a 25 to 30% chance of developing type II diabetes. If both parents have type II diabetes, the risk may be as high as 75%.

How Do I Know If I Have Diabetes?

Diabetes can affect the entire body and everything in it and can produce a vast array of symptoms and problems. It has been called "the great imitator." However, as the level of the sugar in the blood rises, certain classic symptoms usually result which suggest this disease. The classic symptoms include the "polys"—polyuria (frequent urination), polydipsia (frequent consumption of liquids), and polyphagia (increased consumption of food)—as well as weight loss, blurred vision, and fatigue. Other symptoms as discussed below, may also be present. These symptoms may begin gradually and may go unnoticed for a long time. Alternatively, sometimes they begin rather abruptly and increase in severity rapidly. Either way, once these symptoms are recognized, testing for the presence of diabetes should be performed and treatment, if the diagnosis is made, should begin.

ONE OF THE COMMONEST SYMPTOMS OF DIABETES IS PROLONGED AND UNEX- PLAINED TIREDNESS. IT IS MISSED BECAUSE IT IS SO COMMON. EVERYTHING ELSE IS BLAMED!

In addition to the classic symptoms listed above, there are other signs of diabetes that may be less common but are just as important.

Skin Symptoms. Diabetes may produce itching of the skin, usually in the genital (especially vaginal) or anal areas. This can cause severe discomfort. Carbuncles, furuncles, and difficulty in healing wounds also may be found. People with untreated diabetes may have very high levels of lipids (fats) in the blood, which may cause small, raised bumps on the skin called *xanthomas*.

Gynecological Problems. It is not unusual for a gynecologist to be the first to discover signs of diabetes. Women with elevated blood sugar levels are more likely to get a fungal infection, called *candidasis* or *moniliasis*, which causes severe itching of the vagina, sometimes accompanied by a chronic discharge.

Impotence. Men with diabetes can develop difficulties achieving an erection. While this problem develops after diabetes has been present for some time, on occasion, when the blood sugar has been quietly abnormal for some time, this distressing failure may be a first sign of diabetes.

The Nervous System. Nerve damage due to diabetes usually occurs after the disease has been present for a long period, but as in the previous paragraph, when the diabetes is present and unrecognized for some time, signs of nerve damage may be the first sign of diabetes. Frequently there is numbness, tingling, burning, or intense sensitivity in certain areas of the skin, especially in the feet and legs. These symptoms may be worse at night. Nighttime leg cramps are a common example, but not all night cramps are caused by diabetes or neuropathy. Occasionally a temporary paralysis of one of the nerves controlling an eye muscle can result in blurry or double vision, which disappears when one eye is closed. This usually disappears by itself in about 4 to 6 weeks.

Fatigue. Fatigue is probably the earliest and most common symptom of diabetes, but fatigue can be caused by many other things. Those with diabetes with only this symptom are often misdiagnosed. If the fatigue is due to the diabetes, the fatigue usually disappears after treatment. It may take a few months for some people to "feel themselves again."

Blurred Vision. Blurred vision is one of the classic presenting symptoms of diabetes. It is usually caused by glucose seeping into the lens of the eye and changing its shape, which results in blurred vision. Once treatment of the diabetes is started, the glucose slowly comes out of the lens, and eventually the vision will improve. This improvement may take some time, however. The right time for an eye check is after the glucose control has stabilized. New glasses may be necessary. Getting glasses before control is improved is useless and wasteful because the vision may rapidly change.

These are a few of the possible symptoms of diabetes which can make one suspicious of possible diabetes. Awareness of these symptoms, plus knowledge of some of the predisposing factors to

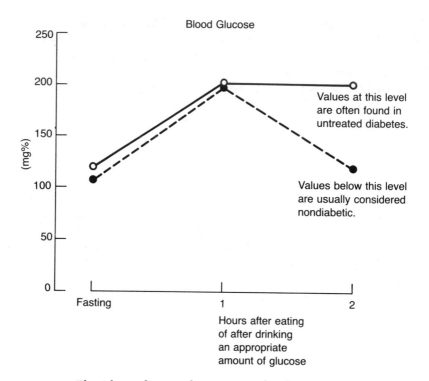

FIG. 1–8. The 2-hour glucose tolerance test. The glucose tolerance test is usually diagnostic of diabetes; it shows the blood glucose response to an appropriate amount of glucose given by mouth. (Values represent blood from the vein, as recommended by the National Diabetes Data Group. Values are higher when blood plasma is used for testing.)

diabetes, should lead the patient and physician to suspect diabetes and confirm its presence if it is there.

Detection of Diabetes: Making the Diagnosis

New cases of diabetes can be diagnosed in a number of ways. It can be diagnosed when one has the classic symptoms and a clearly elevated blood sugar, taken any time of the day. More than one blood test must be done to clinch the diagnosis. Laboratory errors can happen. When the symptoms are less obvious or the index of suspicion is lower, more specific testing needs to be performed.

Blood Glucose. Patients often ask, "Do I have sugar (glucose) in my blood?" The answer is always yes, because everyone must have glucose in the blood at all times. The question is, how much? The abnormality in diabetes is that the blood glucose level is too high. The normal blood glucose level usually falls within a very definite range. When a person is fasting (in the morning before food), this value is usually between 60 and 100 mg%, usually closer to 60 mg%. After a person either eats or challenges the beta cells to produce insulin by drinking glucose, the blood glucose level may become elevated for an hour or so, although it almost never increases above 140 mg%. Normally, the blood glucose drops quite rapidly, so that 3 hours after the meal, the previous fasting blood glucose level is reached.

The Glucose Tolerance Test. The glucose tolerance test challenges the body's ability to use a quick, large amount of ingested glucose. It has become the "gold standard" for the diagnosis of diabetes, although it is now used only if the symptoms are not obvious or if there is any doubt. This test can settle the issue definitely.

For three days before the test, the person being tested should eat large amounts of carbohydrates (starch). If carbohydrates are restricted, the test might suggest that diabetes is present when it really is not. Physical activity should continue as usual during these three days. A glucose tolerance test on a bedridden patient may also falsely show diabetes when none exists.

While the person being tested is still fasting on the morning of the test, a fasting blood glucose level is taken, and then the person drinks a measured amount of a glucose solution (usually 75 grams). Subsequently, blood samples are collected every 30 minutes for 2 hours, and then hourly thereafter (this may vary). To diagnose diabetes, 2 or 3 hours is usually enough, although longer tests may be performed to diagnose certain unusual conditions. Table 1–2 lists the results that are normal, that diagnose diabetes, and that would be called borderline (see also Fig. 1–8).

The glucose tolerance test is not usually needed for diagnosis, but is used for confirmation of questionable cases. Actually, a blood glucose result of more than 200 mg% 1 to 2 hours after a meal is enough to raise suspicion. If the result is during fasting, there is essentially no doubt.

Urine Glucose. Urine testing is not used to diagnose diabetes. While blood glucose levels may be high enough to lead to a diagnosis of diabetes, urine glucose may not be apparent if the *renal threshold* is high enough. If only the urine test were done, the

TABLE 1–2. Interpretation of a Glucose Tolerance Test

	VENOUS BLOOD (FROM ARM)	CAPILLARY BLOOD (EARLOBE OR FINGER)
Normal glucose levels (nonpregnant adult)		
Fasting	under 115	under 100
1/2, 1, or 1 1/2 hrs after glucose	under 200	under 180
2 hrs after glucose	under 140	under 120
Impaired glucose tolerance (IGT) (nonpregnant adult)		
Fasting	under 140	under 120
1/2, 1, or 1 1/2 hrs after glucose	200 or over	180 or over
2 hrs after glucose	140-200	120-180
Diabetes Mellitus (nonpregnant adult)		
Multiple fasting samples	over 140	over 120
or		
1/2, 1, or 1 1/2 hrs after glucose	over 200	over 200
plus		
2 hrs after glucose	over 200	over 200

Note: These values are based on recommendations by the National Diabetes Data Group as published in *Diabetes*, 28 (December 1979): 1039–56.

diagnosis could be missed. Conversely, the presence of glucose in the urine without elevated blood sugar does not mean diabetes. *Renal glycosuria*, in which glucose appears in the urine but the blood glucose level is normal, can be quite common in children. If glucose in the urine is detected, blood testing should be done.

Conclusion

So this is what diabetes is, why people get it, and how you can tell whether you have it. Although many things are not known about diabetes, we now know more than ever before, and more is being found out constantly.

Next we move on to the important part—what you or the friend or family member can do about it!

2

Treating Diabetes Mellitus

Now that diabetes mellitus has been defined and the problems are understood, we must ask, what can be done about it? Actually, considering the complex condition that diabetes is, there are at this time relatively few choices that make up the treatment. In fact, there are just five: education, exercise, diet, oral medications, and insulin.

Treatment of Diabetes
1. **Education**
2. **Exercise**
3. **Diet**
4. **Oral medications**
5. **Insulin**
(**Most people need at least two of these.**)

The changes that have occurred in the treatment of diabetes since the first general use of insulin in 1922 have constituted one of the most exciting chapters in the history of medicine. Within just a few years, the outlook for people with diabetes changed from one of near starvation and mere survival to a life in which survival is taken for granted and the horizons are almost unlimited. Increasing numbers of people have lived for longer than 50 years following the diagnosis of diabetes—50 useful and productive years.

The treatment of diabetes must last a lifetime. Even people who can cope with acute illness are often unprepared to withstand the longterm treatment required by diabetes. Treating diabetes is like waging a prolonged war: it is possible to lose some battles, but the war must be won. Diabetes is ever-present; the treatment is for now and for the future. It requires a constant effort. With modern treatment, diabetes can be well regulated, and this state can be maintained for many more years through constant attention and "upkeep."

Goals of Treatment

There are two main goals of the treatment of diabetes. One is to restore the "physiology" (the chemical workings of the body) of the person with diabetes to as normal a state as possible. The "as possible," however, may sometimes require compromises because our ability to treat diabetes, while improved, is not yet perfect. The second goal is to have the person with diabetes live a life as close to "normal" as possible. Obviously, the tasks and restrictions required to manage a lifetime condition do not permit a "normal life" in the strictest sense. Yet many people adapt and have a happy, useful life that becomes "normal" for them. Normal for most people means not really having to think about anything. Improvements in treatment have permitted much greater personal freedom. To live long is good, but not enough. It should be a happy life as well!

Some people claim to be unconcerned about their blood or urine tests, saying that fate determines whether they will develop the complications of diabetes. They claim that the degree of "control" (how close to the normal physiology they can get) makes no difference. There is growing evidence that this is not so and that control does make a difference (see Chapter 18). The better you treat your diabetes, and thus avoid the extremes of blood glucose levels, the better you feel. Almost every physician has had to struggle to get some patients to accept treatments such as insulin. When such patients finally do accept treatment and reach normal physiologic sugar levels, after a month or two they tell their doctor: "I feel great! I did not realize how badly I felt. I thought that was normal for me. Why didn't you give me this treatment sooner?" It is no wonder that physicians age and gray long before their time! The chances of avoiding many longterm complications of diabetes are also improving with improved glucose control. Good control is not achieved with just insulin or pills. It is obtained by following a carefully planned total program including balanced eating, acceptable blood glucose levels, and activity (*exercise!*). It takes effort,

TABLE 2-1. Goals of Diabetes Treatment

EARLY IN THE COURSE OF DIABETES (OR WHENEVER NEEDED)
Avoid insulin reactions
Prevent ketoacidosis or coma
Avoid dehydration
Improve resistance to disease
Keep lipids normal
Improved, happier life-style

LATER IN THE COURSE OF DIABETES
Avoid or improve complications
Reduce chances of neuropathy
Prevent early cataracts
Maintain excellent control to have normal babies
Prevent vascular complications
Reduce chances of developing tiny blood vessel diseases

but it is worth it. Once good control is achieved, even those who had professed to "feel good with high sugars" often feel even better. They had forgotten how well they *could* feel!

For some people with diabetes, maintaining a "normal" level of blood sugar at all times is difficult. This does not mean they should give up this goal, but that it may take a greater effort. One can often achieve these objectives with other than totally normal values, but the closer to normal (nondiabetic) levels, the better, provided, of course, that you do not overeat.

Throughout this book there are specific discussions on how to achieve the goals of your diabetes treatment. You and your physician and health care team should decide exactly what your treatment goals are and how to achieve them (Table 2-1).

The "Normal" Life

It has sometimes been said that people with diabetes can live a "normal" life. This is not strictly true. Any person who must always think about *what, when,* and *how much* he or she eats, who must test blood and/or urine glucose levels frequently, and who must use tablets or insulin injections cannot be said to live a "normal" life. For most people, a normal life means doing what they please without thought of medicines, diet, or other restraints.

While the life of someone with diabetes is not strictly normal, it can be extremely livable, useful, and enjoyable. It is important to take the attitude that diabetes care is part of your life-style and to

develop a new "normal" for you—a normal that includes the care of
your diabetes. You are not "a diabetic." You are a person who has
diabetes, but the good news about diabetes is improving all the
time.

The Tools for Treatment

The chief tools in the treatment of diabetes are education,
exercise, diet, oral medications, and insulin—no more, no less—
there are no other. Most people need at least two of these.

Education. Although it has been a vital part of diabetes care for
many decades, it is only recently that the absolute importance of
education has been recognized. How do you know what diet to
follow? What insulin dose? How often? How can you know these
things without education? This is the first and probably the most
important item, because without it, some of the others will not be
possible.

> **EDUCATION IS NOT A PART OF TREATMENT
> — IT *IS* TREATMENT.**

Activity. Exercise is one of the original ways of controlling diabetes—perhaps not by itself, but it improves the effect of the other
treatments. It is important because it not only improves general
health, but it may reduce insulin requirements by making the
insulin more effective, probably by improving the function of the
insulin receptors (discussed later). The required level of activity of
each individual is important in designing a diabetes treatment plan.
Exercise, to the extent that it is suitable to a person, can be very
desirable.

The Place of Diet. Control of the type and amount of food ingested
is still the basis of all treatment of diabetes. Of course, it is
important for the nondiabetes world as well, although it is often
ignored. Many patients who develop type II diabetes retain the
ability to make some insulin, and proper diet makes it easier for the
insulin to be effective. For the person with type I diabetes, the
eating plan is also important. While it is often less restrictive than
the program for those with type II, it provides guidelines for wider

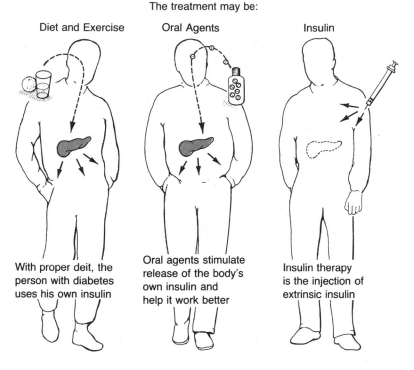

ALL DIABETES THERAPY MUST DEPEND ON *INSULIN*

The treatment may be:

Diet and Exercise   Oral Agents   Insulin

With proper deit, the person with diabetes uses his own insulin

Oral agents stimulate release of the body's own insulin and help it work better

Insulin therapy is the injection of extrinsic insulin

BUT . . . ALL OF THESE TREATMENTS DEPEND ON *INSULIN*

FIG. 2–1. Regardless of the prescribed treatment—diet alone, diet plus oral hypoglycemic agents, or diet plus insulin injections—ultimately all treatments depend on insulin to control blood glucose levels.

and more intelligent food choices. It is a plan for healthy eating that is coordinated with insulin and activity.

Oral Medication. The oral hypoglycemic agents are tablets taken by mouth which lower blood glucose levels. They actually can stimulate the release of more insulin and help reduce resistance to whatever insulin is available. They are used by perhaps 30 to 40% of those with diabetes in the United States and perhaps as many as half the people with diabetes worldwide. Unfortunately, they are not effective for everyone with diabetes. They are effective only when the pancreas itself can make insulin.

Insulin. If the available body insulin is not adequate (type I diabetes), or if more insulin is needed despite proper diet in people

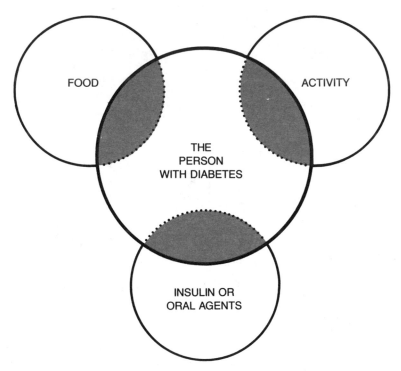

FIG. 2–2. The control of diabetes depends on the triad of food, activity, and insulin or oral agents. All of these however, must be balanced properly by the person with diabetes.

with type II diabetes, then it may be necessary to use insulin. Since it was discovered, *insulin is still the backbone of all diabetes treatment* whether the body makes its own or it is injected (Fig. 2–1).

These are the tools of treatment. Which will the physician prescribe? For people with type II diabetes, the first-line treatments are diet and exercise and perhaps the oral compounds. Failure with these signals the need for insulin. For someone with type I diabetes, diet and exercise are important, but insulin is always necessary.

Many people needing injected insulin ask, "Will I have to take insulin for the rest of my life?" Who knows? For those with type I diabetes the answer is usually yes—not because insulin is habit-forming, but because it is needed for life itself! For those currently making some of their own insulin, however, it is difficult to predict whether a period of good control, coupled with some weight loss if they are overweight, might allow a reduction or even eventual cessation of insulin. Changes in treatment may be necessitated by areduction in insulin production by the pancreas. Such a reduction is usually due to the progression of or change in the disease itself or to the actions of the patient and is usually not an effect of anything used to treat it.

So the treatment of diabetes is a system of balances. The triad of variables—insulin or oral agents, eating, and activity—can all be manipulated by the individual (Fig. 2–2). There are also other factors—the "intangibles" that effect any treatment program. These intangibles are minor, often imperceptible, daily variations in various factors—stress, timing, food absorption, etc.—that can also affect the diabetes. They are all factors that make us human! Humans are not machines and do not live each day as if it were a carbon copy of the day before. However, the more we pay attention to the variables that can affect diabetes, and the more we learn from them and about them, the more effective the diabetes treatment will be. Now, more details of treatment.

3

Learning for Life

Does it surprise you that the previous edition had no chapter on education for diabetes? It surprised us, especially because one of Dr. Elliott P. Joslin's greatest contributions to the treatment of diabetes was the education of the patient. In fact, in the Joslin auditorium, the teaching center of the New England Deaconess Hospital, a wall plaque with the likeness of Dr. Joslin is inscribed with the words, "Gladly he would teach." And chiseled in stone on the front of the Joslin Clinic building, built in 1955, is this statement:

THIS BUILDING
GIVEN BY
THOUSANDS OF PATIENTS
AND THEIR FRIENDS
PROVIDES AN OPPORTUNITY
FOR MANY
TO CONTROL THEIR DIABETES
BY METHODS OF TEACHING
HITHERTO AVAILABLE TO
THE PRIVILEGED FEW

In addition to concentrating research and patient care in one area, the Joslin Clinic was designed to educate people with diabetes—a new idea in the treatment of diabetes in the early part of this century. Patient understanding and self-care was always an obsession with Dr. Joslin since this manual was first published in 1918. His belief was, "The diabetic who knows the most, lives longest!" For many, many decades the person with diabetes was told very little. Now, almost all health care professionals would agree on the importance of education. The World Health Organization recently stated: "Education is the cornerstone of diabetic therapy and vital to the integration of the diabetic into society."

Why Educate the Person with Diabetes?

There are lots of good reasons, but one of the best is that people with diabetes have it every day, every week, and every month of the year. If they see the physician four or five times yearly, they still have it for 365 days.

There are other good reasons. The very best, of course, is survival. Other reasons are:
1. To live longer and happier. Quantity of life is important, but so is quality.
2. To have fewer days of illness and complications.
3. To be able to function and cope with the rigors of modern life.
4. To have more productive and useful lives.
5. To be less costly to oneself, one's family and community, and the health system under which one lives.

These are reasons enough. Can education do this? Well, not by itself, but the more people understand their condition and *know* what to do, the more the physicians and other members of the health team are able to help direct them along the path to continued health.

More Freedom?

Most people think diabetes is a very restrictive condition. To those who know nothing about it or have never accepted it, it could seem that way. Knowing more should give you *more* freedom. Even the Declaration of Independence said that "Life, liberty and the pursuit of happiness" should be our heritage! For the person with diabetes, the freedom to pursue these goals is far more possible than it was even a few years ago. What has allowed this freedom is the growing body of knowledge about diabetes and an understanding of how to apply this knowledge to daily life.

As more and more is learned, it becomes easier to develop treatment plans that are consistent with the needs of various life-styles and that allow people to reach for the life goals they want to pursue and to fulfill them. The diet recommended for people with diabetes is now nearly the same as for those without diabetes, and it has immense variety. Insulins with different action patterns are available, making it possible for people with different life-styles to have their insulin needs met. Similarly, self–monitoring of blood glucose, a most important advance, makes possible a personal, custom-made diabetes management program. Using self glucose monitoring, people can know at once whether to modify their treatment programs. Many activities which a few years ago were frowned upon for people with diabetes are today not only allowed but encouraged as an integral part of treatment.

The best news is that our new knowledge is making possible the avoidance of many complications. Until recently, the threat of impaired vision, kidney failure, and nerve damage hung like a dark cloud over the lives of people with diabetes. Today, the cloud is much less ominous because maintaining near normal blood sugar levels not only helps people feel well now but also offers hope that longterm complications can be avoided or minimized and better treated. Increasingly, people with diabetes can feel hopeful that the pursuit of their goals will not be cut short by debilitating or life-threatening complications.

There is never a good time to have diabetes, but the chances for people who have this condition to live full and satisfying lives are better today than ever before. Dorothea Sims, an author of books and articles about diabetes, says that now is clearly a time when people with diabetes can "reach for health and freedom" with a reasonable expectation of achieving them. But knowledge is an absolute necessity. Unlike most medical conditions, for which a physician prescribes a regimen for the patient to follow until the condition is improved or cured, diabetes is an *ongoing* state with which one must live for a lifetime. The word "ongoing" is crucial. While care by a physician and other members of a health team are critical, it is the patient who must assume responsibility for day-to-day management. This requires a lifetime of learning.

Knowledge, Skills, and Attitudes

The lifetime of learning includes not only *knowledge* but also *skills* and *attitudes*. Knowledge, of course, is understanding what diabetes is, why some people develop it, how the body uses food for energy, how diabetes affects the body's use of food, and the various forms of treatment used to help the body function despite diabetes. Skills include things people with diabetes must learn to do in order to manage it. Attitudes are ways of thinking about themselves and their condition which predispose people with diabetes to reach for that all-important health and freedom.

The three kinds of learning are closely related. One or two without the other are useless. For instance, knowing that monitoring provides information which helps maintain blood glucose levels as close to normal as possible is useless without the skills necessary to actually perform the test for urine and/or blood glucose according to an appropriate schedule. Neither the knowledge nor the skill is helpful, however, unless one's attitudes include a hopefulness that monitoring will help maintain good health, a confidence in one's ability to carry it out, and a commitment to do it.

Stages of Learning

Acquiring knowledge, skills, and a hopeful attitude is an ongoing endeavor. Immediately after diagnosis of diabetes and in the first few weeks that follow, it is critical for people to acquire a beginning knowledge of diabetes and some management skills as well. These are often called "survival skills." With their physician, teaching nurse, dietitians, and others, they must work out a treatment program that includes balancing insulin or oral agent needs with food consumption and normal daily activity. *Skills*, such as urine or blood testing, injecting insulin if needed, care of the feet, and carrying out sick-day procedures, also need to be learned almost immediately. Attitudes toward the new situation are also of enormous importance during the first few weeks after diagnosis. A good attitude will help decrease fears and anxieties associated with the new situation and will help develop confidence in the ability to manage diabetes. This is the first step in being able to reach for health and freedom in the coming months and years.

Once people with diabetes achieve this beginning knowledge, they will want to learn how to manage their condition in the variety of situations that add zest and pleasure to their lives. You could call this stage 2. There is no need to give up family picnics, parties with friends, weekend ski trips, eating at favorite restaurants, or even not-so-favorite fast-food establishments, travel to places near and far, or the myriad other activities people find enjoyable. The growing knowledge about diabetes and its management, along with the accompanying skills and attitudes, keep open almost unlimited options for pleasurable and fulfilling activities. The possibility of reaching for freedom while still having good health are for real!

Many with diabetes will want to explore still other areas of diabetes management in order to pursue life goals they want to fulfill. Some women, for instance, along with their spouse or partners, do not want the presence of diabetes to deny them the delight of having children, nor should it. Here again, newer knowledge about diabetes and its management provides choices which a few years ago were fraught with risks and disappointments. The key, of course, is education.

Choosing an Educational Program

It is vital for people with diabetes to participate in as many educational opportunities as possible, not only in the period immediately after learning they have diabetes, but throughout their lifetimes. By doing so they can continually develop and deepen their knowledge, skills, and attitudes.

Educational programs can be found in physicians' offices, diabetes clinics, local hospitals, health centers, camps, and many other locations. The adequacy and extensiveness of such programs will vary depending on the available resources. A local physician, for instance, can provide the needed education for the first few weeks after diagnosis, but many want to refer the newly diagnosed person to a center specializing in diabetes education for more intensive education.

Next we describe some important considerations for an educational program.

Active Participation. A person can learn a great deal about diabetes by sitting and listening to a lecture, especially if the presenter is a lively and engaging speaker. This is one way to acquire information about diabetes in an organized way. Usually people learn more when they participate actively in their own education and put their own energy and imagination to work to achieve their goals. By using educational resources on their own, they may find answers to questions they have about diabetes, try to solve problems related to diabetes care, or practice needed skills. In one educational program, for instance, people are given the records of blood glucose tests which an imaginary patient has collected over a period of three days. The participants in the education program are asked to look over the records, find patterns of high or low blood glucose levels and make recommendations for adjusting the insulin dose. Sometimes, participants are taken to fast-food restaurants for a meal and asked to select foods from the menu which meet the requirements of their meal plans. Participants also should have opportunities to try various kinds of exercise to determine how their blood glucose levels are affected by them and what they must do to prevent insulin reactions. This type of activity has proven an effective mode of learning and prepares people for dealing with their own actual life situations. A good education program must include many opportunities for people to participate actively in the learning process.

Your Own Needs and Problems. Diabetes education programs are especially valuable if they allow participants to focus on needs and problems of daily living. In one program, for instance, participants are shown slides of various social situations in which they might find themselves. This could be eating out at a restaurant, playing tennis, or spending a day at the beach. Based on their own experiences, participants are then asked to rank in order the situations according to whether they think it would be very hard, somewhat hard, fairly

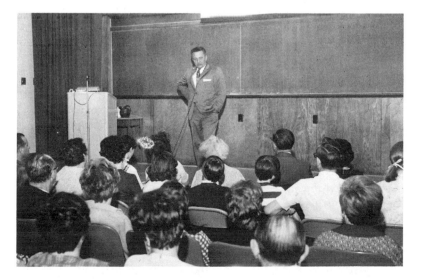

FIG. 3–1. A class at the Joslin Diabetes Center. Education has been the cornerstone of diabetes care at the center for many years.

easy, or very easy to manage their diabetes while doing the things shown in the slides. The group then explores how to manage their diabetes while doing the things they enjoy doing with family and friends when they face situations they have identified as difficult.

Attitudes toward Daily Life. For many the discovery of diabetes is a massive blow to the hopes and expectations they have for how they want to live their lives, to say nothing of their personal pride. At first, the discipline required for eating by meal plan, injecting insulin, testing or monitoring according to schedule, regular exercise, and many other requirements seems to ruin life's spontaneity and replace it with stiff rules and regulations. That it takes a while for most people to come to grips with the concerns, fears, and anxieties of their new situation should not surprise anyone.

A proper diabetes education program must give people an opportunity to face their own innermost feelings, to share these with health professionals, and to discuss these with others who have the same problems. Such discussions will help participants find ways to bring the care of diabetes into their daily living while at the same time fulfilling the hopes and expectations they have for themselves and their families.

Other Available Resources. Physicians and other health professionals such as teaching nurses, dietitians, exercise therapists, and social workers are the primary resource for help in learning to manage diabetes. Other resources are also available, including educational publications and tapes. There are cookbooks especially created to assist people with diabetes prepare appropriate meals. Informative pamphlets about self-care products and medications are often available at neighborhood pharmacies. Opportunities for regular exercise are available in many communities at health spas, the YMCA or Jewish community center, or at the athletic and health facilities of local high schools or community colleges. Dance groups, yoga classes, and sports groups provide other exercise options. Educational programs should put participants in contact with the abundance of resources that have been created to help people help themselves. Foremost among these are the various state and local branches of the American Diabetes Association, whose address is 1660 Duke Street, Alexandria, Virginia 22314.

Talking to Others with Diabetes. An often overlooked source of help in managing diabetes is the others with the same condition. The insights of people who have lived with and coped with diabetes for many years are helpful because they have fought the daily battle and won. They can provide clues about how to put various principles into practice in real life. To facilitate such interactions, many educational programs have adult support groups in which people with diabetes meet regularly to share their experiences.

Becoming Less Dependent. People with diabetes must make daily decisions affecting the care of their diabetes. Determining what to eat during a farewell coffee hour for a retiring fellow employee at the office, planning activities so that they will not have to be interrupted by monitoring their blood glucose level, or deciding whether they have time to feed the baby before their own snack is due are a few of the many decisions affecting diabetes care which must be made daily. Educational programs should give people the guidance they need to make such decisions without constantly having to seek authorities for advice. A part of reaching for freedom and health is becoming as free as possible from constant dependency on anyone else, although those with diabetes should always feel free to call on health-care providers for regular checkups and assistance in emergencies.

The Economics of Education

In this era of cost-consciousness, we must ask whether the cost of education is worth it. You bet it is! Education for diabetes arms you with the tools to prevent problems or to help solve them yourself, and this saves money! For example, good foot care can prevent weeks of hospitalization with its high cost of treatment and lost earnings for you. Learning to monitor allows you to solve problems and improve control at home, preventing hospitalization. Monitoring also makes sick-day management easier and may prevent hospitalization or emergency room visits. There are many more examples.

So, is education worth the cost? It's the best bargain in town!

Conclusion

Education about diabetes, which was once a luxury, is not an addition to treatment—*it is treatment.* Nothing could be more true. Without it, the "reach for health and freedom" is impossible to obtain. How much education is needed? There can never be too much. Dr. Joslin's favorite answer to "How much education?" was a quotation from Isadore, Bishop of Seville (c. 570–636): "Learn as if you were to live forever, live as if you would die tomorrow." In other words, make every day count, but do it in such a way that tomorrow will be as good or better!

4

Nutrition and Diabetes

We have often been told that we are what we eat. Unfortunately, we also are what we don't eat, because if we choose poorly or lose nourishment because of uncontrolled diabetes, we may be building our body structure with inferior materials, or, worse, we may be skipping some materials altogether.

There is much more mystique and confusion about diet than there should be. It is really quite simple. Why do people with untreated or poorly treated diabetes eat so much and yet lose body weight? It is because their body cells are actually starving despite the food eaten. The food cannot be used and is actually wasted, lost in the urine. The situation is much like that of a person sitting on a raft on a freshwater lake dying of thirst and dehydration because he cannot reach the water.

No matter what you eat, it consists of only three kinds of nutrients: carbohydrates (sugars and starches), protein, and fat. These come in endless varieties and choices. None are "good" or "bad." It is not a moral issue. The problem is how they are used or misused.

Body Fuel

Food is the fuel for the body. It provides the energy we need to run our organs, muscles, and tissues, and it supplies the materials that rebuild body structures as they are used up or worn out. The body can use this fuel immediately, or it can store it for future use.

47

Stored energy can be quite important because energy requirements change daily. In fact, these energy needs may change from minute to minute! It is amazing that our bodies can almost always have just enough fuel for use whenever it is needed. The key, of course, is proper, balanced nutrition.

In people with diabetes, the ability to use, store, and retrieve these food fuels is impaired. In treating diabetes, we try to correct this impairment. Food, therefore, is an important part of this treatment. Indeed, the treatment of diabetes consists of three components: (1) the food that is eaten, (2) the level of activity, which affects how much fuel is needed, and (3) the insulin, either injected or made by the pancreas. Therefore it is essential to understand the fundamentals of the "diabetic eating plan" and how the plan fits into overall treatment.

The U.S. Department of Health and Human Services recently issued dietary guidelines for all Americans:

1. Eat a variety of foods.
2. Maintain desirable weight.
3. Avoid too much fat, saturated fat, and cholesterol.
4. Eat foods with adequate starch and fiber.
5. Avoid too much sugar.
6. Avoid too much sodium (table salt). Beware of processed and fast foods with high sodium contents.
7. If you drink alcoholic beverages, do so in moderation.

Eating plans for people with diabetes follow these same guidelines. Good nutrition and good diabetes control can be achieved through very similar eating plans! In fact, a diabetic diet is no longer restrictive and is good for everyone.

Is Diet Obsolete?

With many newer insulins and oral hypoglycemic agents, and with the ability to monitor blood glucose levels at home, daily compensation for variations in blood glucose levels is now possible. This makes some wonder, "Why is diet still necessary? Isn't diet now obsolete?"

"Diet" is one of the most unpopular words in any language: It suggests sacrificing the good things in life that people most enjoy. The idea of dieting attacks our basic instincts. The young enjoy goodies and sweets. In fact the poem "Night Before Christmas" states that "visions of sugar plums danced in their heads." Santa Claus himself is suspect because he is described as "chubby and plump—a right jolly old elf!" He had "a little round belly that shook, when he laughed, like a bowl full of jelly." He was obviously obese and the right age for diabetes!

Older persons (including Santa) like sweets as well. In fact, most parties and holidays are built around food, food, and more food! Many older persons have diabetes at this time of life when other pleasures may be less possible. Restriction of eating habits is never popular.

While some people with diabetes do have to make major diet restrictions, what most lose is the right to overeat or make poor food choices. Free eating should never have been a "right" any more than any other bad habit may be. Proper eating can be good and should be pleasurable itself!

What is really being asked is whether good nutrition is obsolete. The answer is no! Self monitoring provides instant information so that insulin doses can be changed to allow for variations in diet. Nutritional principles, however, and diet, in the sense of eating right, are still important parts of the treatment of diabetes.

It is for these reasons that we encourage the concept of an "eating plan" (or "meal plan") rather than a "diet". A diet is usually a short-term affair to achieve an objective—usually weight loss. Once this is achieved, the diet ends. The purpose of a diabetic eating plan is to be a part of the treatment of diabetes, which is eating for life. We must develop eating habits that are part of daily life-style—permanent habits that you can live with.

Dieting Is Not New

Long before the discovery of insulin, the disease diabetes mellitus, which means "the production of great quantities of sweet urine," was described as being a disorder in which people could not use carbohydrates (sugars). The treatment was elimination of carbohydrates from the diet. Because carbohydrate is the major source of energy for the body, eliminating it caused the body to use other energy sources—fat and also protein. The original treatment for diabetes, before insulin, was marked diet restriction—in fact, almost starvation. It is amazing how many people with diabetes (obviously type II) survived this, sometimes for years.

Carbohydrate is also the major stimulus of insulin production by the pancreas. People with type I diabetes did not survive long in the days before the discovery of insulin. People with type II diabetes, however, usually do not make quite enough insulin to overcome insulin resistance. Carbohydrate is a necessary part of their diet to stimulate as much insulin secretion as possible. Thus for these people, these early low-carbohydrate diets were not as effective as they should have been.

Even after the discovery of insulin, the guidelines for carbohydrate were about one-third of the total daily calories, with protein providing 15 to 20% and fat the remainder. Now it is known that high-fat diets elevate blood cholesterol levels, which contribute to coronary artery (heart) disease. It is also known that people with diabetes can handle more carbohydrate—often as much as 50 to 60% of the total daily calories—without adverse effects on the blood glucose levels. As diabetes itself can increase the risk of developing heart and other vascular diseases, diets with their reduced fat content make much more sense.

Therefore in 1986 the Committee on Food and Nutrition of the American Diabetes Association (ADA) recommended lowering the fat content in diabetic diets. The average American diet today contains about 40 to 45% of the daily calories as fat, which is much too high. Reductions in the fat content of the diets recommended by both the ADA (30%) and Joslin Clinic (30 to 35%) have therefore been made. (The Joslin recommendation is based on what we feel is a practical fat reduction, but would include less fat if the individual had elevated blood fat levels.

The current Joslin recommendation for carbohydrate content is 45 to 60%. These carbohydrates must be chosen carefully to include a significant amount of fiber. They must be "slow-release" carbohydrates such as legumes, rice, pasta, and whole fruits. These cause a slower rise in blood glucose levels, rather than the rapid rise caused by "quick-release" carbohydrates such as sweet sodas, tonics, and other simple sugars.

Now it is known that high-fiber diets are useful. These provide more bulk, which gives a feeling of "fullness," thus allowing people to feel satisfied with less food and lower fat content. Fiber also slows carbohydrate absorption from the bowel. By comparison, most American diets today have almost 40% of the daily calories as fat!

A Diabetic Eating Plan

Three parts must be considered in designing a diabetic eating plan:

1. Quantity (how much food is eaten)
2. Food types (what type of food is eaten)
3. Timing (when the food is eaten)

What we are saying is that to keep the blood sugars under proper control, the proper type of food must get into the body in the proper amount and at the proper time so that the insulin can make sure it is used for energy or stored for later.

Quantity

The basic measure of energy that is derived from the food we eat is the calorie (technically, a "kilocalorie," abbreviated kcal). Energy in the form of calories is used to run the body machine: muscle contraction, the beating of the heart, and the thinking of the brain. The three basic types of nutrients—carbohydrate, protein, and fat—all provide calories, but carbohydrate is the primary source, providing 4 calories per gram (115 calories per ounce). Protein provides a slower, more sustained supply of energy, also contributing 4 calories per gram. Protein, however, must also build muscle and other tissues and is not an optimal energy source. Fat is a very dense, concentrated energy source and functions as a long-term storage depot for energy. It provides 9 calories per gram (258 calories per ounce).

We all need a certain basic number of calories each day to keep the body functioning. Of course, this need differs from person to person, depending on age, sex, activity level, and body size. A simple starting estimate of daily caloric requirements is helpful. The average (although somewhat inactive) adult of normal weight requires about 25 calories per kilogram (2.2 pounds) of *ideal* body weight per day (or 11 calories per pound of ideal body weight per day) for weight maintenance. The ideal body weight is a theoretical weight based on height and body frame size and is not *necessarily* the weight you should be or the goal of any diet therapy. Table 4–1 gives ideal body weight by height.

Prescribing Calories. Once the required level of calories is determined, adjustments in eating can be made to promote weight changes and to provide enough fuel for various levels of activity. If someone is overweight, and weight loss is wanted, the calorie level is reduced to below 11 calories per pound per day (25 calories per kilogram per day)—perhaps to about 9 calories per pound per day (20 calories per kilogram per day). This intake does not have enough calories to meet daily requirements, and energy stored as fat will be used to make up the difference. Weight will be lost. To gain weight, of course, we must do the opposite. More than 11 calories per

Table 4–1. Desirable Weight Ranges—Ages 25 and over*

Height (no shoes) (ft. in.)		Men Weight Range	Weight‡ MRW = 100	Woment Weight Range	Weight‡ MRW = 100
4	9			90–118	100
4	10			92–121	103
4	11			95–124	106
5	0			98–127	109
5	1	105–134	117	101–130	112
5	2	108–137	120	104–134	116
5	3	111–141	123	107–138	120
5	4	114–145	126	110–142	124
5	5	117–149	129	114–146	128
5	6	121–154	133	118–150	132
5	7	125–159	138	122–154	136
5	8	129–163	142	126–159	140
5	9	133–167	146	130–164	144
5	10	137–172	150	134–169	148
5	11	141–177	155		
6	0	145–182	159		
6	1	149–187	164		
6	2	153–192	169		
6	3	157–197	174		

*Adapted from the 1959 Metropolitan Desirable Weight table (weight, in pounds, without clothing; height without shoes).
†For women between the ages of 18 and 25, subtract 1 lb for each year under 25.
‡Midpoint of medium frame range used to compute MRW: MRW = [(actual weight)/(midpoint of medium frame range)] x 100.

pound per day can be given—perhaps 14 or even 16 calories per pound (30 to 35 calories per kilogram).

Other factors can also affect the amount of needed daily calories. Women usually require fewer calories than men because they are smaller in size and frame. Smaller people usually require fewer calories to maintain their weight. Younger people using energy need more calories than older people, especially during periods of growth. Caloric needs also increase with certain kinds of physical stress, such as after severe injury or illness or during pregnancy and lactation (breast milk production).

This calorie prescription (11 calories per pound per day) is useful for relatively inactive individuals. Active young people need more calories than this—about 14 calories per pound (30 calories per kilogram). With increased activity, the body needs more calories, but not more insulin than the usual amount needed to keep glucose control. Thus very active people can eat more than they would have needed if they were inactive to maintain their present weight. A

TABLE 4–2. Tendency to Get Fat Increases With Age

	Age	Percentage of persons who exceed ideal weight by 10% or more	Percentage of persons who exceed ideal weight by more than 20%
Women	20–29	23	12
	30–39	41	25
	40–49	59	40
	50–59	67	46
Men	20–29	31	12
	30–39	53	25
	40–49	60	32
	50–59	63	34

Adapted from Metropolitan Life Insurance Company, studies reported in *U.S. News & World Report*, 6 June 1965, p. 68.

physician or dietitian should be consulted to help determine your actual calorie intake.

Obesity. Obesity is the plague of today's society—among people with and without diabetes. Obese people often look for excuses beyond their control such as a "glandular condition" or "stress," but the basic reason that they are overweight is that they have eaten more calories than they need. In a recent Boston Globe article, Earl Ubell pointed out that eating involves 10 inches of esophagus, 20 feet of small intestine, and 5 feet of large intestine. Of course, there is also the stomach, but there is the potential for trouble all the way. One trouble is that a lot of food is absorbed—often too much. Not enough absorption can also be a problem. So, as with much else in life, there must be a balance.

To lose weight, as stated above, people must either eat fewer calories than they need or use up calories by exercising—preferably both. Exercise alone does not result in significant weight loss; it is effective when accompanied by less caloric intake. Dr. Joslin, in a humorous vein, said that one of the best exercises is pushing yourself away from the table before you are full.

Other forces can affect the ability to achieve a desired weight. Age (Table 4–2), ethnic customs and beliefs, and family habits also contribute. Unfortunately, in many cultures obesity is confused with prosperity and good health. It also runs in families. The chubby child with an obese mother and grandmother (Fig. 4–1) has a greater chance of being an obese adult not only by inherited tendency but also by learned eating habits and ethnic diet preference.

In recent years, "slim is in!" seems to be the fad, and many diets have come and gone. Almost any diet can help you lose weight for a short time, but long term success depends on long term changes in eating habits and life-style. Weight takes time to come on, and time is necessary for it to come off. Unfortunately, the same diet will not perform in the same way for each person. The diet that allows one person to lose weight will make another person gain. Remember, "Jack Spratt could eat no fat, his wife could eat no lean!"

One has to consider why people eat. Loneliness, depression, and anxiety can lead people to seek gratification by eating. Some people eat out of habit while watching television or reading. You must recognize and deal with reasons you overeat before reducing food intake will be successful.

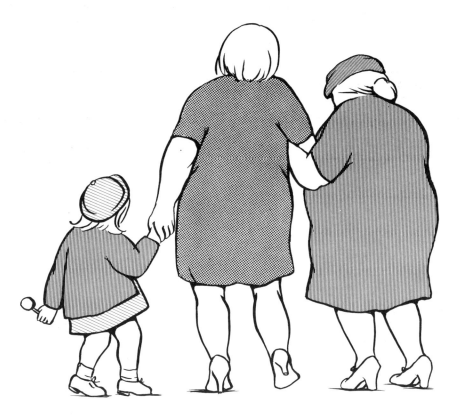

FIG. 4–1. A chubby child who has an overweight mother and an obese grandmother will probably become an overweight adult. This cycle can be broken, but ethnic habits and eating patterns often make changing this type of life-style difficult.

Weight loss is more successful when accompanied by an increase in exercise. The weight loss then is due to decreased fat cell size. With weight loss insulin works more effectively, and less insulin is needed. Triglyceride (absorbed fat) levels also decrease. Overall, the glucose tolerance is improved, signifying improved diabetes control. The energy used and basal metabolic rate decrease with weight loss with a low-calorie diet alone, which can slow down fat metabolism and cause the observed "plateau" in weight loss that sometimes occurs. Adding exercise may make the difference.

> **FOR THE OVERWEIGHT PERSON WITH TYPE II DIABETES, FEWER CALORIES AND MORE EXERCISE TO ACHIEVE WEIGHT LOSS ARE CRITICAL TO DIABETES TREATMENT.**

Food Types

Carbohydrates are the major source of energy for the body's needs and are the major constituents of the "starchy" foods such as breads, cereals, grains, pasta, fruits, vegetables, etc. These carbohydrates have been called complex carbohydrates because they are themselves constructed of long chains of sugar molecules.

Fast or Slow Sugars. The complex carbohydrates are preferred for people with diabetes because they are absorbed more slowly. The absorption is slow because complex carbohydrates must be broken down (digested) into the basic sugar molecules in the stomach and intestines before they can be absorbed into the bloodstream. This process takes time, and therefore they are absorbed and used slowly. Thus, complex carbohydrates are also known as *"slow"* *carbohydrates.* Simple carbohydrates—the sugars—need less digestion and are absorbed more quickly, producing a more rapid rise in the blood glucose levels. They are therefore known as *"quick"* *carbohydrates.*

This simple division of carbohydrates into "slow" versus "quick" provided a good explanation until recently, when studies showed that other factors affect the speed with which certain carbohydrates were taken into the bloodstream.

Glycemic Index. The concept of "glycemic index" was developed by Dr. David Jenkins and coworkers at the University of Toronto and shows how certain food affects blood glucose levels. For example, early studies found that potato (a starch) produced a glycemic response (i.e., a rise in the blood glucose level) similar to that of the same amount of carbohydrate in the form of glucose (a sugar). In contrast, rice or pasta (also starches) result in much "flatter," or more gradual, responses in the blood glucose levels (Fig. 4–2).

Unfortunately, many of the studies were performed in research laboratories on people without diabetes who were eating special test foods. Therefore it is difficult to know just how practical the glycemic index is in everyday use. These studies however, give a new and exciting insight into the way our bodies get needed nutrition. Not all carbohydrates have the same effects on blood glucose levels. Thus while it is not necessary to eliminate potatoes, it is important to choose a variety of starches from day to day and to understand the differences among the various choices.

Fiber. It is important to mention *fiber* in the diet. Fiber refers to a group of foods of plant origin which the human gastrointestinal system (stomach and intestines) cannot digest. Fiber can slow the carbohydrate absorption pattern, making blood glucose curves "flatter."

Fiber may be insoluble or soluble. A typical food that is high in insoluble fiber is wheat bran, as found in bran flakes, bran muffins, or whole wheat bread. *Insoluble fiber* holds onto, but does not dissolve in water, making foodstuffs move faster through the intestinal tract. The fiber is not digested and contributes to stool bulk, occasionally acting as a laxative.

Foods high in soluble fiber include apples, citrus fruits, oat bran, dried beans and peas, and many vegetables. These types of fibers slow down gastric emptying—the speed with which food passes out of the stomach and into the intestines. This slowing down can affect the glycemic response and thus can be useful for people with diabetes. Soluble fibers are also known as "gel-forming" or "gummy" fibers because, when dissolved in water, they become a gummy gel, which slows down glucose absorption and blunts the rise in blood glucose right after meals. They probably do this by disbursing the incoming food into various parts of this gel structure, which slows down the movement of nutrients toward the gut wall to be absorbed. Digestive enzymes may also become caught in the gel, slowing down their movement toward the foodstuffs they should help digest. Slowing down the absorption of carbohydrates is helpful to people with diabetes. Soluble fibers may also be useful in treating certain hyperlipidemias (high blood fat levels). Oat bran (in oat bran cereal and oatmeal), pectin (in citrus fruits and apple peel),

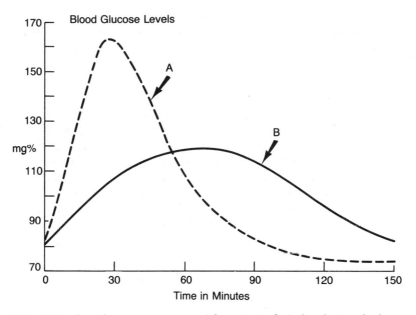

FIG. 4–2. The glycemic response (glycemic index) for fast and slow carbohydrate sources. Curve A, The rapid blood glucose rise that would be seen after consumption of a quick-release source of carbohydrate. Curve B, The "flatter," more gradual and prolonged rise in glucose levels after a slow-release carbohydrate is eaten.

and legumes (dried beans and peas) all contain soluble fibers which help to lower the level of cholesterol in the blood.

Carbohydrate. Once carbohydrate (glucose) gets into the bloodstream, there are three "metabolic directions" it normally takes, and insulin is required for all of them. Carbohydrate can be used to provide for immediate energy needs. As you sit at dinner, however, only minimal amounts of energy may be needed! Therefore, there must be a way for the body to store energy.

One storage form is glycogen (a long chain of glucose molecules). This is stored in the liver and in muscle and is a quickly accessible depot of energy. The glucose that leads to a rise in blood glucose levels after a low-blood-glucose reaction (rebound) comes from the release of stored glycogen. Energy to fuel the muscles for sudden bursts of energy may also come from glycogen.

The storage space for glycogen is limited. If there is too much carbohydrate to be stored as glycogen, the rest of the carbohydrate is converted into fat and is stored in fat (adipose) cells. This storage depot, unfortunately, is seemingly unlimited! Since insulin is required to store this fat in the fat cells, a myth has arisen that insulin makes you fat. This is not true! Insulin does not provide calories! You provide calories that insulin helps the body use when needed.

> When you eat too much and have enough insulin, the body stores the energy as fat for future use. Unfortunately, it is stored in unflattering places, and people see that you are a miser, storing more than you need for the future that may not come!

Protein. The second of the foods we eat is protein. Just as carbohydrate is made up of sugar molecules hooked together into a long chain, proteins are also made up of basic building blocks that are attached together as chain-like molecules called amino acids. Amino acids are the foundation for many important substances in the body such as hormones, antibodies, and various materials for building and rebuilding the body. They also provide energy to the body if carbohydrates are unavailable and can stimulate insulin secretion from the pancreas. In preinsulin days, individuals survived with diets low in carbohydrate by using energy from their fat and protein; their insulin was stimulated by the protein.

When protein is eaten along with carbohydrate as part of a full meal, the protein delays the rise in the blood glucose level. This delay may be caused by the insulin stimulated by protein, (in people with type II diabetes). Also, protein sources such as meat have much fat. Fat slows down carbohydrate absorption by delaying gastric (stomach) emptying.

Fat. The primary role of fat (triglycerides) is also an energy source, either for immediate needs or as a storage form for later use. It is the highest source of calories (9 calories per gram). Because fat delays the emptying of food into the intestines, it may slow down the rise in the blood glucose if included in a meal.

Fats are also needed to make up certain molecules and structures in the body, and not all of the needed fats can be manufactured by the body. Some essential fats (linoleic and linolenic acids) are needed in a normal diet.

Some sources of fat in the diet are butter, oils, margarine, fatty meats, whole milk, dairy products, sour cream, cream cheese, olives, and nuts. Recent dietary advice has recommended less fat in the diet because of its probable role in producing blood vessel

---

TABLE 4–3. Normal Fasting Values for Blood Lipids (Fats)

A. Cholesterol values and their respective risks for complications. The greater the risk, the more important it is to treat the condition aggressively.

Cholesterol Value (mg%) at Which There May Be:

Age (years)	Moderate Risk	High Risk
2–19	over 170	over 185
20–29	over 200	over 220
30–39	over 220	over 240
over 40	over 240	over 260

B. Normal ranges for blood plasma lipid concentrations—triglycerides and high-density lipoprotein (HDL) cholesterol (mg%)

	Male		Female	
Age (years)	Triglycerides	HDL-cholesterol	Triglycerides	HDL-cholesterol
0–19	30–100	30–70	35–105	35–70
20–29	46–165	35–65	40–115	35–80
30–39	50–235	30–65	40–160	35–80
40–49	55–250	30–65	45–180	35–85
over 50	60–220	30–65	55– 95	35–90

NOTE: Values may vary from laboratory to laboratory. It is always best to ask your physician to interpret your values.

Data in part A from National Institutes of Health, Consensus Conference, 1984. Data in part B from Lipid Research Clinic Prevalence Study.

---

diseases and because insulin may be less effective with high-fat diets. It is now recommended that a maximum of 30 to 35% of the daily caloric intake be fats, with even less for people with high blood lipid (cholesterol and triglyceride) levels (Table 4–3).

SATURATED OR UN-? *Triglycerides* are made up of three fatty acid molecules. Fatty acids can be *saturated* (filled with as many hydrogen atoms as possible) or unsaturated (not all the spaces for hydrogen atoms are filled). The choice of fats is important. Saturated fats can increase cholesterol levels and are more harmful than unsaturated fats. Animal fats are mostly saturated fats, which are usually solid at room temperature. Exceptions are palm and coconut oil, which are saturated and liquid at room temperature.

Monounsaturated fats, such as olive and peanut oil, are unsaturated fats that are missing only one pair of hydrogen atoms. They probably have little effect on blood fat levels but they still have calories. It has been suggested that olive oil may help reduce blood cholesterol levels. Polyunsaturated fats have many empty hydrogen atom spaces. They probably lower cholesterol levels, and they are the preferred fats for the diet. The primary sources of polyunsaturated fats are the vegetable oils such as corn, safflower, and sunflower oils. There fats are helpful, but they also contain just as many calories as all other fats, so beware! Remember, too, that if these "good" oils have hydrogen added to them ("hydrogenated" as indicated on the ingredient label), they become more *saturated*.

Fish is a source of a particularly useful fat, eicosapentaenoic acid (EPA, Omega-3). This fat has two to five times the ability to lower serum cholesterol levels as do the vegetable oils. Good sources of this substance include salmon, herring, mackerel, and bluefish.

The goal is to have a diet that is as low as possible in total fat, although some is needed. The current ADA recommendation is for approximately 30% fat in the daily diet. Of this total, 6 to 8% should be polyunsaturated, under 10% saturated, with monounsaturated fats making up the balance of the daily fat intake.

Atherosclerosis (hardening of the arteries) probably occurs when lipids (triglycerides and cholesterol) circulating in the blood are deposited on the inner lining of the arteries. Saturated fats in the diet cause the cholesterol level to be raised, and high blood cholesterol levels may make atherosclerosis more likely. Elevated blood levels of triglycerides probably play a role in atherosclerosis as well, but the link is less certain than with cholesterol.

HIGH- AND LOW-DENSITY FATS. Cholesterol and triglycerides travel in the bloodstream attached to particles known as lipoproteins. Lipoproteins are classified by density and size. *Low-density lipoproteins* (LDL) usually carry cholesterol. High levels of LDL are dangerous because they deposit the cholesterol in the walls of the blood vessels. *High-density lipoproteins* (HDL), however, carry cholesterol away from blood vessel walls, back to the liver, which disposes of it. HDL cholesterol is sometimes called the "good cholesterol."

When eaten, fats are broken down (digested) in the stomach into their building blocks, the fatty acids, which are then absorbed into the bloodstream or stored. When the level of insulin is low, such as during weight loss or ketoacidosis, the opposite occurs—that is, fat comes out of storage and is an alternative source of energy. The byproducts of the use of fat as an energy source are known as ketones. If ketones are seen during weight loss despite well-controlled blood glucose levels, they show that the diet is successful. However, the presence of ketones in a person with type I diabetes with high blood glucose levels due to sickness or missed insulin injections shows a dangerous insulin insufficiency and tells us that more insulin is needed immediately.

REDUCING DIET FATS AND CHOLESTEROL. Fats have been both confusing and controversial for many years, but finally scientific opinions about them are becoming more consistent. Nutritionist Dr. Jean Mayer has been particularly vocal in his criticism of the high fat content in American diets and has said, "It is unfortunate that our federal government, which already dragged its feet to a scandalous extent as regards cigarette smoking, is equally negligent as regards saturated fat."

In general, a diet that controls the total consumption of fat, but especially saturated fat and cholesterol from foods such as red meats, eggs, and dairy products, is a "heart-healthy" diet (Appendix 2). Cholesterol intake should be less than 300 mg per day. Yet the average American consumes 500 to 1000 mg per day! Your dietitian can make certain that your diet has the proper balance of fats.

Timing of Eating

The timing of eating is important. People who do not need insulin for their diabetes should divide their total consumption of calories into three meals and snacks. Spreading out the intake of the calories into consistently timed feedings may make it easier for the pancreas to release insulin.

If insulin therapy is needed, the food intake should coincide with the peak action times of the insulin. For this reason diabetic eating plans often include several snacks which are consumed at insulin peak times.

Variations in the timing of meals affects the blood glucose levels. Home blood glucose monitoring (HBGM) gives people a better idea of what their actual blood glucose levels are and allows adjustments of the insulin or snacks to compensate for timing variations. Consistency in timing and in food quantities is the best way to achieve good diabetes control. Any compromise can be like "shooting at a moving target"!

The Nutrition Prescription

The diabetes eating plan is designed and prescribed as any other medical treatment would be. In designing such a program, we translate the theory discussed above into practical guidelines for individuals to follow.

TABLE 4–4. Dining Out

Once you are familiar with your eating plan, can accurately estimate sizes of portions, and have a knowledge of substitution, you are ready to dine out. Following are the basic guidelines for success:

1. Know your meal plan, or carry a wallet-sized copy with you.
2. Know how the dish you are ordering is prepared.
3. Know the ingredients of the dish.
4. Ask for salad dressing "on the side" to help control portion.
5. Beware of foreign sugar substitutes if abroad. Bring a familiar brand with you if necessary, or if you have preferences.
6. Don't assume anything! If you don't know, ask!

The Role of the Dietitian

It is best to have a registered dietitian (RD) work with you to develop your dietary program. The dietitian can help design a flexible eating plan that insures nutritional balance and is compatible with your diabetes and your life-style.

Your physician may recommend a dietitian. The local American Diabetes Association chapter, other diabetes groups, or your local hospital can find dietitians to work with you. It is best to seek a registered dietitian (RD), which means someone who has completed college and postgraduate study and has passed a national qualifying exam. Beware of unqualified "nutritionists" who often make fantastic claims about their services or prescibe large doses ("megadoses") of vitamins or minerals to cure or prevent your ailments.

The RD translates the physician's recommendations into an eating plan that is tailor-made for you. The physician's prescription will take all the information about your diabetes into account as well as any other medical problems you may have. The RD will make this prescription understandable for you. Your life-style and eating preferences are important and your diet counselor will also discuss your present eating habits so that the plan can be designed with your tastes in mind. Food choice lists and other guidelines will then be prepared and explained to you. By communicating with the physician as needed, you and the dietitian accommodate changes in the eating plan or medical therapy.

There are now many menus, shopping lists, and guidelines for dining out available (Table 4–4). You should also be taught how to properly interpret labeling information and other helpful nutrition data. The dietitian should also advise you on the use of alcohol, sweeteners, dietetic foods, food and exercise, holiday meals, snack ideas, and cooking methods. Proper dietary advice from an RD, and follow-up support as needed, can be the difference between successful diabetes treatment or frustrating failures.

Planning Meals

A meal plan is designed with your life-style and dietary preferences in mind and also helps establish consistency and nutritional balance. How strictly the dietary restrictions should be followed will vary individually and should be determined as one of the goals of treatment.

Life would be quite dull if we did exactly the same things each day and ate exactly the same things. Even foods we like would become tiresome with repetition. Food choice lists provide daily variety to the diabetic meal plan (Appendix 1).

The food choice lists group commonly eaten foods into six categories based on similarities in food value or type. For example, bread, potatoes, corn, and cereal are all in the "bread" (starch) list because they are all high in starch. Foods such as eggs, poultry, and fish are included in the meat list as they are protein sources.

The food lists specify certain *quantities* of a food. The individual may choose whichever food, in the quantity shown, he or she desires that day. For example, a small apple, a whole peach, or one-eighth of a medium-sized honeydew melon may be substituted for an orange. Almost anything on the list can be substituted. There are alternatives within food groups to satisfy even children who may be picky eaters. One tablespoon of peanutbutter is approximately equal in nourishment to 1 ounce of steak or a medium egg, which accounts for why so many children survive despite their impossible eating habits!

The actual food lists are found in Appendix 1. For example, the bread list tells you that 1 slice of bread, 1/2 cup of corn, and 1/2 an English muffin all have the same calories (68), grams of carbohydrate (15), and grams of protein (3), and trace fat. These portions are equal to one "bread" choice.

Having determined the number of calories needed per day and the proper ratio of carbohydrate, protein, and fat, and having divided them up among meals and snacks, the dietitian then outlines the number of choices from each food list for each meal. This automatically keeps calorie and nutrient intake consistent while allowing variety. The Joslin Clinic Food Choice lists and the

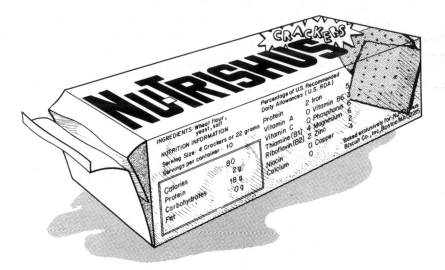

FIG. 4–3. A sample food label. (See text for discussion.)

ADA lists are quite similar. The Joslin lists offer extensive variety and have a great emphasis on high-fiber selections. There are always minor differences in assigned food values between lists from various sources. The food values are actually averages.

Food Labels

People are increasingly conscious of what they eat, and gradually foods are being packaged with better nutrition labeling. This is a boon to consumers. Increasingly, ingredients are being listed, as well as calories per serving and amounts of protein, carbohydrate, and fat.

There are still many pitfalls in tracking through the jungle of labels. Some are difficult to read and hard to understand. Words do not always mean what they say, particularly in the so-called dietetic foods. Knowledge of the jargon on labels is therefore helpful.

Figure 4–3 shows a sample food label. Note the following:
1. *Ingredients.* The major ingredients are listed first, followed by lesser items.
2. *Serving size.* The serving size defines one portion—how

much of the product or how many items. The number of calories, nutrients, etc. will be based on this portion size.
3. *Servings per container.* The label tells how many servings are in a package.
4. *Calories.* This is important because it tells how many calories are in a serving. In this example there are 80 calories in 4 crackers.
5. *Protein, carbohydrates, fat.* The grams of protein, carbohydrate, and fat are useful to know. You can compare them with other foods. This information helps you fit the foods into your eating plan.
6. *The percentage of U.S. recommended daily allowances (U.S. RDA).* The contents of each serving is listed as a *percent* of the minimum daily requirement, not in grams or other measures.
7. *Manufacturer, with address.* Labeling laws require that all packages list the manufacturer and their address. This becomes helpful if a nutrition label is either incomplete or nonexistent. Most companies will provide this information to consumers if requested.

Sweeteners

There are two major categories of sweeteners: "nutritive" (contain calories) and "non-nutritive" (noncaloric).

Nutritive Sweeteners. Nutritive, or calorie-containing sweeteners, should be counted as part of the meal plan. They are usually carbohydrates with names ending in -ose (a sugar) or -ol (a sugar alcohol chemically, but not "liquor"). Examples include sucr*ose* (table sugar), fruct*ose*, gluc*ose* (also known as dextr*ose*), sorbit*ol*, and mannit*ol*. All of these substances contain the same number of calories per gram (4), and, in significant amounts, all can elevate the blood glucose level.

The basic sugars we commonly use are made up of a chain of six carbon atoms hooked up in a row to form a molecule called a hexose. These six carbon sugars are usually found in our diet. One of these sugar molecules is called a "monosaccharide," while two attached together is a "disaccharide." Glucose is a monosaccharide (single molecule of sugar) hexose (6 carbon) sugar. So is fructose.

Sucrose, a disaccharide made up of glucose and fructose, is the commonest sweetener used by manufacturers to sweeten their products, and the one that those with diabetes try hardest to avoid. Compared to most other sugars (other than glucose itself) sucrose causes a rise in blood glucose levels that is most rapid and reaches the highest level.

It is important for people with diabetes to avoid items with high concentrations of sugar, such as pie and frosted cakes. Some products, however, contain a small amount of sugar but are not overly sweet (salad dressing, bread, crackers, etc.). These may be included by the RD in the eating plan. Information on the package labels can help you determine the amount and nature of the sucrose. People can spend enormous amounts at health food stores buying expensive foods that are 100% sugar free but which are not necessarily good for diabetes control.

Recently, there has been a trend toward adding to the diet some forms of sucrose that are more slowly absorbed. Ice cream is one of these foods. Usually, this is allowed as part of a full meal (or as dessert) so that the other foods slow down the absorption. Calories still count, however, and for those on weight-loss diets, these extra calories are not advisable. If such foods are eaten, the blood glucose level should be monitored 1 1/2 to 2 hours after the meal so that the individual can develop his or her own "glycemic index"—the measure of the effect of these foods on the blood glucose levels— and learn to make appropriate adjustments.

Fructose, or "fruit sugar," is found in fruits and honey. It is absorbed into the bloodstream more slowly and appears to cause a slower rise of the blood sugar level for a given concentration of calories in persons with well-controlled diabetes. However, it is still a sugar which needs insulin. People who have high blood glucose levels due to insufficient insulin convert fructose to glucose which results in a further rise in blood glucose level. Fructose may also worsen pre-existing problems with high triglyceride levels. There- fore fructose should be used cautiously after discussion with your diet counselors. In practice, the routine use of fructose as a substitute for sucrose in small quantities such as in cooking and baking is reasonable. Beware of some "high-fructose" corn syrups which are only part fructose, the rest being glucose.

The sugar alcohols are not drinking alcohol! They are basically slightly altered sugar molecules which are classified chemically as "alcohols" but have nothing to do with the beverages! *Sorbitol* is one of these and is found in many products such as chewing gum and "sugar-free" candy and baked goods. Like fructose, sugar alcohols are absorbed into the bloodstream more slowly than sucrose or glucose because they must undergo some chemical changes in the gastrointestinal tract first. Sorbitol causes diarrhea if taken in large

TABLE 4–5. Non-Nutritive Sweeteners Currently Available in the United States		
Brand Names	Sweetener	Comments
Equal, Nutrasweet	Aspartame	Essentially noncaloric. Contains no sugar. 180 times sweeter than sucrose.
Sucaryl, Sugar Twin, Sweet Magic, Sweet'n Low	Saccharin	Noncaloric. Contains no sugar, 300 times sweeter than sucrose.

amounts (over 30 grams daily). It has the same number of calories as sugar and must be calculated or counted into the diet.

Non-Nutritive Sweeteners. Non-nutritive sweeteners provide almost no calories and will not affect the blood glucose level. These include *saccharin* and *aspartame.* (Technically, aspartame is nutritive, as it contains 4 calories per gram, but because it is 180 times as sweet as sucrose, it is effective in such tiny doses as to have no real caloric value.) Cyclamate is also a non-nutritive sweetener, but is currently not available in the United States, although it is elsewhere. While not strictly necessary, these artificial sweeteners have made life more pleasurable for sweets lovers of all ages who must reduce calories or avoid glucose (Table 4–5).

Saccharin was first developed in the late nineteenth century. It is 300 times sweeter than sucrose by weight. Until recently, it was the most widely used non-nutritive sweetener in the United States, being especially popular in soft drinks and as a tabletop sweetener, although many people report a bitter or metallic aftertaste.

Some research on rats suggested a higher incidence of bladder cancer in animals that had been fed enormous, unrealistic doses of saccharin. This research has come into question. Nevertheless, saccharin products have a label warning of this fact. However, many experts disagree with the studies and the conclusions. Furthermore, no relationship between saccharin use and cancer in humans has been found. The American Medical Association condones the cautious use of saccharin and states that it should remain available.

Aspartame, considered a non-nutritive sweetener although it has 4 calories per gram, is made synthetically from the two naturally occurring amino acids aspartic acid and phenylalanine. Because it is made from phenylalanine, people with a disease known as phenylketonuria (PKU) who cannot metabolize phenylalanine should avoid aspartame. By weight, it is 180 times as sweet as sucrose. The Food and Drug Administration approved its use in 1981. It does not have the same aftertaste as saccharin and consequently is found in countless products from cereals to soft drinks to chewing gum. It is added to products under the brand name Nutrasweet, while the tabletop form is marketed as Equal. Equal contains some added dextrose and dried corn syrup to allow its granular form to flow. Each packet is as sweet as 2 teaspoons of sugar, and provides 4 calories (compared to 32 calories for 2 teaspoons of table sugar). Aspartame is unstable at high heat and loses its sugar-like sweetness, and so it is not used in most cooking. Some creative cooks, however, have found ways to add it at the end of the cooking process and the manufacturer has a recipe booklet telling how to cook with Equal.

Like saccharin, aspartame has faced some controversy, based, as usual, on studies with laboratory rats. Because it has been available for only a few years, it is still being watched carefully. Extensive studies have proven no toxicity damage. There have been a very few reports that in some persons it may trigger migraine headaches or diarrhea, but these complications appear to be relatively rare.

Both the American Diabetes Association and the FDA recommend limiting the daily intake of aspartame to 23 mg per pound of body weight (50 mg/kg). For a person weighing 150 pounds, this would be about 3400 mg daily, an amount quite difficult to reach. Remember, one can of diet soda (tonic or pop in some places!) contains 170 to 200 mg of aspartame. (Thus 3400 mg equals 17 cans daily.) A packet of Equal contains 35 mg of aspartame. Even a 60-pound child would need to consume 1380 mg of aspartame to reach the maximum daily intake level.

Some people are "sensitive" to aspartame, and even small quantities make them feel uncomfortable. They must exert some care in choosing commercially prepared foods because aspartame is found in many of them.

Cyclamate was first approved for use in the United States in 1950 and was marketed as Sucaryl. In 1969, the FDA removed cyclamate from the market, first as a food sweetener and then as a diet additive. Enormous amounts of cyclamate (500 times the maximum recommended for human consumption) has been fed to rats in whom an occasional bladder cancer was found. However, the Delaney amendment states, in simple terms, that anything that might even possibly cause cancer in any species of animal, regardless of the relationship to humans, cannot be sold for use as, or in the preparation of, food. As a result, cyclamates were banned. Many medical authorities do not agree with the total ban, although some stated that "unlimited consumption is not warranted." Cyclamates are widely used in much of the world without any apparent problems.

Concerned individuals with diabetes are left with decisions to make regarding sweeteners. Nutritive sweeteners provide unwanted calories and potentially poor diabetes control. The available non-nutritive sweeteners are basically acceptable despite nagging but unproven fears about their safety. The best idea is the same as with many other things—moderation! Eventually, other sweeteners now used in other parts of the world or under development will be made available here.

Dietetic Foods

Many people mistake *dietetic* for *diabetic*. Another common error is to assume that all "dietetic" and "sugar-free" foods are low in calories or have no carbohydrate. Not true!

Some dietetic foods are useful for people with diabetes. These include sugar-free soft drinks, sugar-free gelatin, artificial sweeteners, dietetic jellies and syrups, reduced-calorie dressings, and so on (see lists, Appendix 1). The most important point is to *read the label*. Even if they are lower in calories than the "real" product, such foods still may contain more calories than the consumer bargained for. Also, look out for the nutritive sweeteners (sucrose, fructose, sorbitol) that can cause a rise in the blood glucose level. The labeling laws allow manufacturers to declare an item "sugar-free" in bright, bold print. The "sugar" that they are referring to is sucrose (table sugar), and often they neglect to mention that they have replaced the sucrose with another carbohydrate (such as fructose, sorbitol, or others). These may have as many calories and may raise the blood glucose level just as much. Usually this information is found on the back of the label in small, unobtrusive print!

A man arriving at the treatment unit beamingly unwrapped a box of "diet candy." Everything is relative, and it was true that these contained "only 80 calories per piece" which is less than similar "regular" candy, which had about 150 calories!

Manufacturers frequently lower the carbohydrate content of a product such as dietetic candy. Frequently, they also increase the fat content so that the expected consistency of the product is maintained. Thus the "health" product may end up *higher* in calories than its "real" counterpart!

Food Additives

Much has been written recently about food additives, which are used when foods are processed and shipped thousands of miles for storage or sale. The most common of these is sodium chloride (table salt), some of which is essential to everyone. Usually, sodium chloride is harmless to those with diabetes unless they have a heart or kidney condition or high blood pressure requiring salt restriction. Still, moderation is a good idea. Most Americans consume six to ten times the quantity of salt they really need! Another common additive is monosodium glutamate (MSG), often used in Oriental food. In susceptible persons, this agent may cause an acute illness characterized by headache, weakness, and gastrointestinal distress. Surprisingly, after salt, sucrose itself is one of the most common food additives.

Other additives commonly used in foods are chemicals that are "generally recognized as safe" by the FDA. These include coloring agents, curing and pickling agents, drying agents, enzymes, flavor enhancers, processing aids, and non-nutritive sweeteners.

Additives are probably here to stay. Before their use, the transport of food was fraught with danger, and food poisonings were common. Packaging, shipping, storage, and processing of foods suited to modern convenience require additives. Individuals choosing to avoid these additives must make efforts to find foods carefully shipped and stored. Except for sugar (and salt for those with high blood pressure) the effects of additives are the same for people with and without diabetes.

Again, reading labels is essential if you are to be a conscientious consumer. Do not be fooled by terms such as "natural." A natural food may indeed be prepared without added "sugar," i.e., the white stuff kept in a sugar bowl! The nutrition label may reveal, however, that the product contains a great deal of "natural" sweetening in the form of honey!

The Vitamin Culture

Americans are faddists by nature. New ideas are rapidly embraced, follow a cycle, and then often disappear, displaced by something new. In recent years, many people have become vitamin-conscious. Vitamins get a great deal of attention because of concern over inadequacies in the diet and because they are used as attempted shortcuts to health. True inadequacies are rare, however, although vitamin deficiencies are frequently blamed for a variety of maladies that may well be caused by other factors.

A textbook might define a vitamin as "a substance that is essential for the maintenance of normal metabolic functions but which is not synthesized by the body and, therefore, must be furnished from an exogenous (outside) source." Vitamins do perform necessary functions. In recent years, however, many spectacular-sounding claims have been made about the benefits from the consumption of massive vitamin doses. These claims are largely unsupported by real evidence. Indeed, probably no group of drugs has been as misused as have vitamins. Although daily minimum allowances are known (the United States Recommended Daily Allowance, or U.S. RDA), optimal or ideal amounts are uncertain and indeed may vary for different people.

While poor eating habits and some ethnic dietary customs may result in poor nutrition and inadequate vitamin intake, it is difficult to *avoid* vitamins, and true deficiencies are rare. Vitamins are found in most foods, obviously more in some than in others. Certainly there are deficiencies in undernourished people and in developing cultures.

Table 4–6 lists the various vitamins and their sources and daily allowances and summarizes known uses. Of note for people with diabetes is that vitamin B_6 and B_{12} deficiencies have been blamed as a cause of neuropathy. Indeed, persons taking a daily megadose of 2 grams or more for several months have developed unsteady gait and numbness in the legs and arms. A problem is that many diseases or causes of weakness are self-limited or intermittent, and whatever a person may be taking at a given time is either blamed or blessed!

People with or without diabetes who use a well-planned diet do not require vitamin supplements, yet it is difficult to argue with the improved, subjective well-being many claim to experience with a daily vitamin supplement. Dr. Art Ulene has stated that "a poor diet plus vitamins is still a poor diet." The decision to take supplements should be based on factors such as need, safety, and cost. Many people take a multiple vitamin supplement "to be sure that they are covered," especially if they rely on "fast" or prepared foods in which vitamin content may be reduced, or if they do not like vegetables and fruits, which have high vitamin contents. These multivitamins are usually harmless. Most people need between 1200 and 1800 well-selected calories per day to meet their daily requirements. Women (especially if they have eliminated dairy products to cut calories) or people with intolerance to milk products may need supplemental calcium as well. Of course, men need calcium as well, but they are less likely to have dietary insufficiencies.

TABLE 4–6. The Vitamin Lineup

Vitamin	U.S. RDA[1]	Functions	Sources
A (retinol)	5000 IU[2]	Helps maintain eyes, skin, linings of the nose, mouth, digestive and urinary tracts	Liver, whole milk, butter, cheese, fortified margarine, carrots, spinach, other vegetables
Thiamin (B_1)	1.5 milligrams	Helps convert carbohydrates into energy	Yeast, rice, whole-grain and enriched breads and cereals, liver, pork, lean meats, poultry, eggs, meats, fish, many fruits and vegetables
Riboflavin (B_2)	1.7 milligrams	Helps energy release; helps maintain skin, mucous membranes, and nervous structures	Dairy products, liver, yeast, fruits, whole-grain and enriched breads and cereals, vegetables, lean meats, poultry
Niacin (B_3)	20 milligrams	Helps convert carbohydrates, fats, and protein into energy; essential for growth; aids synthesis of hormones	Liver, chicken, turkey, halibut, tuna, milk, eggs, grains, fruits and vegetables, enriched breads and cereals
B_6 (pyridoxine, pyridoxal, pyridoxamine)	2.0 milligrams	Aids in more than 60 enzyme reactions	Milk, liver, lean meats, whole-grain or enriched breads and cereals, vegetables
Folic acid	0.4 milligram	Aids blood-cell production; helps maintain nervous system	Liver, many vegetables
Biotin	0.3 milligram	Aids in intermediary metabolism of fats, carbohydrates, and protein	Widely distributed in foods
Pantothenic acid	10 milligrams	Aids in metabolism of carbohydrates, fats, and protein	Eggs, liver, kidneys, peanuts, whole grains, most vegetables, fish

TABLE 4–6. The Vitamin Lineup (Continued)

Vitamin	U.S. RDA[1]	Functions	Sources
B_{12}	6.0 micrograms	Helps synthesis of red and white blood cells; aids many other metabolic reactions	Liver, meat, eggs, milk
C (ascorbic acid)	60 milligrams	Helps maintain and repair connective tissue, bones, teeth, cartilage; promotes wound healing	Broccoli, brussels sprouts, citrus fruits, tomatoes, potatoes, peppers, cabbage, other fruits and vegetables
D (cholecalciferol)	400 IU[2]	Helps regulate calcium and phosphorus metabolism; promotes calcium absorption; essential for development and maintenance of bones and teeth	Fortified milk, fish-liver oils; sunlight on skin produces vitamin D
E (tocopherol)	30 IU[2]	Protects and maintains cellular membranes; protects fats and vitamin A from destruction by oxidation	Vegetable oils, whole grains, leafy vegetables; smaller amounts widespread in foods
K	70 to 140 micrograms[3]	Used in synthesis of prothrombin (essential for blood clotting)	Green leafy vegetables, soybeans, beef liver; widespread in other foods

[1]U.S. RDA for adults and children 4 or more years of age.
[2]International Units. [3]Estimated safe and adequate intake.
From *Consumer Reports*, March 1986, p. 174. Used with permission.

Vitamin deficiencies usually should be treated with specific vitamin doses. Supplemental vitamins may be useful and indeed necessary with extremely rigorous or unbalanced diets, in pregnancy, in malnutrition, and in situations of debilitating stress. When used as supplements in this manner, vitamins are considered in the same light as any other medication that is prescribed. In deciding which product to take, choose one whose label states that it provides 100% of the U.S. RDA of the ingredient(s) you are concerned about replacing. The nationally advertised vitamin supplements and the generic store brands are usually comparable in all ways, except in price! When in doubt, a dietitian can advise you whether you need supplemental vitamins.

> **Many people use vitamins with the same rationale as the notorious chicken soup: "It can't do any harm!"**

Vitamin preparations now have a sales volume of about 3 billion dollars yearly in the United States. Many are harmless, because excess is destroyed or eliminated from the body. However, some vitamins can be harmful in very large doses. Vitamins are of two types: (1) water-soluble vitamins, such as those in the B complex and vitamin C, and (2) fat-soluble vitamins, such as A, D, K, and E. When large doses of the water-soluble vitamins (B and C) are consumed, much of the excess is either not absorbed at all or is lost in the urine. In extremely high doses, however, they may be stored in the liver and can cause toxicity. Certainly high doses of fat-soluble vitamins are deposited in the fat and may become harmful. High doses, such as 25,000 IU of vitamin A taken daily for several months can be risky, particularly for pregnant women and their fetuses. In pregnant animals, huge doses of vitamin A produce central nervous system changes and birth defects in the offspring.

Vitamin D preparations must also be used with caution. Mild toxic effects can be observed in children given 50,000 IU daily. Massive doses may produce calcifications (calcium deposits) in many parts of the body, including the kidneys. Other possible effects include convulsions, acute pancreatitis, elevations of triglyceride (a blood fat) levels, nausea, diarrhea, blurred vision, headache, and bone depletion.

Vitamin C. Vitamin C has an important and proven function. A lack of this vitamin causes scurvy, the scourge of seafarers in sailing-vessel days. English sailors on long voyages took lime juice to prevent this and became known by the slang term "Limeys." Vitamin C is readily found in foods, especially in citrus fruits and juices, cantaloupe, strawberries, raw cabbage, and green peppers. Recently there has been controversy about the use of massive doses of vitamin C for the alleged cure of many conditions, but chiefly for prevention of colds. This theory was put forth enthusiastically by Dr. Linus Pauling, a respected two-time Nobel Prize winner, who has been quoted as saying that large doses of vitamin C (up to 10 grams a day) not only are harmless, but also greatly reduce your chances of getting the common cold. This theory has not been verified, and some studies question it.

Some reports have suggested that vitamin C may someday prove helpful in the cellular metabolism of people with diabetes, but this is not proven. Some people claim they "feel better and have fewer colds" when using vitamin C. Yet in locations in which diets are naturally very high in this vitamin, the number of colds does not appear to decrease. If you do feel better, certainly an extra bit of vitamin is not harmful. Smokers need more, probably 250 mg per day as compared with the recommended daily allowance of 60 mg for others. Large doses should be avoided by patients with a history of gout or uric acid kidney stones. In addition, ingestion of large doses of vitamin C may cause unreliable results in some of the urine glucose dip and tape tests. People using large doses of vitamin C should compare urine testing results with home blood glucose test results.

The Vitamin E Fad. Another darling of faddists, users, and sellers, is vitamin E, also called the "antiaging vitamin." For some time after vitamin E was discovered, no specific function could be found. More recently, research has uncovered roles for this vitamin (Table 4–6) in maintaining health of cell membranes and in helping metabolic pathway function. Vitamin E is commonly found in foods and there appears to be no evidence of a deficiency in the population as a whole. There is also no evidence that supplements of vitamin E are necessary or especially helpful to persons with diabetes, but they are probably harmless in ordinary doses (400 IU per day).

Minerals   ·

Minerals are involved in many body functions. Copper and iron are necessary for blood building. Sodium, chloride, and potassium are constituents of the blood and body cells; that is, they maintain the electrical balance that is so important to the function of nerves and muscles. Manganese, zinc, and other so-called trace elements are widely found in foods, and almost no one needs to take supplemental amounts. Some have suggested that supplemental chromium may help control diabetes, but there is no evidence for this.

Calcium. There has been much discussion recently about calcium and its relationship to osteoporosis, a thinning of the bones seen primarily in women past menopause. A physician or RD may suggest calcium, along with other medications, if you are at high risk to develop this condition. If enough is not provided in the diet, supplemental calcium is available in tablets or in certain antacids. Other than foods themselves, the most readily absorbed forms of calcium supplements are calcium carbonate and calcium citrate.

Iron. Iron supplementation may be necessary for people with certain types of anemias in which insufficient iron stores are to blame. The most common such anemia occurs in women who lose a great deal of blood during menstruation.

Mineral Excesses. Sometimes it is necessary to reduce intake of a specific mineral. This is most common in people with high blood pressure (hypertension), in which high amounts of sodium (salt) in the diet can worsen the condition. High blood potassium levels are seen in conditions such as kidney failure. These levels can predispose the heart to rhythm disturbances. In such cases dietary restriction of minerals is necessary.

Special Weight-Loss Diets and Other "Specialty" Diets

Next to the promise of "Get Rich Quick!" the promise of "Lose Weight Quick!" draws the most attention. In this era of "slim worship" many of us are unhappy with what we see in full-length mirrors unless we see Madison Avenue perfection. Overweight is neither healthy nor attractive, especially for persons with diabetes, but it is also unhealthy to become neurotic about weight and try "quick fix" weight-loss programs. While weight loss may be important, a sensible weight-loss program should be used. Each year book stores show many diet books and systems named after physicians, movie stars, good or bad habits, athletes, and vices. They appear like a shooting star, sell many thousands of books, and then fall out of sight to be replaced by others. The fact that none of these remains in view for long should tell you something. The truth is that any diet or deprivation, including plain starvation, will cause weight loss for a period of time. What is needed for many is a complete change in life-style, and that is not easy!

Weight Loss: Group Therapy

For many people wishing to lose weight, a diet planned by a dietitian combined with personal motivation and support from friends and family can help. Some people are more comfortable in a group. There are many advantages to a well-run diet group that can promote successful weight loss. Just joining a group does not insure success, however. Only about 30 percent of those who take part in a group weight-reducing program lose 20 pounds or more. Another third lose less than that, and the remaining individuals fail to lose weight at all. Unfortunately, many of those who lose weight gain it back once the program is completed. A short-term program is not enough.

Failure of the group approach is often due to the attitude "I've joined your group—now you lose weight for me." Yet for a sizable number of people willing to work actively at weight loss, groups do work. Many find comfort seeing others struggling along with them. It is also helpful to have frequent checks by a disinterested party (i.e., not a nagging spouse!) to monitor progress and give positive encouragement or negative feedback as needed. Furthermore, when one has to pay for something, it is often taken more seriously.

The weight-loss diet should satisfy all nutritional needs except calories. It should be realistic—something you can live with. The program should suggest that you consult your physician or dietitian, particularly regarding your daily insulin or oral agent dose. Using insulin does not mean you cannot diet; it means adjustments must be made. Exercise should be encouraged as well. The program's eating plan should take your own habits and ethnic food preferences into consideration. The program should also prevent extreme between-meal hunger or dangerous lows in blood glucose levels, and it should give you a feeling of well-being, rather than tiredness. There should also be a variety of food choices to stave off boredom. Finally, the diet should be the framework for appropriate lifelong changes in eating habits to maintain good weight and health.

No diet is going to work for *everyone*. Actual guarantees of weight loss are almost impossible. Watch for marketing buzzwords designed to grab your attention, such as *new, revolutionary, secret, startling, amazing, quick, melts fat away, burns fat*, etc. Be suspicious of programs that are really just trying to sell expensive diet products. Avoid diets using one or just a few foods or one that completely eliminates a food group. Be suspicious of diets that are designed by anyone who is not in the field of nutrition and not a member of, or approved by, either the American Medical Association, American Diabetic Association, or American Dietetic Association.

Many successful diet groups have been useful for motivated people. Weight Watchers has been quite helpful for many, encouraging participants to discuss their efforts with each other in a "group therapy" type session. Members are weighed periodically, and longterm changes in eating habits are encouraged. Other successful programs are run by hospital outpatient departments, HMOs, or clinics. Usually no fewer than 1000 to 1200 calories per day for women and 1500 to 1600 calories per day for men should be prescribed, although there are exceptions.

Pills for Weight Loss

Because modern living demands pills to fix everything, many people who want to lose weight approach their physician with the plea, "Doc, please give me some pills to make me lose weight." Unless a person has fluid accumulation or an underactive thyroid needing treatment, there is no pill that will "melt fat away."

The only pills that might affect weight are appetite suppressants. These are basically amphetamines (also known as "pep pills" and "uppers"), and as such they have been condemned by most physicians because they may be habit-forming, can elevate the blood pressure and blood glucose level, can overstimulate the nervous system, and are helpful at best only briefly. No magic pill can take the place of a sensible, well-balanced diet. There are no "easy fixes" in life.

Vegetarian Diets

Vegetarian diets, practiced wisely, can be very healthy. Vegetarian populations and groups (such as Seventh-Day Adventists) have a lower morbidity and mortality from the diseases known to be promoted by the fats in animal meat, especially coronary heart disease. In addition, one of the staples of the vegetarian diets, the legumes (dried beans and peas), have been found to have a very low glycemic index and the fiber in them may help lower cholesterol levels. People following a "lacto-ovo" diet can get protein from milk and eggs. However, people who follow a strict vegetarian ("vegan") diet (eliminating all animal protein including dairy and eggs) must combine their protein sources from cereals and grains carefully to maintain an adequate intake of protein. The complementary protein concept should be employed in any vegetarian diet. This means that one item deficient in certain amino acids is combined with another food that provides them. It is important to be well informed when choosing this type of diet, especially when feeding children. Remember, vegetarian diets are inherently higher in carbohydrate, but planned carefully, they can be well tolerated. Furthermore, real vegetarianism requires intelligent choices and extraordinary culinary abilities to be successful. Healthy vegetarianism is possible, and dietitians at the Joslin Diabetes Center can use vegetarian food choice lists to develop eating plans for people that wish them.

Organic Diets

"Organic" foods, fancied by some people, are grown with the aid of fertilizers of animal or vegetable origin. Nutrients are actually in the seed, and what is in the soil usually affects only the yield (quantity) of what is being grown. There is no solid evidence that foods grown in this manner make much difference nutritionally, although not much is known yet about the longterm effects of chemical fertilizers and additives. In fact, many "organic gardens" still have residues of chemicals from the atmosphere, water, or past fertilizers. The effects of these foods are the same for people with and without diabetes, but certainly if this concept helps you enjoy eating—great!

Fasting

Fasting is not recommended for anyone with diabetes, especially those people treated with insulin. Fasting for the purpose of weight loss can be dangerous for anyone and should not be done except under strict supervision by a physician.

Some people wish to fast for religious purposes for periods of about a day, such as for the Jewish holiday Yom Kippur. Many rabbis have suggested that an individual's health takes precedence over religious observance and have condoned the decision not to fast for health reasons. For those wishing to live the "spirit" if not the letter of the law, there are ways to compromise. Priscilla White, M.D., used to suggest a drink of sugar-containing liquid (such as juice or soda) every hour or two, to equal one ounce for every hour of fasting. Various modifications of this program are being recommended today. In response to this approach, some rabbis have commented that while a full meal would be a big sin, many small snacks would be just tiny sins and in total would not be very much of a sin at all!

The fast of Ramadan, observed by those of the Moslem religion, actually represents a one-month shift in the time that meals are eaten to hours of darkness. Using the results of home blood testing, your physician can give you advice on how to adjust your diabetes treatment to compensate for this time change.

The decision to fast is a personal one, but fasting can be difficult for people with diabetes. Nevertheless, if you feel strongly about fasting for religious occasions, you should always consult your physician before the fast for specific advice on how to adjust your treatment program.

Summary

A proper eating plan is not merely important, but vital for most people, particularly for people with diabetes. Diets of one type or another are becoming increasingly commonplace. Not all of them are being used for medical reasons. More and more restaurants are following the practice of offering healthful foods such as low-fat and low-salt selections. Many even list the calories.

> The problem with many "diets" is that they tell you what you should *not* eat instead of telling you what you *should* eat and *enjoy!*

With recent advances in many areas of diabetes care, the eating plans for people with diabetes are more enjoyable—yes enjoyable! —to follow. All it takes is some interest and creativity. The purpose of a diabetic eating plan is not to deprive someone of food; rather it is to provide good health. To quote Julia Child, "Bon Appetit!"

5

Exercise with Diabetes

Exercise is probably the earliest form of treatment of diabetes, although it was not always recognized as a form of therapy. In fact, primitive man had to exercise to find food before he even began to eat, so one could say it came *before* diet!

Exercise, whether at work or play, is as much a treatment of diabetes as any other form of therapy. From the beginning of the modern era of diabetes therapy, which began in 1921 with the discovery of insulin, it was recognized that the treatment of diabetes had three components: insulin (manufactured by the pancreas or injected insulin), diet, and exercise. In fact, Dr. Elliott P. Joslin listed exercise as one of the three mainstays of treatment in the original Joslin emblem! Each item is important in the treatment of diabetes, and if improperly used or ignored, makes diabetes treatment unsuccessful.

Why Exercise Helps

Exercise is good for you, whether or not you have diabetes, and it should be fun as well. While there is no firm evidence that physical fitness itself directly prevents complications of diabetes, it is known that in people without diabetes, exercise reduces the risk of vascular problems such as heart disease and peripheral vascular disease (hardening of the arteries). Sustained endurance exercises reduce blood lipid (fats, such as cholesterol) and blood pressure as well, while promoting blood circulation and strengthening the heart. While it is reasonable to assume that a person with diabetes would enjoy the same benefits to the cardiovascular system, exercise also has special importance to blood glucose metabolism, not only by lowering the blood levels, but also by improving the body's sensitivity to the effects of insulin. First, let's understand why exercise is important, and then let's decide how you can find the exercise program that is best for *you*.

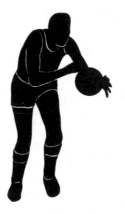

Exercise without Diabetes

Normal muscle uses two fuels, glucose and free fatty acids (i.e., fat!), to generate energy needed to make a muscle contract for movement. The glucose can come from various sources: the blood, the liver, and the muscles. It is stored in liver and muscle as glycogen, which can be converted back into glucose by a process known as "gluconeogenesis". During short bursts of activity, most of the fuel for the cells comes from either blood glucose or the muscle glycogen. After about 15 minutes of activity, however, the glucose used for fuel comes increasingly from glucose newly made in the liver from glycogen. It can also come from protein breakdown products, the amino acids (especially alanine). After about 30 minutes of exercise, the body begins to get more of its energy from the free fatty acids.

When we exercise, the body begins rebuilding the glycogen stores in the muscle and liver. This process may take 4 to 6 hours, but can take 12 or even 24 hours after extreme exertion. Insulin must be available to direct this process, but there also must be enough glucose in the blood from which to make the glycogen. In people with diabetes, if the blood glucose levels are too low after exercise, the rebuilding of the glycogen stores can result in hypoglycemic reactions over the next few hours ("lag" effect).

Exercise with Diabetes

The manner in which the metabolism of someone with diabetes copes with exercise is determined by the amount of insulin available, the level of diabetes control, and the state of hydration. In theory, and often in reality, the person with well-controlled diabetes, whose insulin and food/fuel are in proper balance, can handle activity just as well as someone without diabetes. If the control is poor, however, there are certain differences in the metabolism.

If the diabetes is under only fair rather than good control, the body runs out of the available glucose fuels earlier and begins to burn the free fatty acids for fuel, producing ketones, the metabolic waste product. Of course, there are often great amounts of free fatty acids in the circulation of people with poorly controlled diabetes, due to the reduced levels of insulin.

With very poor control, the problem of getting proper fuels is even worse. Blood glucose levels are high, but the lack of insulin prevents this fuel from getting into the cells to be used for energy. This short insulin supply also allows the liver to make more glucose. It is as if the body tissues, starved for sugar, "think" that more is needed. Stimulated by the increased demand from the exercising muscles, the body tries to make more glucose by pouring it out from the liver. However, this glucose (fuel) cannot get into the muscle cells because of the insulin lack. The body then turns to its alternative fuel—free fatty acids—which are used instead of glucose to fuel the muscles. The use of the fat for energy results in the production of ketones. (Remember—insulin helps deposit free fatty acids in the adipose or fat cells, while insufficient insulin allows the free fatty acids to circulate for use as an alternative fuel.) What happens during exercise by a person with poorly regulated diabetes is that glucose levels keep rising along with ketones from the use of free fatty acids for fuel. It becomes a high and very undesirable tide!

There is another interesting change that occurs with exercise in people with diabetes. As long as the diabetes control is good and enough insulin is present, the additional glucose needed to fuel this increased activity does not require any additional insulin. In addition, working muscle is more sensitive to insulin action than is muscle at rest. As a result, more glucose can be used for fuel per unit of insulin by working muscle than by resting muscle. For these reasons, activity is one of the three major factors affecting blood glucose levels, along with food and insulin.

Exercise is known to effect glucose tolerance in people without diabetes, too. When people without diabetes are at bed rest, they have impaired ability to metabolize glucose and show slightly higher blood glucose levels. By contrast, endurance training improves glucose tolerance in people without diabetes and people with non-insulin-dependent diabetes. Improvements in glucose metabolism have been seen in obese individuals as a result of a regular exercise program, probably because the cells of the body become more sensitive to the effects of the insulin.

Therefore exercise is a useful way to reduce blood glucose levels in the short term, but regular exercise also increases insulin sensitivity in persons with both type I and type II diabetes and helps reduce insulin resistance found in non-insulin-dependent diabetes. (see Chapter 1).

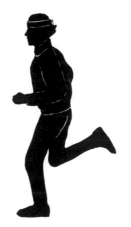

The Exercise Program

There are two types of exercise programs: endurance and strength training. *Endurance training* is exercise requiring great use of energy. It stimulates the heart and lungs and uses most of the body muscles for at least 15 minutes each session. *Strength training* is exercise such as weight lifting. This applies heavy resistance to specific muscle groups. Most physicians and exercise physiologists recommend endurance exercise as the most useful activity for adults because of the beneficial stress effect on the cardiovascular and metabolic systems. This is the training most recommended for people with diabetes.

Evaluation before Starting. Before starting an exercise program, anyone, including people with diabetes, must first be evaluated by a physician. This evaluation is important at *any* age. The older individual needs medical clearance to reduce the risk of heart, lung, or circulatory damage. In fact, many young people with long-term diabetes still have a potential for circulatory or heart damage. It is better to be safe than sorry! Sometimes an exercise electrocardiogram ("stress test") helps determine the safety of endurance exercise, as people with diabetes can have coronary artery disease and ischemia (insufficient blood flow to the heart) without warning signs.

Certainly, for everyone with diabetes, the degree of diabetes control needs to be assessed and, if poor, should be improved before the exercise program begins. Any possible complications of the diabetes must be monitored during the exercise program. People with retinopathy, for example, should discuss the activity with an ophthalmologist (eye doctor) so as not to increase the blood pressure in the small vessels in the eye which might lead to a small bleed in the retina of the eye. People with diabetes must also be careful about their feet and avoid circulation and stress risks.

Prescribing Exercise. A prescription for an exercise program should take into account four things: (1) the type of activity, (2) the intensity, (3) the duration of each session, and (4) the frequency of the sessions.

The type of activity should require that the person expend 5 to 7 times as much energy as would be expended by resting. Table 5–1 lists some appropriate activities for people with diabetes. Obviously, choices will vary depending on personal interest, climate, and available facilities.

The intensity of exercise is determined by monitoring the heart rate and other signs of stress. Heart rate is measured by taking the pulse at the carotid artery in the neck, the temple, or the wrist or by placing the hand on the chest. A fairly accurate estimate can be obtained by measuring for 10 seconds and multiplying by 6, which gives the heart rate per minute. This should be taken within 5 seconds of stopping activity. In addition, the new exerciser should monitor his or her pulse rate four or five times during an exercise session. Remember, if you are on a medication that affects the heart rate, such as some cardiac medications used to treat high blood pressure, or if you have a neuropathy that your doctor said affects

TABLE 5–1. Physical Activities Beneficial to People with Diabetes

Individual Activities

Brisk walking	Running or jogging
Swimming	Bicycling (including stationary)
Dancing	Skipping rope
Rowing	Skiing (downhill and cross-country)
Badminton	Skating (ice and roller)
Wrestling	Golf (with brisk walking only!)
Fencing	Stair climbing
Calisthenics	Tennis
Handball	Squash
Racquetball	

Team Activities

Soccer	Volleyball (vigorous only!)
Basketball	Hockey (ice and field)
Lacrosse	

Other activities, if done at the proper intensity

Digging	Wood cutting and splitting
Lawn Mowing	Farming

TABLE 5–2. Levels of Intensity of Exercise
This table should be used as a guide to gauge your exercise effort. Goals should be set in consultation with your physician.

Pulse Rate (beats per minute)	Rating of Perceived Exertion (RPE) (How hard the exercise is)	Comments
60–70	Very, very light	This intensity is of little value.
80–100	Very light	
100–120	Fairly light	GO! This intensity is just right.
120–140	Somewhat hard	
140–160	Hard	
160–180	Very hard	STOP! This intensity is much too hard.
180–200	Very, very hard	

your heart rate, the rate of your pulse may underestimate the actual stress on your body, and caution must be taken. Other signs of stress include labored breathing, light-headedness, or a very pale face. Table 5–2 suggests various levels of intensity based on heart rate and the rating of perceived exertion. The activity should feel fairly easy

TABLE 5–3. The Exercise Prescription. This table lists the various levels of activity by frequency, duration, time, and intensity. Unless you are currently more active than the "sedentary" level, you should start at that level and work your way up.

Activity Level	Frequency (sessions per week)	Duration (minutes per session)	Total Time per Week (minutes)	Intensity (heart rate during exercise)
Sedentary	4–6	10–20	40–80	100–120
Somewhat active	4–6	15–30	90–120	100–130
Moderately active	3–5	30–45	120–180	110–140
Very active	3–5	30–60	180–300	120–160
Athlete	5–7	60–120	300–840	140–190

most of the time. However, age and some medical conditions will change actual target pulse rates. In general, when exercise becomes uncomfortable, reduce the intensity.

The duration and frequency of activity sessions depend on age, time you can spare, and level of endurance fitness. In general, three to five exercise sessions per week of 15 to 30 minutes each would be ideal. To begin, estimate your present level of activity. Start with that level of exercise with the intention of slowly increasing it. Table 5–3 gives estimates of various activity levels. Unless you are above the "sedentary" level at the start, you should begin there and work up. The activities used for this estimation are those listed in Table 5–1.

A workout time of 15 to 30 minutes, 3 times per week, reaching 60 to 90% of the maximal heart rate, should be the minimum to achieve health and fitness benefits. People with poor fitness should start more slowly and increase frequency and duration gradually. The elderly, or those with limited exercise potentials due to other medical conditions, will still get some benefit from even limited exercise. Taking walks three times weekly can be beneficial to almost anyone.

The Daily Routine. Regardless of the type of activity, a good exercise program consists of (1) the warm-up phase, (2) the cardiovascular phase, and (3) the "cool-down" phase.

The *warm-up* should include stretching exercises and muscle strengthening such as sit-ups, push-ups and half-knee bends, to get the body properly heated up and stretched out to prevent injury.

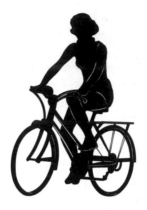

The *cardiovascular*, stimulatory phase should start slowly, reaching a peak about half to three-quarters of the distance and/or time into the session. It should be followed by a gradual slowdown over the remaining portion of the activity session. The final *cool-down* phase may include light walking and some arm, leg, and abdominal exercises. This helps restore the energy expenditures and the blood flow to the resting state.

Motivation! Once you decide to start an exercise program, it takes motivation to continue after the first enthusiasm wanes. Here are some suggestions to help keep you going, whatever your program of activity.

The program works better if it is designed for you alone and is written down. Goals should be short-term—two weeks, for example. A sedentary person whose goal is to run in the Boston Marathon in three years is much less likely to succeed than if the goal is half a mile in two weeks! Let family or friends know of your plans. They can encourage you to continue, perhaps exercise with you, and give you the added push of the "someone is watching" syndrome! Do activities that you enjoy! Alternate activities should also be included in the plan so that bad weather, equipment failure, etc., will not give you an excuse to skip exercise. The intensity and duration of the activity must be realistic, and you should not overdo it—a bad experience can turn you off to exercise altogether. Get a partner to exercise with you. Having an appointment with another person helps motivate you not to miss sessions. The place of exercise should be easily reached so that time, weather, or laziness do not prevent exercise. Written schedules also help, especially in integrating exercise with eating and insulin. Small rewards for reaching goals are helpful too, but often the best reward is *just feeling good!*

Adjusting Diabetes Treatment to Exercise

For people with diabetes, exercise lowers the blood glucose levels. While this is a very beneficial effect, it is important to adjust properly the two other major factors controlling blood glucose levels—food and insulin—so that diabetes control remains in proper balance.

Type II Diabetes. Endurance training is of greatest benefit to the person with non-insulin-dependent (type II) diabetes, as it lowers insulin resistance and improves glucose tolerance. Over time, the right endurance program may allow the dose of insulin or oral hypoglycemic agent to be reduced.

Monitoring blood glucose levels can help you or your physician decide on medication adjustment. For the person with type II diabetes, the goal may include weight loss or reduced medication dose. People using oral medication should monitor their glucose levels and discuss the possibility of dose reduction with their doctor if self monitoring tests show improved control. Remember that even oral hypoglycemic agents may cause hypoglycemia. Therefore look for evidence of blood glucose level drops, and if hypoglycemic symptoms occur during or after exercise, the treatment may be reduced. For occasional exercise with resulting hypoglycemia, when the dose of oral agent needs to be at a given level for nonexercise days; lowering the dose on the occasional exercise days is not effective in preventing the glucose drops. Instead, small snacks before or after exercise on the occasional active days may be useful to prevent hypoglycemia despite efforts at weight reduction.

People with type II diabetes using insulin therapy should follow the guidelines for people with type I diabetes outlined below.

Type I Diabetes. Exercise is an important part of therapy for persons with insulin-dependent (type I) diabetes. With proper thought and adjustment of eating and insulin dose, diabetes control can be maintained at target levels, and the person with this type of diabetes can perform as well in sports or other activities as others without diabetes.

There are a number of things the person with type I diabetes must remember when exercising. First, no exercise should be performed if the diabetes is out of control. A blood glucose level over 240 mg%, and especially the presence of ketones, should be a warning not to exercise unless the abnormality is corrected. Exer-

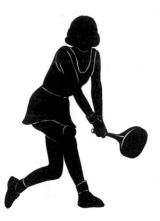

cising with hyperglycemia and with the presence of ketones, which suggest an insulin lack, may lead to increases in blood glucose levels or a worsening of the ketosis.

Food and insulin dose may need to be changed to prevent low blood sugar reactions during or after an exercise session. To determine exactly how much to adjust, keep careful records of the blood glucose levels and find out for yourself how much change of food and/or insulin is needed for any amount of exercise. Blood testing before and after exercise is a minimum requirement, and it is helpful to test blood during an exercise session and a few hours afterwards, looking for low blood glucose levels.

The time of day that the exercise is being done can influence the blood glucose levels. Late afternoon exercise or exercise during the peak time of the morning insulin (see Chapter 7) may cause different blood glucose changes than exercise just before breakfast or an hour after supper, when the insulin action may be different. The best time for exercise is at least an hour after a meal.

Exercise is fueled by increased glucose metabolism. Hypoglycemia occurs when the body cannot provide the muscles with this increased glucose, either because it cannot use the glucose present (not enough insulin) or because the amount of glucose is already too low (too much insulin has used up the glucose in the blood, or not enough carbohydrate has been eaten). If there is proper diabetes control, insulin should be decreased or food increased in anticipation of activity, and perhaps, for some, after activity as well.

Low-Level Exercise. Some insulin dose reduction may be necessary at the start of an exercise program. Once the program is a routine,

TABLE 5-4. Snack Foods for Exercise ("Exersnacks")

Dried fruit and nuts
Plain cookies
Granola bars
Yogurt (plain or fruit-flavored)
Pretzels
Various sandwiches
Nuts
Milk and muffins (corn or bran)
Junior baby foods
Cheese and graham crackers, rye
 wafers, Triscuits, Rye Krisp
Trail mix
Cheese or peanutbutter crackers
Beef Jerky and fruit

people with ideal body weight who are not trying to lose weight should need no change in insulin dose for occasional, moderate exercise of short duration (under 30 minutes). For intense exercise, a snack may be needed, especially if the activity is performed more than 1½ or 2 hours after a meal. One fruit or one bread exchange should be enough for 30 to 60 minutes of moderate exercise such as "friendly" tennis, leisurely biking, or walking. It may be helpful to get into the habit of testing the blood glucose level before each exercise session and adjusting the snack based on the result of that glucose test. The lower the blood glucose level at the start of activity, the more food may be needed.

More Vigorous Exercise. More vigorous activity requires more food, perhaps half a sandwich (one bread and one meat) plus a piece of fruit for the first 1½ hours of activity. Table 5-4 lists exercise snack foods. Some of these are higher in fat than those for use on a daily basis. Fat slows the emptying of foods from the digestive system. Slower absorption produces a more prolonged and even energy supply during your activity. Of course, these foods should be low in saturated fats and cholesterol! For unexpected activity (the fire fighter who drops his playing cards to rush to a fire), it is certainly acceptable, indeed recommended, to consume "quick" carbohydrate such as sugar-containing tonic or juices in anticipation of sudden bursts of activity.

Longer Exercise. For longer activity, you may require additional snacks at intervals (perhaps every 30 to 60 minutes) during the activity. These may be a piece of fruit plus a meat and a bread exchange. Such snacking is essential for all-day activities such as

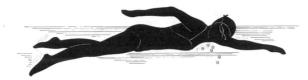

cross-country skiing or hiking—you should bring food along for the occasion. Remember, snack quantities may vary depending on the time of day and the insulin that is having its peak activity, so "trial and error" with good record keeping will help determine the actual quantities that are best for you. Of course, for some very vigorous all-day activities, you may need many more calories. Backpacking, for example, may require 5000 to 6000 calories per day, and the increase should be spread over the meals as well as the snacks. Unless all-day backpacking is your usual daily activity, vigorous exercise of this nature may also demand a reduction of the insulin dose as well. Regardless of your anticipated adjustments, however, you should always have some "quick" carbohydrate handy, "just in case . . . !"

Fluids are important! You may lose a great deal of fluid as sweat, so be sure to drink enough before starting. Water is the best fluid because it is most easily absorbed. Fluids are especially important for prolonged activity on a warm day or for activities that cause much sweating. Dehydration can worsen diabetes control.

Activity that lasts more than 30 to 40 minutes should be followed by an additional snack, consisting of protein and fat in addition to the carbohydrate, especially if the blood glucose levels are in the normal range. This is to provide fuel for the body to use to replenish its glycogen supplies and therefore to prevent hypoglycemia a number of hours after the activity.

An overweight person with type I diabetes may undertake an exercise program to lose weight. When weight loss is the goal, one should obviously try to avoid the additional calories of snacks before and after exercise. Thus insulin reduction would be the major adjustment made. Again, trial and error, with frequent testing of blood glucose levels, will help train you to know how much to reduce the insulin for a given amount of activity and help you and your physician design an adjustment program. Remember, too, that the "lag" effect may lead to hypoglycemia after the exercise session is complete, so that more than one insulin dose may need to be lowered.

The site of insulin injection is important. It may help cause hypoglycemia during exercise. If insulin is given into an exercising arm or leg, the increased blood flow through that limb during exercise may cause the insulin to be absorbed more rapidly than it would otherwise. The higher insulin levels in the blood would lower the blood glucose levels too much during exercise. Therefore, it is recommended that insulin be injected into the abdomen or sides when exercise is anticipated.

Exercise is important not only to prevent poor health, but also to improve the health you have!

6

The Oral Hypoglycemic Agents

For many, the development of a treatment of diabetes that can be taken by mouth is one of the most exciting advances since the discovery of insulin.

It is not only that many people can avoid, at least for a time, insulin injections; there is even greater importance. Anything that simplifies treatment for a significant number of people is a great public health measure. When the tablets were first announced about 30 years ago, many people who suspected that they had diabetes or actually had the disease and were afraid of the insulin injections were encouraged to see their physicians in hope of the new treatment. Furthermore, there are whole areas of the world where insulin is either scarce or not found at all. The fact that many in these areas have type II diabetes (non-insulin-dependent) means that treatment is now available for them.

Looking Back

These pills for diabetes are not new at all. Actually, German scientists found compounds to lower blood sugar in 1920. The compound called Synthalin did lower blood glucose levels, but it had problems with toxicity which caused its removal. Nevertheless, it stirred hopes for better future treatments. Dr. Elliott P. Joslin said at that time that while this particular agent was not useful, others in the future would be. At any rate, insulin was announced a year later and everyone forgot everything else until the 1950s, when the forerunners of today's oral agents were developed.

Natural Remedies

In many parts of the world, certain plants have been used as medications for generations. Nearly everyone has heard of someone who said that various herbs and plants lowered blood sugar levels. This is true except that most of these plant and tree substances are quite toxic, and while they do diminish blood sugar levels, they often damage or destroy the liver and other organs. Pharmaceutical companies and even the World Health Organization have had teams scouring remote areas of the world in the search for more effective medications for many years.

What Are the Oral Agents?

Perhaps it is better to start by saying what they are *not*. *They are not insulin!* When they are effective, they help the body make or release its own insulin, and they have other actions as well. Not only is there evidence that they increase the sensitivity of the receptors on the cells (Chapter 1), but there is even more evidence that they help to combat insulin resistance (Fig. 6–1). This means that even though insulin output may be diminished, in many patients it might be enough insulin. Since most people with diabetes do, at least early in their diabetes, put out some insulin, the potential target group for oral agent use is quite large.

Who Can Use Them?

The person must have live and active beta cells that will respond to the stimulation of the tablets. This eliminates the person with true type I diabetes, the person with juvenile-onset or "brittle" diabetes, and others with insufficient insulin response. This also eliminates those who have required insulin for many years.

There is, however, a mistaken idea about diabetes which has made the oral agents unsuccessful for many people. Some have the idea that the oral tablets practically eliminate diabetes and that

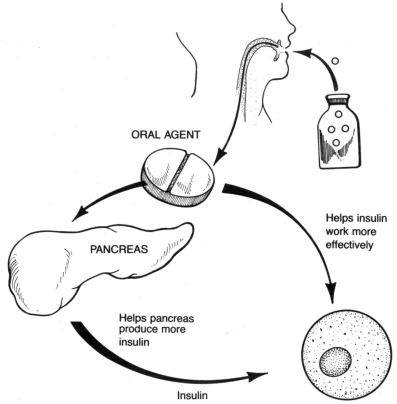

ORAL AGENT

PANCREAS

Helps insulin
work more
effectively

Helps pancreas
produce more
insulin

Insulin

FIG. 6–1. The mechanism of action of the sulfonylurea oral hypoglycemic agents. These medications work to improve glucose metabolism by helping the pancreas produce more insulin in response to the presence of glucose in the blood, and they help the insulin work more effectively to get the glucose from the blood into the cells of the body.

therefore no diet treatment is necessary. This is not true. As effective as the oral agents may be, they are not as potent at lowering glucose levels as the ordinary amount of insulin would be. For this reason, some diet discipline is even *more* important than ever. In fact, the difference between success and failure with this simple means of treatment depends on whether a sensible eating plan is followed.

Best of all, *if the oral tablets are effective, they enable the person to use his or her own insulin* steadily through the entire day. An individual's own insulin should not provoke antibodies as would insulin from foreign species. So it is safe to say that *when effective,* this method of treatment can be very useful. However, it is certainly not for everyone. In fact, oral agents are most effective in people whose diabetes started after age 40 and whose diabetes is of less than 10 years duration, although as with all general rules, there are exceptions to these.

Another thing to remember is that most physicians will consider treating you with diet first. If diet is effective, then you are living in the best of worlds because you will be keeping weight down and supplying enough of *your own insulin,* which is the way it should be. Sometimes if the diabetes has been poorly controlled, the pancreas may not be able to respond to the oral compounds, and your physician may find it necessary to give you insulin for a time until the pancreas is well enough rested to respond to the pills with insulin release. Sometimes people who start with insulin, have lost weight, and achieved effective control with diet can later go to treatment with oral agents. Some patients who start with the tablets can later respond to diet alone, so hope always springs eternal, especially if you follow the rules to diabetes.

How Do the Oral Agents Work?

This is much simpler to explain than it was in the previous editions because there is only one general type of oral compound—sulfonylurea. Previously, there were biguanides available (Phenethyl-biguanide, phenformin, DBI). These are no longer available in the United States, although they are still widely used in one form or another in most of the rest of the world. Research has started with another methyl-biguanide in the U.S.A.

What has gone wrong to cause type II diabetes in the first place? There are a number of possible places that problems can occur along the complex pathway from insulin secretion to the use of glucose by the cells of the body.

1. There could be a malfunction of the insulin secretion by the beta cells of the pancreas so that they are not triggered as usual by the glucose in the bloodstream.

2. Other hormones or antibodies may make insulin ineffective.

3. There could be a defect in the receptors on the cells which tells these cells to let the glucose in through their cell membranes.

4. The liver, which usually maintains balanced blood glucose levels, may be the culprit. It is possible that the liver either does not take in enough glucose or pours too much back out into the bloodstream.

TABLE 6-1. Oral Hypoglycemic Medications in Use in the United States

GENERIC NAME	TRADE NAME	MANU-FACTURER	TABLET SIZES & COLOR	USUAL DAILY DOSE
"FIRST-GENERATION" AGENTS				
Tolbutamide	ORINASE	Upjohn	White 250 mg / White 500 mg.	500–2000 mg
Tolazamide	TOLINASE	Upjohn	White 100 mg / White 250 mg / White 500 mg	100–1000 mg
Chlorpropamide	DIABINESE	Pfizer	Blue 100 mg / Blue 250 mg	100–500 mg (occ. 750 mg)
Acetohexamide	DYMELOR	Eli Lilly	White 250 mg / Yellow 500 mg	250–1500 mg

"SECOND-GENERATION" AGENTS

Glipizide	GLUCOTROL	Roerig Div. of Pfizer	White 5 mg (PFIZER 411) White 10 mg (PFIZER 412)	2.5–40 mg
Glyburide (glybenclamide)	MICRONASE	Upjohn	White 1.25 mg Pink 2.5 mg Blue 5 mg	1.25–20 mg
	DIABETA	Hoechst-Roussel	White 1.25 mg Pink 2.5 mg Light Green 5 mg	1.25–20 mg.

Indeed, the causes of type II diabetes are more complex than those for type I diabetes, which is caused by the inability to manufacture enough insulin.

So where do sulfonylureas act? It seems that they work not only at the pancreas but also at the other locations, the liver and the various other cells of the body, where potential problems may exist. They (a) help the pancreas release insulin, (b) possibly increase the sensitivity of the insulin receptors on the cells, (c) prevent the release of too much glucose from the liver, and (d) most of all, help decrease the resistance to insulin in the cell (Fig. 6–1).

Most recently the focus has been on the phenomenon known as "insulin resistance." Normally, insulin attaches to an "insulin receptor" on the surface of the cell somewhat as a key fits into a lock. This interaction between the insulin and the receptor causes a chemical reaction which allows the glucose to enter the cell. Insulin resistance takes place when this interaction does not work properly. What results is an increase in the blood glucose levels because the glucose cannot get into the cells. This mechanism is thought to be a major cause of type II diabetes. Some of the hypoglycemic agents seem to be very effective in reducing insulin resistance, allowing this hormone to work more effectively.

It is interesting that high levels of insulin in the blood seem to make insulin resistance worse! High levels of insulin can be seen in people with type II diabetes who are overweight or who may be unnecessarily treating their diabetes with large quantities of insulin. These large doses are an attempt to overcome the resistance, but are often ineffective. There is already too much insulin with no place to go.

Let's assume that there are twenty boats on a huge lake. There are only four piers or docks. A tremendous storm comes up. Those boats that get tied to the few available docks are safe. The others go round and round with no place to land. That is what happens to the person with diabetes who has tremendous amounts of insulin but no receptors to tie to!

Sometimes oral agent therapy *may* be more effective than large doses of insulin because oral agent therapy is less likely to *worsen* the resistance and, indeed, may actually decrease insulin resistance.

Available Oral Agents

The oral hypoglycemic agents currently available in the United States are of the sulfonylurea class and are listed in Table 6–1. There

TABLE 6–2. Contrasting the First- and Second-Generation Oral Agents for Diabetes

SIMILARITIES
Both generations need workable pancreas beta cells.
Both lower blood glucose levels by:
  Increasing insulin secretion, and
  Decreasing insulin resistance
Both have minimal side-effects.
Both generally free from toxicity (although individuals may react differently)

DIFFERENCES in the second generation:
Much more potent per dose
More effectively decreases insulin resistance
Remains in body for shorter period and is destroyed rapidly
Less fluid retention
Less likely to combine with other medications
Almost no Antabuse (facial flushing) effect
Often used in once-daily doses
Greater potential for hypoglycemic reactions because these are more effective

are two types of these medications. Those that have been available for many years are known as "first-generation" agents, while a group of agents made available more recently are known as the "second-generation" agents. These latter compounds were given FDA approval in May, 1984, although they have been used in the rest of the world for almost 15 years. In fact, the second-generation oral agents are the most widely used hypoglycemic agents worldwide. Although the two generations are similar, they do have differences that help choose which agent is best for a particular individual. These differences are summarized in Table 6–2. Variations among agents differentiate them and can affect the choice of medication. For example, tolbutamide (Orinase) is rapidly destroyed in the body, and most of it is excreted in the urine in 24 hours. On the other hand, less than 1% of chlorpropamide (Diabinese) is destroyed by the body's metabolism, and only 60% is excreted from the body in a 24-hour period. This is why the latter compound has a much longer duration of action, perhaps 36 hours or more. Tolazamide (Tolinase) and acetohexamide (Dymelor) are intermediate in the duration of their action.

Of the second-generation agents, glipizide (Glucotrol) has a duration of action of about 12 to 16 hours, while glyburide (Diabeta, Micronase) is effective for 18 to 24 hours. All of these second-generation agents are highly effective in lowering blood glucose,

TABLE 6–3. A Comparison of the Two Available "Second-Generation" Oral Agents		
	Glipizide (Glucotrol)	Glyburide (Diabeta or Micronase)
Action	Both may effectively lower blood glucose levels	
Daily dose	2.5–40 mg daily, often once daily	1.25–20 mg daily, usually once daily
Eliminated	Mostly urinary tract	50% urinary tract, 50% gastrointestinal

and, as shown in Table 6–1, are given in much lower quantities. Five or ten milligrams of glyburide would have the same effect as 500 to 1500 mg of tolbutamide. These agents have certain other advantages over the first-generation agents. For example, they have fewer side effects and are less likely to interact with other medications. They may also be given in a wide range of doses, which allows a great deal of dose adjustment without the need to switch agents. Table 6–3 contrasts the two second-generation medications.

Table 6–1 lists the agents available in the United States. For people who travel, Appendix 3 lists various brand names of these agents abroad, as well as agents such as gliclazide and the biguanides, which are not available in the United States but are widely used elsewhere.

Possible Undesirable Sulfonylurea Effects

Low Blood Glucose Reactions. Anything that lowers blood glucose levels effectively may cause symptoms of hypoglycemia (hunger, trembling, sweating, etc.—see Chapter 15). Exercise without eating can do this, and insulin is the greatest cause of "insulin reactions." If a sulfonylurea compound causes the increased release of, and more effective response to, insulin, and there is not enough glucose present, then an "insulin-like" hypoglycemic reaction is possible. Some of the longer-acting hypoglycemic agents can bring on these reactions, especially in people who may have variations in their eating or activity habits or in whom removal of these drugs from the system is decreased because of reduced kidney function. Shorter-acting agents may be preferable in these situations. In general, prevention and treatment of these reactions are the same as it would be for reactions with insulin (Chapter 15).

Side Effects. This is a term that is applied to symptoms that may result from taking any medication. While these are not desirable, they are usually unexpected symptoms that cause no real harm or permanent damage and disappear when medication is discontinued or the dose reduced. Even common medications such as aspirin can sometimes cause an upset stomach, for example.

The sulfonylurea compounds may cause side effects, but these are infrequent. Among these are gastrointestinal upsets, appetite loss (which, to some degree, might be beneficial!), skin rash, itching, and other unexpected symptoms that are really quite rare. Many of these disappear after one "adjusts" to the medicine, but occasionally the dose needs to be reduced or the medication stopped.

Toxicity. Toxicity is something else. It generally refers to something more lasting and possibly damaging. Perfectly good medications are occasionally "toxic" for certain individuals. For example chloromycetin, an antibiotic that is lifesaving when used to treat typhoid fever and certain severe urinary tract infections, has occasionally caused severe anemia. Physicians, the pharmaceutical industry, and the Food and Drug Administration are eternally vigilant against toxicity. Oral hypoglycemic medications have been used by millions of people with diabetes around the world for more than 25 years, and they have been extraordinarily free of toxicity. The sulfonylureas are particularly remarkable in this respect.

The biguanides, no longer available in the United States, have a higher incidence of side effects than the sulfonylureas. Among these are lactic acidosis (an excessive accumulation of lactic acid) in some people who were treated with phenformin. Only several hundred patients out of a quarter of a million who used that particular medication daily for several decades developed lactic acidosis. Still, because effective hypoglycemic agents such as insulin and sulfonylurea compounds were available and because lactic acidosis is a serious complication, the FDA took the phenformins off the market as "an imminent hazard." However, phenformin is still available to some patients under special conditions. By FDA regulation, phenformin may be dispensed only by physicians who obtain IND (investigative new drug) certification and only in carefully prescribed circumstances. Phenformin, Buformin, and Metformin are in fairly general use abroad.

Physicians are aware of side effects and other possible problems with any medication, and for this reason, patients should report any unusual symptoms or circumstances to their physicians as soon as possible.

The University Group Diabetes Program (UGDP) Report

Physicians and their patients with diabetes became quite disturbed in the early 1970s by a series of sensational reports, often featured in the news media, stating that oral hypoglycemic agents available at that time could be ineffective as well as possibly damaging. These reports and the surrounding furor was discussed much more extensively in the eleventh edition of this book, but things have changed. While the UGDP report was useful in emphasizing the importance of careful observations of all treatment methods, the importance of the findings of this study was blown out of proportion. In essence, investigators from 12 university groups studied a total of 200 patients who received either a standard dose of tolbutamide (doses were not adjusted), a fixed dose of insulin, adjusted doses of insulin, or a placebo (an inactive tablet with no medication). At the end of an observation period, it was found that there was a higher number of deaths, presumably from cardiovascular disease, in those using tolbutamide. These deaths were found in a few—3 of the 12 centers. Because these groups were small (about 16 people were studied by each of the 12 universities), any problem from whatever cause would seem common because the total number of patients was so low.

At the time, there was an enormous medical outcry for or against the findings. Among the objections were that the groups were too small, that they were poorly chosen, that they contained many people who had significant cardiac findings *before being enrolled as study subjects*, that the tolbutamide doses were not adjusted, and that a significant number of people studied were being "undertreated" and thus were not really "controlled." After considerable debate, most medical organizations nationally and internationally did not accept the report's findings. The oral agents were not taken out of use. As the years went by, what should have been a scientific discussion became very political. Eventually, package inserts acceptable to the Food and Drug Administration, the medical profession, and diabetologists were adopted.

Essentially, these package inserts, now found in all prescription items, warn about all the potential problems that any medicine may cause, whether common or remote. The insert mentions the UGDP study and states that physicians and patients should be aware of this. It also states that only one of the first-generation compounds was used in the study. Quite properly, it states that diet and exercise are mainstays of diabetes treatment, and that the oral agents may be used if diet and exercise are not effective. If the oral agents fail, then the obvious recourse is the use of insulin.

The study was useful in pointing out that good control, no matter how attained, is good for persons with diabetes. Also, many people who use the oral agents neglect diet and exercise, expecting that the pill will do miraculous things for their diabetes. In fact, diet can mean the difference between successful treatment or failure for many. When people eat "anything they want," these agents are often not effective. We now have a better focus and a commitment for better use of these therapeutic tools.

The Good and the Bad of Oral Medications

The oral agents have some obvious advantages for people in whom they are effective. Many patients find it difficult or impossible to use insulin. For a handicapped or older individual, improper use of insulin poses a greater risk due to possible hypoglycemia than any risk from the proper use of oral hypoglycemia agents. Indeed, for many, these tablets may actually be a better treatment for the specific problems that cause type II diabetes. Also they use the individual's own insulin.

There are also some disadvantages. Patients who start with oral agents often resist treatment with insulin, postponing this treatment to their own detriment. Oral agents also lack the flexibility of insulin therapy and do not permit daily adjustment for eating or activity variations.

Looking Ahead

Medicine is a dynamic field. Many medications bring early enthusiasm that later becomes tempered by reality. The really useful treatments continue while others fade into obscurity, to be replaced by something newer and better. Diet is the very best oral agent. The latest are improved and "state of the art," but certainly newer oral agents are continually being investigated.

The oral treatment of the future may not be the same as today's. The first-generation agents provided hope to some but were ineffective for many. The second-generation agents are probably a step in the right direction, with greater effectiveness for more people. The ultimate oral agent will probably be insulin by mouth. As exciting as this prospect may be, there are too many formidable obstacles to "oral insulin," and it is not expected to be available in the near future. If the first-generation agents released more insulin, the second-generation agents probably decreased insulin resistance so that a little insulin meant more, and the third generation, when it arrives, may have an even greater effect in decreasing insulin resistance. Just think: some place, in some laboratory, someone is working on new things to help simplify the treatment of diabetes.

Summary

The presently available oral hypoglycemic agents are very useful for an enormous number of people with type II diabetes around the world. They are not miracle drugs that will wipe out disease or change the course of diabetes history. However, they are available for people who need diabetes care but do not need insulin, and they are used in many places where insulin is a rare or unavailable commodity. *If effective,* an oral agent uses the person's own insulin in a gradual process during the entire day. The second-generation agents are an improvement over the first-generation in many ways. They are used in smaller doses, often taken once daily and effective for 24 hours. In much of the world they have superseded the first-generation agents. If the first-generation compounds are really effective, however, there is no need to change. While the oral agents are helpful, nothing will replace the education-motivated person who works with his or her physician and other health team members in the constant care of a lifelong problem.

7

Insulin

Few developments in medicine have so changed the course of a disease and given life to so many as the discovery of insulin.

Drs. Banting and Best of Toronto are credited with the discovery of insulin in 1921. This was all the more remarkable because neither of them was a researcher in the modern sense. Frederick Banting was a surgeon and Charles Best a graduate student at the University of Toronto using borrowed equipment in a borrowed laboratory. Such an accomplishment would be near impossible today because they did not have the qualifications, background, or equipment to qualify them for a research grant (Fig. 7–1)!

Others, of course, had prepared the ground for them. The German scientists von Mering and Minkowsky, for example, had found that laboratory animals in which the pancreas had been surgically removed developed diabetes. And indeed, in several parts of the world, others were on the verge of the great discovery. However, these two young Canadians got there first.

Upon hearing the reports from Toronto, Dr. Elliott P. Joslin said, "With the bright news from Toronto, a hope for life." The first insulin was known as "isletin" because of its origin in the islets of Langerhans of the pancreas. Later the term "insulin" was adopted because it had been used by earlier investigators. Reviewing the charts of the first patients who received insulin is like reading about a dramatic moment in history. Initial words of gloom for an individual's chances of survival change to glimmers of hope as the shipment from Toronto arrives, tempered by uncertainty about how to use the stuff. Finally, the comments turn more jubilant as the

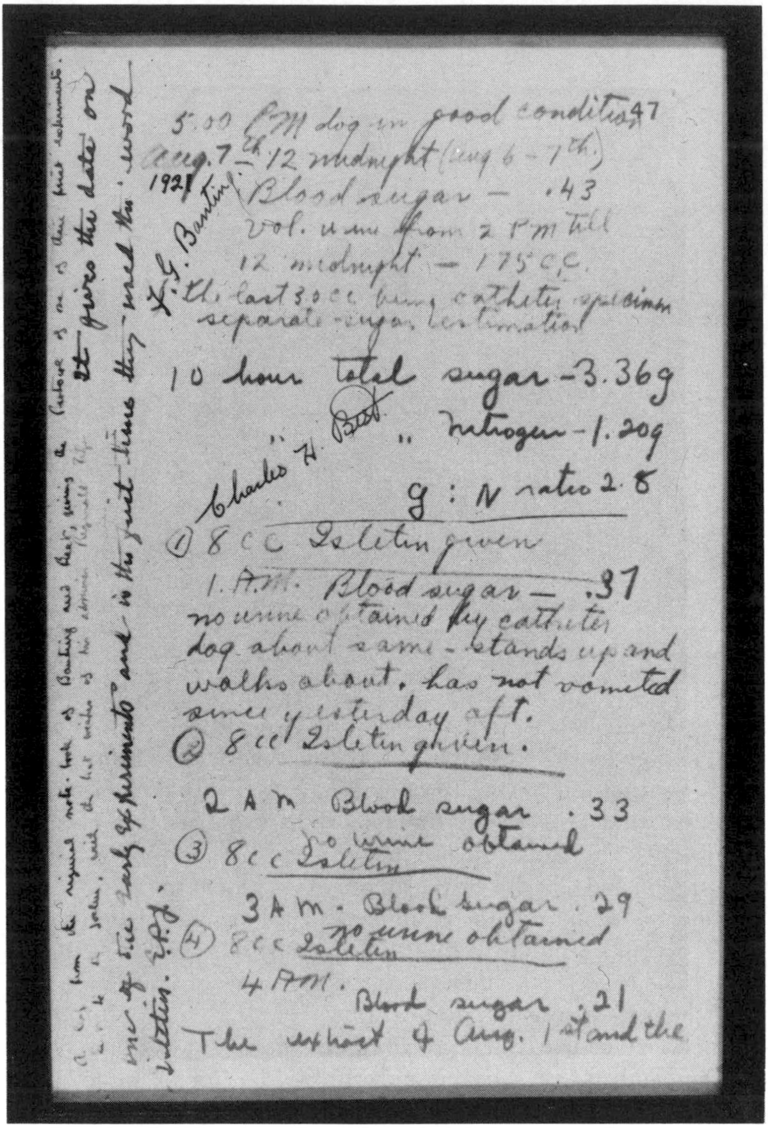
5.00 P.M. dog in good condition .47
Aug. 7th 12 midnight (Aug 6–7th)
1921
Blood sugar — .43
Vol. urine from 2 P.M. till
12 midnight — 175 c.c.
the last 30 c.c. being catheter specimen
separate sugar estimation
10 hour total sugar — 3.36 g
" " nitrogen — 1.20 g
G : N ratio 2.8
(1) 8 cc Isletin given
1. A.M. Blood sugar — .37
no urine obtained by catheter
dog about same — stands up and
walks about, has not vomited
since yesterday aft.
(2) 8 cc Isletin given.
2 A.M. Blood sugar .33
(3) 8 cc Isletin no urine obtained
3 A.M. Blood sugar .29
(4) 8 cc Isletin no urine obtained
4 A.M. Blood sugar .21
The exhaust of Aug. 1st and the
F. G. Banting
Charles H. Best
It gives the data on
one of the early experiments and is the first time they used the word
isletin. E.P.J.

FIG. 7–1. The original laboratory worksheet used by Drs. Banting and Best at the time that insulin was first found to be effective. Notice how the blood sugar in the depancreatized dog started at 430 mg% (stated as .43), with a 10–hour total urine glucose of 3.36 grams. Then 8 cc of isletin (insulin) was given. The strength of this insulin was about 1 unit per cc. (This is as if the insulin were "U-1"—we use U-100 today!) The next blood glucose level was 370 (.37), then 330 (.33), then 290 (.29), and finally 210 (.21) with successive insulin injections of 8 cc (8 units) each. This sheet is signed by Drs. Charles Best and F. G. Banting. The comments on the left side by Reginald Fitz and Dr. Joslin (E. P. J.) read as follows: "A leaf from the original note-book of Banting and Best, giving the protocol of one of their first experiments. Sent to Dr. Joslin, with the best wishes of his admirer Reginald Fitz. It gives the data on one of the early experiments and is the first time they used the word isletin. E.P.J."

physicians realize that the isletin is working, and the patient is surviving and gaining weight.

Because the preinsulin treatment was essentially starvation, the survivors were slender ghosts of persons. Among these was a young man who was surely doomed to die but was saved by the discovery of insulin. He survived and lived to later win a Nobel prize for his discovery of liver as a treatment for pernicious anemia. His name, still engraved on the outer wall of the Joslin Clinic, was George Minot.

What Is Insulin?

Insulin is a hormone secreted by the pancreas. It is a protein and therefore must be injected for use. The original insulin, of course, was what we now know as crystalline or "regular" fast-acting insulin. For many years it was the only available insulin. There were numerous attempts to make a longer-action insulin, and finally in 1936 the Danish physician Hagedorn developed long-acting protamine zinc insulin. Later, in 1946, his group developed

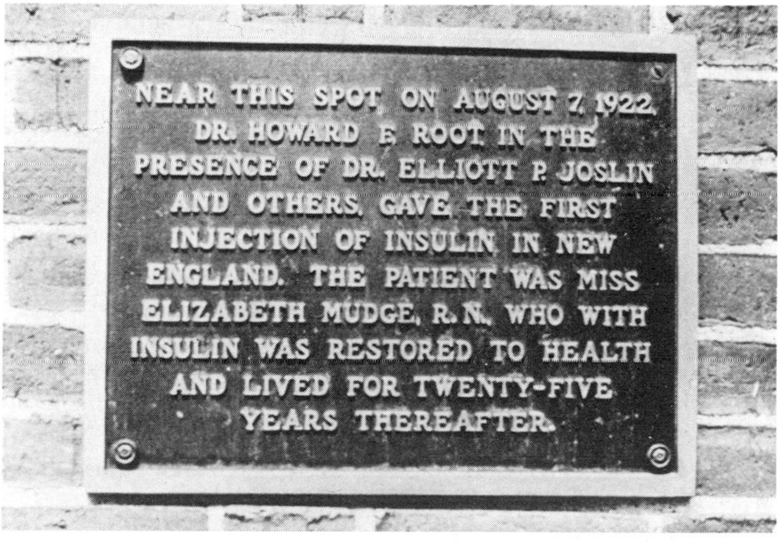

FIG. 7–2. The bronze plaque on the wall of one of the New England Deaconess Hospital buildings marks the place where, in the old building, the first insulin in New England was given. One can imagine the tension as the physicians watched the first injection.

isophane insulin, which we now know as NPH, for "Neutral Protamine Hagedorn." In the 1950s, Hallas-Moller developed Lente, another insulin with similar action. Progress in extracting the insulins and purifying them led to "single-peak" insulin (insulin with fewer byproducts and side-products from the pancreas) in 1972 and highly purified insulins in 1980. In 1984, the human-like insulins became available—some made by altering pork insulins, others synthesized anew in specially prepared bacteria. It has been a long trip from 1921!

Fortunately, the insulin marketed for injection is a stable protein and fairly easy to transport, store, and use. Even after a year at room temperature, a very small percentage of its potency is lost—possibly a dozen units per vial (1000 units total). However, any reserve supply of insulin should be refrigerated (40°F). At constant high temperatures (greater than 86°F) the loss of strength is only 2.3% in 2 months, but after constant high heat (104°F), about 10% of its strength is lost.

The normal fasting blood level of insulin in humans varies from 1 to 30 microunits in 1 cubic centimeter (1 milliliter, or 1/1000 of a U.S. quart and a quarter) of blood. A microunit is 1/1,000,000 of a unit of insulin. Obviously, even in people who do not have diabetes, the amount of insulin actually circulating in the blood at one time is very small. The amount increases after each meal and returns to the normal fasting level in about 3 hours. In people who do not have diabetes, insulin is supplied in exactly the amount needed moment by moment.

Characteristics of Insulin

It is important that people who use insulin injections know certain basic characteristics of the insulin they use so that they can understand its effects on their bodies and more precisely inform physicians, either their own or another physician who may not know them as well, what treatment they have been using. Insulin has four basic characteristics: (a) concentration, (b) type, (c) purity, and (d) species. In addition, the brand of insulin should also be known, because there may be some differences among the available products.

The Unit. Insulin is measured in units. This measure appears on the label as "U," which means "clinical unit." A unit is always constant because it measures a specific amount of insulin activity, and *always* represents the same amount of activity for *every* type of insulin. The unit is an international measure and is consistent throughout the world.

Concentration. An additional factor, however, is the concentration. Insulin concentration is designated by the number after the "U," such as U-40, U-80, or U-100. The differences between these insulins is not the strength of the unit—a unit is always a unit! The difference is the concentration. The numbers tell the total number of units of insulin found in 1 milliliter (commonly referred to as cubic centimeter, or cc), which is equal to 1/30 of an ounce, of solution. U-100 insulin is insulin concentrated such that 1 cc of insulin fluid contains 100 units of insulin. The standard syringes used for these insulins are designed so that they contain 1 cc of insulin solution (Fig. 7–3). However, there are some low-dose syringes that contain only ½ cc and some large ones containing 2 cc. The reason for the ½-cc syringe (with only 50 units if filled) is that some people take very small doses, and in this low-dose syringe the marks are spread apart making it easier to read. Recently an even smaller syringe holding 0.3 cc. has become available. Those using more than 100 units per dose need the 2-cc syringe. The markings on the syringe indicate the number of units. Therefore, U-100 insulin should be used with a U-100 marked syringe, which would divide a 1-cc quantity into 100 1-unit increments. U-40 insulin would be used with a syringe marked off with 40 unit markings per cc, etc.

In the past, U-40 and U-80 were the primary insulin concentrations used, although others were available. Recently, U-80 (80 units per cc) insulins have been discontinued in the United States in favor of U-100, which is the standard in this country and increasingly abroad. An advantage of the more concentrated insulin is that a smaller amount of fluid is injected. However, insulins are still available in the United States as a U-40 concentration, although it is possible that these too will be phased out so that only one concentration will be available, reducing the chance for errors or confusion.

Insulin Type. As mentioned, originally only *regular* insulins, known as "Toronto" insulin in Canada, were available. They are rapidly effective and have a short duration of action in the body. Originally, three or four daily injections were necessary. Their speed of action still makes them the best emergency insulins. *Protamine zinc insulin* was made, as described, by adding protamine, a simple protein, and zinc in a certain concentration, making its duration somewhat longer than 24 hours. This is referred to as a long-acting

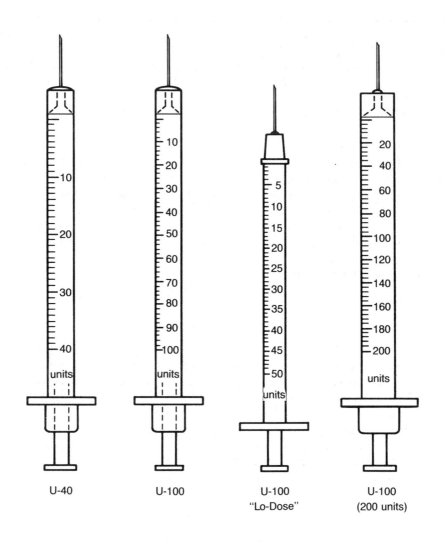

| U-40 | U-100 | U-100 "Lo-Dose" | U-100 (200 units) |

FIG. 7–3. U–40, U–100 standard, U–100 "Lo-Dose" (50-unit), and U–100 200-unit capacity insulin syringes. A UNIT OF INSULIN IS STILL A UNIT REGARDLESS OF WHICH TYPE OF INSULIN IS USED. To get the proper number of units, the syringe used must correspond to the concentration of the insulin. For example, both the U–40 and the U–100 syringes hold 100 cc of fluid. However, the amount of insulin in a full U–40 syringe would be less than the amount in a U–100 syringe because U–100 insulin is more concentrated than U–40 insulin. For people using lower amounts of insulin, the 50–unit ("Lo-Dose") syringe, which is marked off in 1-unit intervals, may be easier to use. The 200–unit syringe is for people using large insulin doses.

TABLE 7–1. TYPES OF INSULIN COMMONLY USED
TODAY AND THEIR ACTION TIMES

Type of Insulin	Onset of Action (in hours)	Peak of Action (in hours)	Duration of Action (in hours)
Short-acting (rapid)			
Regular (clear or crystalline)	About ½ hour	2–4	6–8
Semilente	1–2	3–8	10–16
Intermediate-acting (slower)			
NPH (isophane)	1–2	6–12	18–26
Lente	1–3	6–12	18–26
Prolonged-acting (very slow)			
Ultralente	4–6	18–24	28–36
Protamine zinc (PZI)	4–6	14–24	26–36

NOTE: Figures are estimates, and actual action times may vary
among brands or species, with amount of insulin used, or among
individuals.

insulin. It also starts acting some hours after injection. By changing
the mixtures of protamine and modifying the zinc concentration,
NPH was developed. The action of NPH insulin is intermediate
between the regular and the longer-acting *PZI*, and thus is called an
intermediate-acting insulin.

Later modifications led to the Lente family of insulins called
Lente, Semilente and *Ultralente*. Lente is also an intermediate-
acting insulin, like NPH in its overall effect. These are, for most
patients, generally interchangeable, although there may be some
subtle differences between the two, especially in the newer human
forms. *Semilente* is an insulin with a short duration, although longer
than regular insulin. *Ultralente* has a prolonged duration, much like
PZI. *Globin*, almost unheard of today, was longer-acting than
regular and shorter-acting than intermediate insulins. PZI is still
available but is used infrequently. The primary insulins in use are
regular, Semilente, NPH, Lente, and Ultralente (Table 7–1). How
these insulins are used to control diabetes is discussed in Chapters
9 (standard insulin therapy) and 10 (intensive insulin therapy).

Insulin Purity. Until recently, all insulins used were from
pancreases of animals used for food. The pancreases usually come
from beef and pork. However, insulin has been made from sheep,

from tuna fish in Japan, and during World War II from whales in some countries. This is one of the few medications that depends in part on the dietary habits of different countries. If, for example, dietary practice changed and people stopped raising cattle (unlikely), there would be a dearth of beef insulin, which is one reason the new synthetic and genetic programmed insulins are important for the future.

Pancreases, however, contain much material that isn't insulin—cell components, digestive enzymes, other hormones, and hormone-like substances, so it is necessary to separate ("extract") the actual insulin from these other substances. The non-insulin but "natural" substances are known as "impurities," which differ from foreign substances, which should not be in insulin at all and are referred to as contaminants. Common impurities seen in animal insulins include insulin-like substances, glucagon, and proinsulin (the precursor of insulin).

Over the years, techniques for purification have improved. The measure of impurities is parts per million, or ppm. Proinsulin, a major impurity, is often used as a gauge of the level of impurity. As of 1972, the purity of the "single-peak" insulins was 3000 ppm proinsulin (0.3%), with an overall purity of 99%. The designation "single-peak" was used by Eli Lilly and Company and refers to a single peak on a chromatograph, indicating no impurities. E. R. Squibb & Sons used the name "high purity" or "single-peak quality."

In 1980, even purer insulins became available. This level of purity, 99.99% pure, is the level for most standard animal species today. Also available are purified pork or purified beef insulin known as "monocomponent" insulins. They have levels of proinsulin impurities under 10 ppm. More recent human-like insulins are the purest yet; they have less than 5 ppm impurities and are overall 99.999% pure.

Impurities can cause the formation of antibodies, as explained below. However, with the purer insulins of 99.99% and 99.999% purity, the antibody problems are almost nonexistent.

Species. The amino acids in insulin are linked together in a specific sequence that differs slightly among species. Strangely, the insulin most like that of a human is from the pig; the amino acid chains are identical with the exception of only one amino acid on the end. Insulin from almost any animal is effective in humans, but the slight differences may cause antibodies to be formed, which in turn make the insulin less effective.

Having to depend on animal sources for insulin caused great concern some years back because the number of people with diabetes increases proportionately just a bit faster than the world population but much faster than the supply of animal pancreases. It was feared that the world would run out of insulin. Indeed, in some parts of the world, there is a shortage of available insulin. However, the recent development of synthetic and other genetically programmed insulins will avert this threat.

Insulin Antibodies

In recent years, more and more has been learned about the effect of insulin antibodies on insulin action. The body's immune system can recognize any foreign protein and manufactures an antibody to it. Antibodies are part of the mechanism that fights off "foreign" proteins such as viruses—and, of course, animal insulins. Antibodies bind to the protein and may inactivate or destroy it. Even though some animal insulins have only a tiny difference from human insulin, they are still a foreign protein, and the body makes antibodies to them. These bind to the insulin, holding onto it and preventing it from functioning. After years of using animal insulins, some people may have as much as 5000 units of insulin bound to these antibodies, floating through the bloodstream. Because they never all let go at once, there is no problem with sudden hypoglycemia, however!

Nevertheless, the antibody-bound insulin can cause some mischief. When new insulin is injected, instead of working as it should, some of it is bound to antibodies, while meanwhile the antibodies continually release small amounts of insulin. This constant interchange—insulin being bound and insulin being released—causes the actual insulin peak to be less exact and to occur at a less predictable, often much later, time than it theoretically should. The duration of action can also be longer than it should be. That is why an intermediate insulin, supposedly acting for only 12 to 16 hours, actually can be effective for 18 to 30 hours. Many of the original studies determining peak times and the duration of action were done in people without diabetes or with newly discovered diabetes without insulin antibodies.

Antibodies to different species' insulins as well as to impurities have been blamed for other problems as well. These include lipodystrophies: the fatty buildup (lipohypertrophy) or wasting (lipoatrophy) at the site of the injections. They also may be the cause of insulin allergies and occasionally of insulin resistance.

The Newer Insulins

For these reasons, efforts have been made to develop insulin that is as human-like and pure as possible. A first attempt was the purified pork, with only one amino acid different from human and as pure as could be, but some people were still allergic to this. Later, purified beef was tried.

Recently, two types of human-like insulins have become available. Squibb-Novo changed pork insulin so that the one different amino acid was now identical to human. This insulin is a semi-synthetic insulin. Eli Lilly produced a synthetic insulin through a recombinant DNA process. Bacteria were "programmed," by changing the messages on their DNA molecules, to manufacture insulin identical to that of humans. This insulin was then extracted from these bacteria and purified. This method may help solve the world insulin shortage because the supply is theoretically limitless. These insulins can reduce the levels of insulin antibodies and thus peak more predictably, have a shorter and more precise duration of action, and reduce the possibility of antibody-induced problems. With the more exact action, subtle differences have been noted between NPH and Lente insulin types when used as human species insulins. These two insulins were thought to be identical; however, as human insulin, NPH may peak more sharply and at a higher insulin level and may have a slightly shorter duration of action when compared with human Lente. This information may be useful in tailoring dosage programs to individual needs.

The technology for the preparation of insulins will continually change and improve. Human insulin may be synthesized as human proinsulin and then broken off into insulin, which may have manufacturing advantages. Proinsulin may someday be used by itself, as it may benefit persons with some types of diabetes. It will likely behave in a manner similar to that of NPH. Change, and improvements, are inevitable!

Available Insulins

In the United States, most insulin is manufactured by Eli Lilly & Sons; Nordisk USA; or E. R. Squibb & Sons, Novo Laboratories. Table 7–2 lists the various products available in the United States, but as with all medications, this will change constantly.

The choice of a brand of insulin may or may not influence eventual diabetes control. There are subtle differences between

TABLE 7-2. Brands of Insulin Available in the United States

PRODUCT	SPECIES	MANUFAC-TURER	STRENGTH	PURITY (IN PPM)
RAPID-ACTING		*(REGULAR)*		
Regular Iletin I	B/P	Lilly	U- 40 U-100	<10
Regular	P	Sb-Novo	U-100	<10
Regular Iletin II, purified beef	B	Lilly	U-100	<1
Regular Iletin II, purified pork	P	Lilly	U-100 U-500	<1
Velosulin	P	Nrdsk	U-100	≤1
Regular, purified pork	P	Sb-Novo	U-100	≤1
Humulin Regular	H-DNA	Lilly	U-100	0
Velosulin, human	H-Pr	Nrdsk	U-100	≤1
Novolin Regular	H-Pr	Sb-Novo	U-100	≤1
Humulin BR (for insulin infusion pump)	H-DNA	Lilly	U-100	0
		(SEMILENTE)		
Semilente Iletin I	B/P	Lilly	U- 40 U-100	<10
Semilente	B	Sb-Novo	U-100	<10
Semilente, purified pork	P	Sb-Novo	U-100	<10
INTERMEDIATE-ACTING		*(NPH)*		
NPH Iletin I	B/P	Lilly	U- 40 U-100	<10
NPH	B	Sb-Novo	U-100	<10
NPH Iletin II, beef	B	Lilly	U-100	<1
NPH Iletin II, pork	P	Lilly	U-100	<1
Insulotard NPH	P	Nrdsk	U-100	≤1
NPH, purified pork	P	Sb-Novo	U-100	≤1
Humulin N (NPH)	H-DNA	Lilly	U-100	0
Insulotard NPH, human	H-Pr	Nrdsk	U-100	≤1
Novolin N (NPH)	H-Pr	Sb-Novo	U-100	≤1

Table 7–2.   Brands of Insulins Available in the United States (continued)

PRODUCT	SPECIES	MANUFAC-TURER	STRENGTH	PURITY (IN PPM)
		(LENTE)		
Lente Iletin I	B/P	Lilly	U- 40	<10
			U-100	
Lente	B	Sb-Novo	U-100	<10
Lente Iletin II, beef	B	Lilly	U-100	<1
Lente Iletin II, pork	P	Lilly	U-100	<1
Humulin L (Lente)	H-DNA	Lilly	U-100	0
Novolin L (Lente)	H-Pr	Sb-Novo	U-100	≤1
		(MIXED)		
Mixtard (30% regular + 70% NPH)	P	Nrdsk	U-100	≤1
Initard (50% regular + 50% NPH)	P	Nrdsk	U-100	≤1
Novolin 70/30 (30% regular + 70% NPH)	H-Pr	Sb-Novo	U-100	≤1
LONG-ACTING				
		(ULTRALENTE)		
Ultralente Iletin I	B/P	Lilly	U-40	<10
			U-100	
Ultralente	B	Sb-Novo	U-100	<10
Ultralente, purified beef	B	Sb-Novo	U-100	≤1
Humulin Ultralente	H-DNA	Lilly	U-100	0
		(PZI [PROTAMINE ZINC])		
Protamine Zinc Iletin I	B/P	Lilly	U- 40	<10
			U-100	
Protamine Zinc Iletin II	B	Lilly	U-100	<1
Protamine Zinc Iletin II	P	Lilly	U-100	<1

KEY: B = beef; P = pork; B/P = mixed beef and pork; H-DNA = human made by recombinant DNA process; H-Pr = human made by pork rearrangement. Lilly = Eli Lilly & Sons; Nrdsk = Nordisk-USA; Sb-Novo = E. R. Squibb & Sons, Novo Laboratories.

brands that may make a difference for some individuals and not others. Your physician should be consulted to help you select the brand that you will use. If there is no preference, price or availability can be your guide. If a particular brand is recommended, however, it is wise to use that brand and not switch around each time you purchase insulin.

Be familiar with the labels on the insulin bottles. Color codes, letter symbols, and bottle shapes have changed over the years. The only real protection is to read the labels and know what is on them. When someone asks what insulin you use, you should know the brand, concentration (if not U-100), types, purity, species, and, of course, the doses!

Emergency Insulin

For emergencies, regular is the only insulin to use. It is effective almost immediately after injection and has a short duration of action. Every insulin-taking patient should have a bottle of regular insulin on hand for emergencies, whether they need it daily or not. It will retain potency indefinitely if kept in the refrigerator.

Storage

Storing insulin is not a problem. The expiration date on every bottle of insulin has a large safety margin, just as with photographic film. This is the earliest date before which there is absolutely no question about the potency of the insulin. After the expiration date, the insulin may start losing some strength, slowly.

Always have at least one or two extra bottles of each insulin you use on hand. Unopened insulin should be stored in the refrigerator at about 40°F, but not in the freezer compartment. Frozen insulin loses its strength. The bottle in current use may be kept at room temperature if under 75°F. If extremes of temperature are avoided, insulin currently in use can be kept at room temperature for 6 to 8 weeks without a significant loss in strength. Your physician may recommend that you discard insulin that has been out at room temperature longer than this.

Recently there has been some concern about the formation of crystals in an occasional vial of human insulin. Manufacturers have been working to determine the exact cause of this problem and to correct it. The temperature at which the insulin was stored, or severe vibration or agitation, may be among the factors involved. Although manufacturers hope to resolve this problem soon, it is still important that insulin currently in use (especially human insulin) be stored at temperatures under 75°F. If room temperature is frequently above this level, refrigeration is recommended. Even when the current crystallization problem is solved, it is good practice to check the insulin solution carefully. If crystals (little white flecks that stick to the inside of the bottle or appear above the surface of the solution) or any other abnormalities appear, the bottle should be replaced. Although the crystals are harmless, crystallization may reduce the amount of insulin you are actually injecting and may cause your diabetes treatment to be less effective.

Any bottle of *regular* insulin that is cloudy or discolored should be discarded. This type of insulin should always be clear. Inadvertent freezing, crystallization, or contamination of any insulin may cause it to lose potency. If there is any question, the safest step is to discard such insulin.

Insulins Abroad

Patients sometimes worry about obtaining insulin when traveling in foreign countries. Insulin units are standardized throughout the world, regardless of the manufacturer. However, various concentrations (U-40, U-80, even U-20) are used. In many parts of the world, insulins manufactured in the United States are available.

Insulin Syringes

Many types of syringes are available for use with insulin. This variety may be confusing. The most commonly used and those approved by the American Diabetes Association have a unit scale on each syringe with the numbers marked in color according to concentration: U-100 is black, U-80 is green, and U-40 is red. U-100 syringes contain 100 units for the 1 milliliter (or cubic centimeter, "cc") contents of the syringe. As noted, syringes are available in capacities of 50 units ("low dose"), 100 units (standard), and 200 units (Fig. 7–3). *Only in an emergency,* syringes for insulins with unit concentrations different from the insulin actually being injected may need to be used. Simple mathematics will allow proper conversion (see Table 7–3). Of course, mismatches of insulin and syringes should be *avoided* if at all possible.

TABLE 7–3. USE OF SYRINGES THAT DO NOT MATCH THE INSULIN BEING USED		
If your insulin is	And your syringe is	Then if you draw up one unit of liquid in the syringe, it actually contains (units) of insulin
U-100	U-40	2.5
U-100	U-80	1.25
U-500	U-100	5
U-40	U-100	.4
U-80	U-100	.8
U-40	U-80	.5

Many patients now use disposable syringes and needles. These syringes are made of plastic and cannot be boiled to sterilize. They usually come with preattached needles, most commonly 26 gauge, which are made of a much softer metal than stainless steel and cannot be resharpened. While the long-term cost of these disposables is higher than the reusable varieties, their convenience and sterile cleanliness is so great that most people prefer them.

Some people still use a glass, reusable syringe with disposable needles. These needles can vary in length from ⅜ to ⅝ of an inch. The gauges may also vary, but 25 or 26 gauge is recommended (the lower the gauge number, the thicker the needle).

Reusable syringes and needles can be kept in alcohol between injections. Before the syringe is filled with insulin, the alcohol must be expelled by pushing the plunger in and out a few times. Reusable syringes and steel needles should be sterilized by boiling approximately once weekly.

In many parts of the world, modern disposable syringes and needles are not available. In addition, some government health plans permit only a certain number of syringes per week. Some people have stated that they use the injection equipment several times, rinsing it in alcohol between uses. This, of course, is not ideal because it may increase the chance of infection, and the needles lose their sharpness rapidly. In one remote Asian country, a physician reported that people with diabetes sometimes used disposable syringes and needles for several weeks or a month using this alcohol technique! He was asked didn't it hurt and wasn't there some danger. "Of course," he replied, "but what choice do we have?" The practice is not encouraged if there is any other choice, but it has been done.

HOW TO INJECT A SINGLE DOSE OF INSULIN

(See also text on page 127)

The following steps should be taken to inject a *single* (not a mixed) dose of insulin (Fig. 7–4).

1. Turn the bottle upside down and roll between the hands. (Fig. 7–4A). Shaking the bottle creates bubbles.

2. Wipe the insulin bottle top with cotton and alcohol or a prepackaged alcohol wipe.

3. Pull the plunger to the unit markings on the syringe which correspond to your dose (Fig. 7–4B). Put the needle through the top of the insulin bottle. Push the plunger down, forcing air into the bottle (Fig. 7–4C).

4. With the needle in the bottle, turn the bottle upside down and pull the plunger halfway down the syringe. This draws insulin into the syringe. Push the plunger toward the bottle. This pushes insulin back into the bottle (Fig. 7–4D).

5. Pull the plunger halfway down the syringe. Check for air bubbles in the syringe. If bubbles are present, repeat step 4. If no bubbles are present, push or pull the plunger to the unit markings on the syringe which correspond to your recommended dose (Fig. 7–4E). Remove the needle from the bottle. The syringe is now loaded with the correct amount of insulin.

6. Place the syringe on a flat surface. Make certain that the needle does not touch that surface.

7. Choose an injection site. Wipe skin with cotton and alcohol.

8. Grasp fold of skin and body tissue beneath it.

9. Pick up the syringe as you would a pencil. Push the needle straight into the skin (Fig. 7–4F). Push the plunger down, injecting the insulin.

10. Release the fold of skin. Press cotton and alcohol around the injection site and pull the needle out.

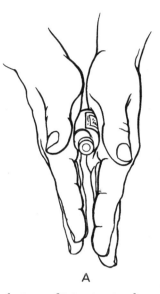

A

FIG. 7–4. A. The technique of injecting insulin accurately must be mastered by everyone who uses insulin. Slight errors can be serious. Begin by turning the bottle of insulin upside down and rolling it between the palms. The purpose of this step· is to mix the insulin thoroughly.

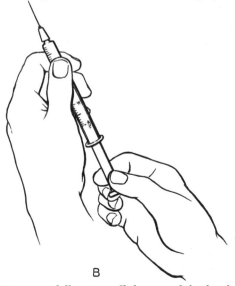

B

FIG. 7–4. B. Next, carefully wipe off the top of the bottle with alcohol-soaked cotton. The next step is vital. Draw air into the syringe in the same amount *as the insulin dose* to be taken. In other words, if you need 20 units of insulin, you fill the syringe with 20 units of air, which is left in the syringe temporarily. The reason for this is that a vacuum exists in the insulin bottle, and in order to remove the insulin, you must first inject the same amount of air.

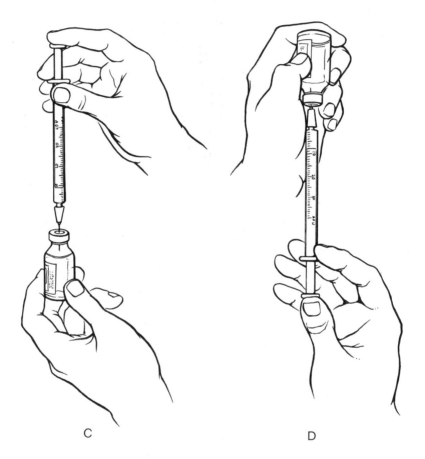

C

D

FIG. 7–4. C. With the air still in the syringe, carefully insert the needle through the diaphragm top into the bottle. Push the plunger down. D. Turn the bottle upside down and pull back the plunger halfway down the syringe. Push the insulin and air back into the bottle. The purpose of this step is to push all of the air bubbles back into the bottle of insulin.

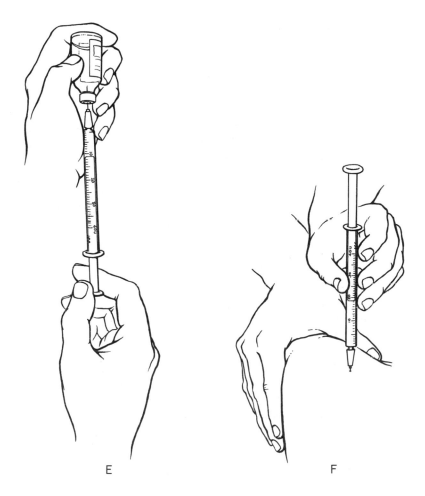

E   F

FIG. 7–4. E. Now that all the air bubbles are out of the syringe, carefully pull the plunger down to the correct amount of insulin. F. The syringe now has the precise amount of insulin required. Wipe the spot to be injected with cotton and alcohol, and pinch the skin. Holding the syringe like a pencil, push the needle straight into the skin and push the plunger down. Release the pinched skin, press the cotton ball next to the needle, and pull out.

HOW TO MIX INSULIN

The following instructions are for preparing a *mixed dose of insulin* (two types of insulin in the same syringe) (Fig. 7–5):

1. Turn the bottle of "cloudy" insulin upside down and roll between the hands (refer to Fig. 7–4A).
2. Wipe off the tops of both "cloudy" and "clear" bottles with cotton and alcohol or a prepackaged alcohol swab.
3. Pull the plunger to the unit markings on the syringe which correspond to the dose of intermediate-acting insulin (refer to Fig. 7–4B). Put the needle through the top of the "cloudy" (intermediate-acting insulin) bottle. Push the plunger down, forcing air into the bottle (Fig. 7–5A & 7–4C). Remove the needle from the bottle.
4. Pull the plunger to the unit marking on the syringe which corresponds to the dose of short-acting insulin (Fig. 7–4B). Put the needle through the top of the "clear" (short-acting insulin) bottle. Push the plunger down. Leave the needle in the bottle (Fig. 7–5B).
5. With the needle in the bottle, turn the bottle upside down. Pull the plunger halfway down the syringe, drawing insulin into the syringe. Push the plunger toward the bottle (refer to Fig. 7–4D). This pushes insulin back into the bottle.
6. Pull the plunger halfway down the syringe. Check for bubbles. If bubbles are present, repeat step 5. If no bubbles are present, push or pull the plunger to the unit markings on the syringe which correspond to your recommended dose of short-acting insulin. Remove the needle from the bottle. The syringe is now loaded with your dose of short-acting insulin (Fig. 7–5B).
7. Turn the bottle of cloudy (intermediate) insulin upside down. Put the needle through the top.
8. Pull the plunger slowly to the unit markings on the syringe which correspond to the *total* dose of the insulins that you are taking (clear + cloudy). Remove the needle from the bottle. The syringe is now loaded with your dose of both short-acting and intermediate-acting insulin (Fig. 7–5C).
9. Place the syringe on a flat surface. Make certain that the needle does not touch the surface.
10. To inject the insulin, follow steps 7 through 10 under the section on the use of a single insulin dose.

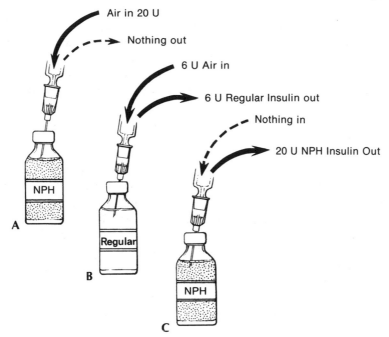

Air in 20 U

Nothing out

6 U Air in

6 U Regular Insulin out

Nothing in

20 U NPH Insulin Out

NPH

A

Regular

B

NPH

C

FIG. 7–5. Technique for mixing short- and long-acting insulins. In this example, 6 units of regular insulin and 20 units of NPH insulin are required.

How to Inject Insulin

The injection of insulin is one of the most important techniques that many people with diabetes must learn. It is important to learn each step of the injection routine in detail and practice it carefully. Eventually it may become almost "automatic," but at first it requires great attention to each detail.

Keep in mind the following points while injecting insulin. It is best to grasp some tissue firmly between the thumb and one finger of one hand, holding the syringe in the other hand. Grasp a large amount of skin and tissue beneath the skin, although not too tightly, so that the injection will be well beneath the surface of the skin. (If using an arm, push it against a solid object to push up the skin, similar to a "grasp.") Don't be disturbed if a small amount of blood appears after the needle is withdrawn. Simply press the spot gently and briefly with cotton soaked with alcohol. It is very important to keep a clean technique to avoid infection at or around the site of injection. Infections and boils can occur when people are careless about injections.

How deep should the injection go? Some people newly learning to inject insulin are afraid that they will pierce some vital organ. This is almost impossible, considering the short length of the needle used.

Avoiding or Removing Bubbles. People worry about the tiny bubbles that sometimes appear in the syringe before giving insulin. To avoid bubbles, do not shake the insulin bottle, but roll it gently between the palms of the hands for mixing. Then, after the insulin is in the syringe, hold the syringe vertically, tip up, and draw back a bit to unite all the bubbles into one big one. Then slowly push the air and bubbles out. However, do not worry if very small bubbles still remain, because it takes an enormous amount (100 cc) of air to do any damage to the person and even then, the air would have to be put directly into a vein. The biggest danger is that if you get some bubbles instead of insulin, you will be cheating yourself. With the small bubbles, however, the error is usually very small and insignificant.

Automatic, Button, and Jet Injectors. Some people with diabetes, squeamish about injecting themselves directly, use a small automatic injector to insert the needle beneath the skin. The use of these devices may be satisfactory if the injector is simple enough. The syringe is filled with insulin as usual and placed into the injector. Then the injector is spring-cocked. After the area to be injected is sterilized, the injector is set against the skin. Touching a small trigger forces the needle through the skin and then the person pushes the plunger down, injecting the insulin. This device is not necessary for most people, who become very adept at self-injection. Diamatic (Ulster Scientific) is just such a device. A similar device, the Injectomatic (Monoject), for ½ and 1 cc syringes, will stick the needle into your skin for you, but you have to push the plunger (Appendix 4).

Button infusers are made up of little injectable discs attached to a catheter that leads to a needle which is inserted beneath the skin. These infusion sets must be changed every 2 days. They are useful for people who require multiple daily injections and wish to avoid the discomfort of repeated punctures and prefer the limited puncture but the inconvenience of maintaining the ever-present hardware on and beneath their skin. One must need many daily injections for this to become a viable alternative.

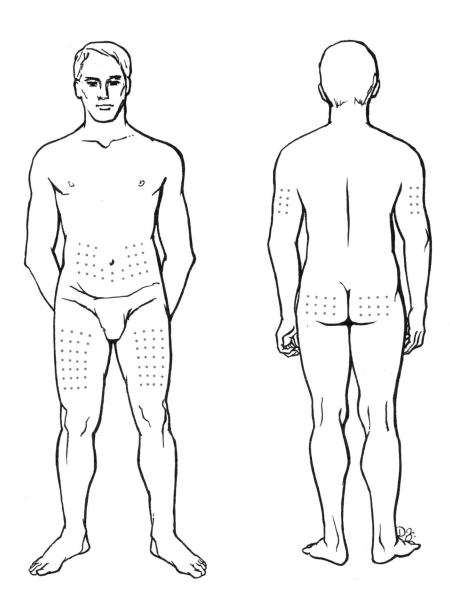

FIG. 7–6. Possible sites for insulin injection. Rotating injection sites helps to prevent the formation of atrophy, scarring, or hypertrophy. By using all the available sites, it may be possible to inject the same area no more than once a month.

"Jet injectors" are also available. These use no needles but force insulin through the skin with air under great pressure. Disadvantages are the cost of the supplies, the cumbersome sterilizing process, and the inability to actually see the insulin in the injector. Also, some injectors lack flexibility to vary doses and use mixtures of insulin types which many people need, although newer ones have overcome these deficiencies somewhat. The injection is not totally without sensation either. These devices are being improved technically and are an alternative for people who are completely unable to bear the trauma of injections. However, consistency of delivered insulin dose is still a concern. The rate of absorption of the insulin is often increased when one of these devices is used, so the insulin dose(s) may need to be changed. No one should start using one of these devices without first consulting the doctor, and for most people, after the initial period, injecting with the newer sharp needles is no problem.

WE'VE COME A LONG WAY!
Until recently, when the new sharp disposable needles became available, people used steel needles over and over again. In time, the needles would develop a hook or a bent place at the tip. People then had to take the needle and resharpen it on a special abrasive stone to get the point sharp. It was no fun.

Insulin infusion pumps are another way to deliver insulin to the body. These pumps supply insulin through a catheter by way of a needle inserted beneath the skin, in a manner similar to that of the button infuser. A discussion of these pumps is found in Chapter 10.

Injection Aids for People with Low Vision. Aids to insulin injection for people with low vision are available. Syringe magnifiers can make reading gradations on the syringes easier. Insulin gauges and click-count syringes (clicks count out unit measures) are available to help draw up the proper amount of insulin if reading the scale is difficult.

Injection Sites. The most common site for insulin injection is the thigh. Most people have enough flesh in this area, and it is easy to reach. However, it is not desirable to continue injecting into the same site constantly, because the skin can become thickened and scarring can delay absorption. Also, lumps of fat may form underneath the skin (known as lipohypertrophy or "insulin hypertrophy").

Injection sites should be changed daily and rotated. If one places the injections in a straight line a little further down the thigh each day and then starts a second and third column, then moves to the other thigh, it will be several weeks before the injection returns to the first site. As Figure 7–6 shows, other possible injection sites are the upper arms and across the front of the abdomen as well as toward the sides. The abdomen is a good choice because it is easy to reach, is a vast area, and many patients have extra fat tissue there. Abdominal tissue is easy to grasp, and if hollows caused by atrophy should occur, they are ordinarily not exposed to public view. The upper buttocks may be hard to reach, but other members of the family could give injections there. Another way of reaching the buttocks is to lean back against a table edge or dresser so that the tissue is compressed firmly and is available as well. One should avoid injecting close to or below the knee or into the very outside of the thigh where the heaviest tissue is found. Some feel that with purer insulins, rotation is not needed. However, constant injection into the same site will thicken the area and change absorption rates.

The important thing is that injection sites are rotated so that any area, within an inch diameter, is not used more often than once monthly if possible.

8

Monitoring Your Diabetes

This chapter is a result of one of the exciting new developments in diabetes treatment, the ability to be in charge of your own diabetes management on a daily basis! In previous editions, this phase of treatment came under the heading "Testing." There is a difference, however, between "testing" and "monitoring." "Testing," still very important, means taking samples of blood or urine at specific intervals to measure how much glucose it contains. Testing is like taking photographs of something—it freezes the action. "Monitoring" means constantly being on top of the situation as a whole, rather than focusing on only one test result. It is like looking at the whole series of photographs.

There is an argument whether Thomas Jefferson or Wendell Phillips first said "Eternal vigilance is the price of liberty!" In either case it applies to diabetes in that "eternal vigilance is the price of good health," especially with the lifelong problem of diabetes. The development of the ability to truly monitor the control of diabetes is one of the reasons this new edition of this manual was written.

Why Monitor?

The answer is simply that a person with diabetes, unlike most other chronic conditions, must always know where his or her blood glucose level is at a given time. In previous chapters, the importance of being as close to normal as possible has been explained. This chapter tells how to tell if you are doing it.

Although continuous testing and monitoring are helpful to your physician, they are even more important for you. For some people with diabetes, *occasional testing* is still sufficient, but for many, especially those with blood glucose changes that are difficult to regulate, monitoring can help prevent the disturbing "ups and downs." This "eternal vigilance" also will warn the patient of an oncoming severe hypoglycemic reaction at one end of the scale or acidosis at the other end.

The goal is always blood glucose levels as near normal as is realistically possible. Recently two new ways have been developed to measure how close to "normal" your glucose levels are: (1) *glycohemoglobin* (also called *glycosylated hemoglobin*) measures longterm management results, and (2) *self blood glucose monitoring* tells you how things are going on a day-to-day basis and helps you make the daily adjustments required to achieve good longterm results.

Of course, glucose and other blood and urine testing in the physician's office are a vital part of your care, but all of these together will help you determine what changes in your treatment may be needed.

A Brief History of Monitoring

There has been a series of revolutions in the treatment of diabetes since the days of starvation treatment prior to the discovery of insulin. Of course, insulin was the greatest of these revolutions. The oral blood-sugar-lowering compounds were another such breakthrough. One of the greatest advances was the acceptance, mostly since World War II on a large scale, that education is essential to the survival of people with diabetes. The concept of constantly measuring your own blood glucose levels is one of the latest and perhaps most important advances. This development not only has revolutionized the treatment of diabetes, but also has taken many in the health profession by surprise. Who would have believed that people who, like the rest of us, frequently quiver at the thought of a needle puncture, would actually draw and test their own blood several times daily? It is estimated that possibly 1 million people with diabetes in the United States alone do this form of monitoring from occasionally to frequently.

With this blood testing, people can truly "take control" of their diabetes. They know their metabolic status immediately, and they are a *part* of the treatment and management team, rather than being passive participants. In short, they are part of the action. In the past when the visit to the physician's office was made, a blood glucose sample was taken. The result might not be known for several days. The assumption was that the glucose level(s) measured on the day of the visit was also what the level was at that time on *every other day*. Unfortunately, this assumption was often misleading. On the day of the visit to the doctor the person's routine may have been different from the usual. Also, it is human nature to try to do as well as possible in self-care just before "inspection" by the physician. Diet, timing, and other aspects of diabetes management were often more exacting just prior to the visit, and thus the office glucose level often gave a falsely optimistic picture of the diabetes control.

Past methods of daily monitoring also failed to give a good picture of the diabetes control. The home urine testing methods had serious limitations, both in helping the doctor measure longterm control and in giving the individual with diabetes daily information about his or her control. The urine tests are dependent on the renal threshold—the blood glucose level above which glucose begins to spill into the urine to produce a positive urine test. This is usually about 150 to 170 mg%, but may be much lower for youngsters and much higher for older persons. This renal threshold is well above the target blood glucose levels for most patients. The only information urine testing usually gives is whether the glucose levels are too high—way too high! They tell nothing about the actual patterns of blood glucose levels—information vital to properly adjusting treatment—especially insulin doses.

When urine sugar testing was, for many years, the only available method, of course it was better than no testing at all. Even now, it is often sufficient for many individuals with type II diabetes that is either very stable or does not require insulin. However, blood glucose levels performed with self testing materials can now provide a clearer picture of what is actually happening to glucose levels on a daily basis. In addition, the glycohemoglobin measurement represents the average level of "control" better than the occasional office blood glucose test. With the glycohemoglobin, the person is also less likely to make a last-minute attempt at improving the level of control than with doctor's office testing.

The Glycohemoglobin Measurement

The blood has many kinds of cells. The white blood cells, for example, help fight disease. The red cells that give blood its color have the important function of carrying oxygen to the cells throughout the body and carrying away a waste product, carbon dioxide, to the lungs, where it is exhaled out of the body. The substance in these cells that carries this life-giving oxygen is called hemoglobin. The most vital part of this hemoglobin molecule is called hemoglobin A. The cell is protected by a covering, but if there is too much glucose in the blood, the glucose can get through this protective cover and attach to the hemoglobin molecule. There is a small percentage of the hemoglobin A—a "subfraction" of it—that is in a slightly different form and is known as hemoglobin A_1. Hemoglobin A_1 forms when the extra glucose in the blood attaches to the hemoglobin A. This hemoglobin A_1 fraction can be measured in a laboratory. In addition to the A_1, some laboratories measure a slightly different portion of the hemoglobin known as the hemoglobin A_{1c}. These hemoglobins with sugar molecules attached are known as "glyco-" (for glucose) hemoglobins: "glycohemoglobin!"

GLYCOSYLATED HEMOGLOBIN
This test gives you an average of blood glucose levels over the last 2 months. If there were some high blood glucose levels and many low or normal levels over that time, the average will show fairly good regulation.

Red blood cells live for an average of about 120 days, after which time they die and are removed from the circulation. New red blood cells are manufactured to replace them. "Glycosylation" (the process whereby the glucose becomes attached to the hemoglobin) occurs continually during the whole lifetime of the red blood cell. At any given time, there are red blood cells that have just been born and those that are about to die. Thus, the *average* age for a red blood cell is 2 months, or half the total life span. Because the amount of glucose that sticks to the hemoglobin molecule depends on the level of blood glucose—the higher the blood glucose level, the more glucose will stick to hemoglobin molecules—the measure of the amount of glycohemoglobin shows the average blood glucose level. As the average age of all the red blood cells at any one time

TABLE 8–1. Glycohemoglobin Ranges, Estimated Average Daily Blood Glucose Values, and Interpretation

Glycohemoglobin* (%)	Average Blood Glucose Level (mg%)	Interpretation
5.4–7.4	<120	Nondiabetic
7.4–8.5	120–150	Excellent
8.6–10.5	150–200	Good
10.6–13.0	200–300	Fair
>13.0	>300	Poor

*Glycohemoglobin values are measures of hemoglobin A at the Joslin Clinic. Values may vary at other laboratories and institutions with varying methods of testing the glycohemoglobin.

is 2 months, the average glucose measured represents what took place during a 2-month period. The measurement of this glycohemoglobin test is given in a percent: what percent of the hemoglobin is glycosylated into hemoglobin A_1 or A_{1c}.

There are various laboratory methods for measuring glycohemoglobin levels, and the range of "normal" values varies from laboratory to laboratory. As a general rule, however, the higher the test level, the poorer the degree of control during the past month or two. Table 8–1 shows the ranges and their interpretation for the hemoglobin A_1 method used at the Joslin Clinic. It also shows the *average* blood glucose levels that the glycohemoglobin represents. Remember, these are *average* glucose levels, reflecting both pre- and post-meal levels. They also say *nothing* about how the blood glucose may vary in a single day. Thus, a "good" glycohemoglobin value may be obtained by having many high and many low glucose levels—not a desirable goal of treatment at all!

The test for glycohemoglobin is very useful, but, like other tests, it is not perfect. For example, people with unusual hemoglobin molecules, such as those with sickle cell anemia, may have false test results. It may also be in error in early stages of pregnancy because the fetus produces its own red blood cells. Nevertheless, it is still a very useful tool in managing diabetes during pregnancy. Anemias occur when there are fewer red blood cells, which may also not live as long, and will make the glycohemoglobin measurement inaccurate as well.

Despite these limitations, the measurement of the glycohemoglobin is still a very powerful tool! It is now thought that many of the complications of diabetes result from the glycosylation of (the sticking of glucose to) various tissues of the body (not just hemoglobin). What happens to hemoglobin is probably what happens to many of the other tissues of the body as well. Therefore, in measuring the glycohemoglobin, we may be actually measuring the process that can lead to the complications of diabetes. The glycohemoglobin is better at assessing overall control than the occasional office glucose measurement, although there is much to be learned from the measurement of blood glucose in the physician's office as well.

What Does Measuring the Blood Glucose Tell Us?

It is important to remember that glucose levels are constantly changing. Think of them like the ocean tides, rising and falling over the post of a wharf. If you look closely at that post sticking out of the water, and watch the water line against it, the water level will appear to rise and fall. However, although the tides rise and fall, they do not reach exactly the same spot each day. In addition, a photograph of the water against the post will not tell you anything about how the tides have risen and fallen in the past; nor will it tell you where the water level will be at any time in the future. It just tells you where the water was at one instant in time. So how does this snapshot—the single blood glucose level—help?

It is just these changing blood glucose levels that can be so confusing to many people. When told that their blood glucose is 135 mg%, they will be alarmed and state, "Why last week it was 120 mg%! What went wrong?" Nothing, really. The blood sugar is usually lowest during fasting and highest half an hour to one hour after eating. It then slowly drops as glucose is used by the body. Similarly, many people do not understand that the blood pressure may also vary. For example, when faced with an emergency or severe sudden stress, both blood glucose and blood pressure may rise abruptly as a normal preparation by the body to handle the emergency or stress. In medical school, physicians are taught that it is adrenaline that is produced to prepare you for this "fight or flight." When the emergency ceases, things should return to normal. If they do not, only then must the physician probe to determine why!

The Office Blood Glucose Measurement

There is still much value in performing the office blood glucose tests. Of course, for those not routinely doing home blood glucose testing, the office test is vital. When correlated with a urine glucose level, it can help the physician to determine the renal threshold as well as provide a picture by which the current state of diabetes control can be evaluated. The office glucose measurement also helps determine the precision of the home testing that the individual has reported. Many physicians now have a rapid office laboratory that gives almost immediate results, allowing "on-the-spot" treatment decisions.

Blood testing results may vary according to the site from which the blood sample was taken. The fingertip or earlobe sample is from tiny arteries (capillaries). This blood has glucose in it that is on the way to the tissues and is often 20 to 30 mg% higher than that from a vein. Veins return the blood to the heart and lungs, and some of the blood glucose has been used. At fasting levels, the results are pretty much equal, but in samples drawn after eating, this difference may be seen. Table 8–2 lists the expected normal venous blood glucose levels, as well as suggested target levels.

TABLE 8–2. TARGET BLOOD GLUCOSE LEVELS

How to Use This Table

The following are "ideal" and "target" blood glucose levels, but they must be individualized for each person. Your physician should help you choose yours. They are set a bit high to avoid insulin reactions.

People with type I (unstable) diabetes aim for values somewhat higher to avoid reactions, but ask your physician for guidance.

Time	Ideal (Normal) Levels (mg%)	Target Levels (mg%)
Before breakfast	70–105	70–120
Before lunch, supper, and bedtime snack	70–110	70–140
1 hour after meals	<160	<180
2 hours after meals	<120	<150
2:00 AM to 4:00 AM	>70	>70

Self Monitoring of Blood Glucose (SMBG)

A recent "miracle" in diabetes treatment is the development of methods of monitoring blood glucose at home. Previously the only way to get serial readings, or a profile of daily blood glucose patterns, was to hospitalize the person being tested. Of course, the routine of the person differed from normal home and work routines. Now a more accurate picture of the patient in normal life-styles—a picture that can better target treatment needs—can be obtained through self blood glucose monitoring (SMBG).

Self Blood Testing Materials. There are two methods of SMBG. (1) using test strips that can be read by the naked eye and (2) using test strips that are read by a glucose meter. The test strips are small strips of plastic with a patch of chemical material on the end. This material reacts with the glucose in blood to produce a color change, which indicates the amount of glucose present. The test strips that are read by themselves may be less accurate, giving an approximate rather than actual glucose level. However, this accuracy is good enough for most, and these methods have the advantage that they can be performed almost anytime or anywhere. People with diabetes have become quite clever in measuring their blood glucose levels on planes, in meetings, or in other previously inconvenient locations—whenever they feel the need of it! The strips may also be saved for as long as a week to be read later by others if the patient has difficulty doing so himself. Table 8–3 lists the currently available test strips that can be used alone. New tests are appearing constantly, and probably before this book reaches you, several others will be available.

SELF MONITORING OF BLOOD GLUCOSE
If several tests are done each day, an accurate and clear picture of diabetes control is available. It can be a basis for adjusting insulin doses.

The strip-reading meters for self use have been greatly improved during the last few years of this "electronic age." Originally they were cumbersome, expensive, and difficult to use. Newer models are smaller—often the size of a pocket calculator—easier to use, and less expensive. They give more accurate results than strips alone, and their use is increasing, primarily when intensive insulin therapy (Chapter 10) is used, when there are visual difficulties, or

TABLE 8–3. **TEST STRIPS FOR SELF MONITORING OF BLOOD GLUCOSE (USABLE WITHOUT METERS, NONWASH STRIPS ONLY)**

Name and Manufacturer	Package Quantity	Instructions for Use	Comments
Chemstrip bG (Boehringer Mannheim)	25	Wait 1 minute, blot, wait 1 minute, read. If over 240, wait 1 more minute, read.	2 color pads. Range 20–800 mg%. Reading stable for 7 days. Can be used with Accu-chek II, Diagen, Diatron Easy Test, or Glucochek SC meters.
Glucostix (Ames)	50 or 100	Wait 30 seconds, blot, wait 90 seconds, read.	2 color pads. Range 20–800 mg%. Must be read immediately. Can be used with Glucometer II meter.
TrendStrips (Orange Medical Instruments)	50	Wait 1 minute, blot, wait 1 minute, read. If over 240, wait 1 more minute, read.	2 color pads. Range 20–800 mg%. Stable for later reading. Can be used with TrendsMeter, BetaScan Audio, or BetaScan B meters.
Visidex II (Ames)	25 or 100	Wait 30 seconds, blot, wait 90 seconds, read.	2 color pads. Range 20–800 mg%. Must be read immediately. Cannot be used with a meter.

when more accuracy is desired. Various meters are listed in Table 8–4, although newer models are constantly appearing. Some models actually have memories that recall the glucose levels at various times of the day over a period of time to help determine glucose patterns, and meters are now available that can feed their stored data into a home computer for analysis!

The overall cost of self blood glucose testing over the course of the year may be somewhat high, but with the growing appreciation of the importance of these test methods, many health insurance policies cover all or some of the costs if the materials are prescribed by a physician. For many, the cost of self monitoring is money well

TABLE 8-4. BLOOD GLUCOSE METERS FOR SELF USE

Name and Manufacturer	Time for Test	Measurement Range	Comments
ACCU-CHEK II (Boehringer Mannheim)	2 minutes	10–500 mg%	Manual calibration. Dry wipe system. Uses Chemstrip bG test strip packaged specifically for this meter. 2-year warranty.
BETASCAN AUDIO (Orange Medical Instruments)	2 minutes	0–400 mg%	Manual calibration. Dry wipe system. Uses TrendStrips. Electronic voice indicates test result. 1-year warranty.
BETASCAN B (Orange Medical Instruments)	2 minutes	0–400 mg%	Manual calibration. Dry wipe system. Uses TrendStrips. 1-year warranty.
DIAGEN (Seton Products)	2 minutes	18–360 mg%	Manual calibration. Dry wipe system. Uses Chemstrip bG test strip. 2-year warranty.
DIASCAN (Home Diagnostics)	90 seconds	10–600 mg%	Manual calibration. Dry wipe system. Uses Diascan test strips. 10-reading memory. 2-year warranty.
DIATRON EASY TEST (Diatron Biomedical)	2 minutes	9–450 mg%	Manual calibration. Uses Diatron Easy Test and Chemstrip bG test strips (dry wipe systems) and Destrostix test strips (wet wash system).

BLOOD GLUCOSE METERS FOR SELF USE (continued)

Name and Manufacturer	Time for Test	Measurement Range	Comments
DIRECT 30/30 (CPI/Lilly)	30 seconds	40–450 mg%	Blood measured directly—no test strips. No self timing; uses replaceable sensor cartridge lasting 30 days. Uses special battery from manufacturer with 1-year life. 1-year warranty.
EXACTECH (Baxter)	30 seconds	40–450 mg%	Manual .calibration. Uses Baxter ExacTech blood glucose strips. Nonreplaceable battery with 2-year expected life. Pen-shaped. 2-year warranty.
GLUCOCHEK SC (EquiMed Medical Products	2 minutes	10–400 mg%	Manual calibration. Dry wipe system. Uses Chemstrip bG test strip. Stores 400 readings. 2-year warranty.
GLUCOMETER II (Ames)	50 seconds	40–399 mg%	Manual calibration. Dry wipe system. Uses Glucostix test strip. 2-year warranty. Also available in memory model and "M" computer-compatible model.
GLUCOSAN 2000 (LifeScan)	1 minute	25–450 mg%	Factory calibration. Dry blot system. Uses Glucoscan test strips. 3-year warranty.

BLOOD GLUCOSE METERS FOR SELF USE (continued)

Name and Manufacturer	Time for Test	Measurement Range	Comments
GLUCOSAN 3000 (LifeScan)	1 minute	25–450 mg%	Same as Glucoscan 2000 plus 29-reading memory.
ONE TOUCH (LifeScan)	45 seconds	0–600 mg%	Factory calibration. No wiping. Uses One Touch test strips. 3-year warranty.
TRACER (Boehringer Mannheim)	2 minutes	40–400 mg%	Manual calibration. Dry wipe system. Uses Tracer bG strips. 2-year warranty.
TRENDSMETER (Orange Medical Instruments)	2 minutes	0–396 mg%	Manual calibration. Dry wipe system. Uses TrendStrips. 1-year warranty.

spent. In the long run, the improvements in diabetes control that can result from SMBG should reduce the costs of health care and lost earnings.

Some people attempt to lower the cost of monitoring by carefully cutting and splitting the test strips lengthwise to make two strips out of one. Strips cut in this manner should be used within a day of being cut. Split strips will not be accurate for some meters, but some meter manufacturers are adapting their machines to this practice. Scissors are often sufficient for cutting strips, although strip splitters (such as Strip Splitter II, manufactured by Larken Industries) are available.

Whichever method is used, the blood for SMBG is obtained by pricking the finger with a lancet. These are special needles used only for this purpose. While some people can prick themselves freehand, others prefer using one of various finger-pricking devices (Table 8–5). Each device holds a lancet which you position over a finger. When you press the trigger button, the lancet springs forward, pricking the finger quickly and with little pain. Some of the devices come equipped with various sizes of "guards" or "platforms," which can be used to adjust the depth to which the lancet enters the finger.

> **DOS AND DON'TS IN USING BLOOD GLUCOSE METERS**
>
> Do learn proper lancing technique or use an autolancer to minimize sore fingers.
>
> Do learn proper testing technique to maximize accuracy.
>
> Do be sure to get a proper blood sample to test.
>
> Don't drop or mishandle meter.
>
> Don't freeze or overheat the meter: leaving a meter in a cold auto or in the sun can be damaging.
>
> Do keep the strips tightly sealed in the container to maintain freshness.

These devices may be purchased without a prescription in some states. Other states require a prescription for them.

A large drop of blood can be obtained by pricking the finger with the lancet, usually on one side of the fingertip, which is preferable to the center, which has painful nerve endings. This drop of blood is transferred to the test strip. The strip changes colors depending on the amount of glucose in the blood. The strip can be read by visual comparison of the color of the test strip to the color chart on the container, or by use of a meter. While SMBG may seem difficult to some individuals, many people feel it is actually less difficult to do than urine testing, and it is far more accurate.

The blood glucose meters are remarkable little instruments, much like a pocket laboratory. These measure reflected light

TABLE 8–5. FINGER-PRICKING DEVICES AND LANCETS

NAME	MANUFACTURER	COMMENTS
Devices		
Autoclix	Boehringer Mannheim	Flat design; comes with 3 platforms to vary depth of penetration. Lancet triggered by pressure on guard.
Autolance	Becton Dickinson	Flat design; lancet triggered by pressure on guard. Uses only Micro-Fine lancets.

FINGER-PRICKING DEVICES AND LANCETS (continued)

NAME	MANUFACTURER	COMMENTS
Auto-Lancet	Palco Laboratories or Orange Medical Instruments	Comes with 1 adult, 1 juvenile tip (guard). Guard screws on, making it less likely to fall off. Button release.
Autolet	Ames or Ulster Scientific, Inc.	Comes with 10 platforms (regular depth). Button release. Comes with 20 platforms (10 each of 2 different depths).
Autolet-DTV	Ulster Scientific, Inc.	Same features as Autolet, plus a digital clock with a seconds display.
Glucolet	Ames	Comes with Unilet lancets and endcaps. Button release.
Monojector	Sherwood Monoject	Comes with 3 caps; puncture depth controlled by amount of pressure applied by user. Lever release.
Penlet	LifeScan, Inc.	Clear guard; puncture depth controlled by amount of pressure applied by user. Allows user to vary depth more than Monojector. Button release.
Lancets		
Easy Stik Lancets	Diabetes Supplies	Can be used alone or in each of the above units except Autolance.
Glucosystem Lancets	Ames	Can be used in either Autolet or Glucolet.
Micro-Fine Lancets	Becton Dickinson	Fits only Autolance or can be used alone.
Monolet Lancets	Sherwood Monoject	Can be used alone or in each of the above units except Autolance.
Trends Lancets	Orange Medical Instruments	Can be used alone or in each of the above units except Autolance.
Unilet Lancets	Ulster Scientific, Inc.	Fits Autolet or Autolet-DTV or can be used alone.

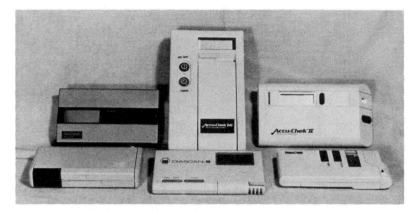

FIG. 8–1. Meters for self monitoring of blood glucose. Top, left to right: Glucoscan 2000, Accu-Chek, Accu-Chek II. Bottom, left to right: Glucometer II, Diascan-S, Tracer.

bouncing off the strip and put it into numbers that give you reasonably accurate blood glucose levels (Fig. 8–1).

Testing Urine for Glucose

There is still a role for testing urine for glucose despite the growing use of self blood testing. The section on self testing methods on page 151 outlines how urine testing fits into an overall home monitoring program.

Testing for the amount of glucose in the urine is possible because the body will allow glucose to spill into the urine once the glucose level in the blood rises above the "renal threshold." Normally, the kidney retrieves any sugar that is filtered out into the urine so that it can be used for nourishment. If there is more glucose than the kidney is able to recover, the excess spills over into the urine. To determine what the renal threshold is for a given person, it is necessary to obtain urine and blood glucose levels at the same time on a number of occasions and compare values, looking for the highest blood glucose value for which there is a negative urine glucose reading.

Urine glucose is somewhat "historical," showing the blood glucose level from a past time. To obtain more current information, a "second voided specimen" of urine is sometimes tested. This is especially important first thing in the morning or after other long periods of not urinating. Samples collected in the urinary bladder

TABLE 8–6. NONSTRIP URINE GLUCOSE TEST PROD-
UCTS FOR HOME USE

CLINITEST (AMES)
2-drop method or 5-drop method

Advantages	Disadvantages
1. 2-drop method has upper reading of 5%	1. 5-drop method has narrow range of results—¼% to 2%
2. Colors easy to read	2. 5-drop method has lower limit of ¼%; 2-drop method, trace
3. Damage by humidity is easily detected	3. Inconvenient (requires test tubes)
4. Less expensive once initial kit is purchased	4. Vitamin C, aspirin, and antibiotics cause test to indicate glucose when none is present
5. 2-drop method useful for people with low renal thresholds	5. Can cause burns if mishandled
	6. Less accurate during pregnancy

BENEDICT'S SOLUTION

Advantages	Disadvantages
1. Lowest cost, especially when purchased in large quantities	1. Clumsy; almost impossible for travel
2. Colors easy to read	2. Positive for sugars other than glucose—can cause false-positive test result

over a long period of time mix the different amounts of sugar that enter the urine at different times during the night and may give an inaccurate reading of the current glucose level. The test using a second sample (the "second voided specimen"), collected half an hour after the first morning urine, reflects more recent blood glucose levels.

The methods of testing commonly used today are listed in Tables 8–6 and 8–7. The methods vary in accuracy, difficulty of performance, cost, and interpretation. The most commonly used tests at the present time are Chemstrip uG and Diastix, but some of the nonstrip tests are still in use here, and some are widely used elsewhere in the world.

Twenty-Four Hour Urine Test. Before the advent of the glycohemoglobin measurement, 24-hour collections of urines were measured for glucose content to gain some measure of the average level of control over a 24-hour period. A person who does not have diabetes should not lose very much sugar, if any, in the urine over a 24-hour period. Ideally, a person with diabetes should not lose sugar either, but, practically speaking, good regulation of diabetes

---

TABLE 8–7.   URINE GLUCOSE TEST STRIPS FOR HOME USE

CHEMSTRIP UG
(Boeringer Mannheim)

Advantages	Disadvantages
1. Wide range of results—1/10% to 5%	1. Difficult to read if strips have been damaged by humidity
2. Convenient	2. Large doses of vitamin C may cause false-negative results.
3. Colors easy to read	
4. Accurate during pregnancy	
5. Not affected by the presence of ketones in the urine	
6. Useful for people with high or low renal thresholds.	

DIASTIX
(Ames)

Advantages	Disadvantages
1. Convenient	1. Vitamin C may cause falsely lowered glucose results
2. Colors easy to read	2. Highest reading is 2%
3. Reading in 30 seconds	3. Reading can be affected by the presence of ketones in the urine

TES-TAPE
(Lilly)

Advantages	Disadvantages
1. Range of results starts at 1/10%	1. Highest reading is 2%
2. Convenient	2. Colors difficult to interpret
3. Less expensive	3. Limited accuracy
	4. Spoilage cannot be detected

---

in an adult should result in a loss no greater than 5% of the total carbohydrate intake for the day. With glycohemoglobin measurements, however, 24-hour urine collections are rarely used. An exception, perhaps, would be for a child if there were concern over inadequate growth due to the undernourishment of poorly controlled diabetes. Another use of this measurement might be for someone who had poor control (especially with weight loss) but was getting negative urine test results.

Urine Testing for Acetone. The urine test for acetone does not need to be performed with each blood test or urine test for glucose. Ketones appear in the urine when fat has been metabolized as a source of energy. Fat metabolism occurs when someone, with or without diabetes, is on a weight-loss diet or is undernourished in the face of physical activity. With reduced caloric intake, reduced amounts of insulin are secreted into the blood by the pancreas (both

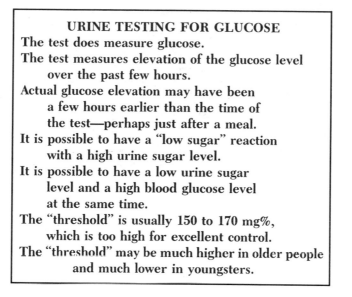

URINE TESTING FOR GLUCOSE
The test does measure glucose.
The test measures elevation of the glucose level
over the past few hours.
Actual glucose elevation may have been
a few hours earlier than the time of
the test—perhaps just after a meal.
It is possible to have a "low sugar" reaction
with a high urine sugar level.
It is possible to have a low urine sugar
level and a high blood glucose level
at the same time.
The "threshold" is usually 150 to 170 mg%,
which is too high for excellent control.
The "threshold" may be much higher in older people
and much lower in youngsters.

for a nondiabetic and for someone with type II diabetes). Low insulin levels allow the body to use fat from the fat (adipose) cells as an alternative source of energy if needed. In such a situation, the blood glucose level is normal. The production of ketones is a sign that fat is being burned and weight is being lost.

However, the presence of ketones and high blood glucose levels in a person with type I diabetes represents a potentially dangerous lack of insulin. When the body lacks insulin, it will also turn to fat as its fuel, but the blood sugar, in this case, will be high!

In general, a urine ketone (acetone) test should be done whenever there is significant glucose in the urine (greater than 1%, especially if SMBG is not also being performed) or the blood glucose level is significantly elevated (usually above 240 mg%). Testing for acetone in this situation is especially important in youngsters.

Another time when ketones may be found is after a hypoglycemic reaction. When this occurs, the blood glucose may be "*rebounding,*" (see Chapter 15 for a discussion of hypoglycemic reactions and rebounds) but is generally not extremely high. There may be a trace amount of ketones present when this occurs. Ketones may also be found in the urine during a fever or in minor amounts during physical overactivity on a hot day without adequate carbohydrate intake.

The methods for testing acetone are listed in Table 8-8. The section on sick-day rules in Chapter 15 discusses other important times when urine acetone testing should be performed.

TABLE 8–8. URINE KETONE TESTING PRODUCTS FOR HOME USE
ACETEST (Ames) Method: Place a drop or two of urine on a tablet and observe the change in the color of the tablet.
KETOSTIX (Ames) Method: Test strips. Place urine on strip, wait, read by comparison with color chart. Strips are foil wrapped and keep for longer periods—an advantage for people who test for urine ketones infrequently.
CHEMSTRIP K (Note: Chemstrip uGK measures both ketones and glucose) (Boeringer Mannheim) Method: Test strips. Place urine on strip, wait, read by comparison with color chart.

Self Glucose Monitoring Programs

Whenever a laboratory test is performed, the person on whom the test is being performed should know *why* it was done and *what to do* about the test results. Yet despite this rule, many respond to the question "Why are you testing for sugar?" with "Because my doctor told me to" and have no idea what to do with the test results.

The basic reasons why home monitoring is important are: (1) It can provide feedback on how well the individual is following the daily routines of eating and activity, (2) it provides data from which the patients and their physicians can make decisions about medication dose changes, and (3) it provides data with which people can make daily decisions on dose adjustments when necessary.

Record Keeping. It is impossible to remember the results of every home test of urine or blood glucose, and therefore proper records must be kept. Good records help guide the physician during office visits and allow you to notice subtle changes in your condition. Also, by examining the results, you can gain an understanding of patterns of blood glucose values and thus an insight into the action, and interaction, of insulin with the other factors that control blood glucose levels.

The preferred form of record keeping is a sheet or booklet that allows test results from a given time of day to be recorded in a column. With this form, you can scan up and down a column to get a sense of what the glucose level has been at a given time of day over many successive days. Avoid graph sheet records. They prevent scanning and imply that the blood glucose level "went from point A directly to point B," or that "point A was the lowest level that the blood glucose reached that day," both of which may not have actually been the case. Remember to bring the records to all physician visits.

Frequency of Testing. The exact frequency of testing, which methods to use, and how to use the results are subjects that should be discussed in detail by each person with his or her physician. Self testing programs tend to work better and be better accepted if they are tailored to the needs of each individual. At the Joslin Clinic, testing programs are grouped into three levels, each for a different type of therapy. These three levels are discussed below.

LEVEL I: PRIMARILY URINE TESTING. People using this program usually test their urines. Of course, occasional self blood tests, performed at specific times—before meals, randomly, or in response to high urine glucose tests—may also be done. How often should these urine tests be performed? This may vary somewhat, but once daily is not sufficient for many. Twice daily is a minimum and is useful for people with type II diabetes treated with diet alone or with an oral hypoglycemic agent. The first test is usually performed with a second voided specimen before breakfast. The time of the second urine test can vary based on the desired level of control and/or the renal threshold. For example, testing after supper can tell you how well you have followed the meal plan at what is often the largest meal of the day.

Anyone using this approach should use the results to check on his or her diet program and to provide the physician with information about diabetes control between office visits. Each person should be instructed about the possible variability in the test results and about what types of results should cause immediate concern. Some people may be instructed to adjust the dose of their oral hypoglycemic medication based on test results.

More frequent urine testing, usually before meals and at bedtime, can be used in a manner similar to the twice-daily test program. People taking insulin who refuse to or are unable to do self blood glucose monitoring may use urine testing in this manner, before meals and at bedtime. Remember, the function of urine testing is to tell when the glucose levels are getting too high. They tell very little about patterns or low blood glucose levels. Thus, this program is ideal for determining when glucose levels are too high for people not taking insulin, and providing them with feedback on diet and activity habits.

LEVEL II: BLOCK TESTING. A block of blood tests consists of 4 blood tests performed during a given day, usually before meals and at bedtime (although other appropriate times may be used) for 4 days in a row. These 4 × 4 blocks should be performed at specific intervals, which are determined by the needs of the patient. Often, blocks are performed when attempts to establish control are under way. In that situation, the testing may be done for 4 days, followed by 4 days off. Once the diabetes control has stabilized, one 4-day block can be performed 1 to 3 times per month, depending on how unstable the diabetes is. The purpose of the block testing is to find glucose patterns. Between blocks of blood-testing days, the objective may be just to watch for evidence of trouble using one or two daily blood tests, or even using urine testing.

This level of monitoring is used for people with type I or type II diabetes treated with standard insulin injection programs, although it may be used for patients who do not use insulin but who have high renal thresholds. It is a good program for longterm monitoring of diabetes control for all but those people with the most unstable blood glucose patterns.

People may be instructed to adjust their insulin dose in response to consistently high or low glucose levels at specific times. Each person should also know what glucose level variations are acceptable and which levels warrant treatment adjustments. When insulin adjustments are to be made, specific instructions should be given (see Chapters 9 and 10).

OCCASIONAL SELF BLOOD GLUCOSE TESTING
This tells what is happening at that time with no relationship to what happened before or later.

LEVEL III: DAILY BLOOD TESTING. This approach to self monitoring consists of testing the blood 4 or more times per day, every day. Urine testing for acetone is done when glucose levels are high or on sick days. This approach is for those with type I diabetes using either conventional type therapies or one of the intensive therapies. Frequently, daily insulin does adjustments are made based on the results of the tests. Detailed adjustment instructions (sometimes called "algorithms") are often used. This approach to testing is discussed in greater detail in Chapter 10, on intensive insulin therapy.

Conclusions

Self monitoring is the key to achieving excellent control of blood glucose levels in a safe and effective manner, allowing careful tailoring of dosages of insulin or oral agents to the needs of each person. It is especially useful when insulin therapy is used. A proper self monitoring program combined with a thoughtfully designed treatment plan can eliminate the frequent, severe hypoglycemia of years past while achieving excellent control. The old fears that "tight control means lots of hypoglycemic reactions" are no longer valid if self monitoring is used. The success of a self monitoring program is dependent primarily upon the motivation of the self-tester. Better, safer diabetes control is the reward for these efforts. Someone once said that the only reward for good care of diabetes is survival. Survival, however, should not be enough! The true reward should be healthy, happy, and comfortable survival!

9

Conventional Treatment of Diabetes with Insulin

Before 1921 the usual treatment for diabetes was a form of starvation. Then came the great breakthrough—insulin—that enabled millions to live. At that time, physicians were rightfully so dazzled by the new life-saving miracle that they thought it was a complete cure for diabetes. One prominent physician said to his staff, "Now that we have cured diabetes, what will happen to my practice of medicine?" As we now know, that physician had nothing to worry about. Indeed, he was busier than ever, because millions of people could now *live* with diabetes!

People facing the prospect of taking insulin often ask, "Will I have to take this for the rest of my life?" The answer is, "Who knows?" Insulin is not habit-forming. Some patients with type II diabetes are able to improve their glucose tolerance so that eventually they can use diet alone or along with oral agents. If insulin is needed permanently, it is because it is needed for health and life.

Another common question is, "Do I need it more than once daily?" Again, one cannot tell without a trial. In some, one injection per day does it; for others, several daily injections may be needed. In answer to "How much will I have to take?" there is only one word, "enough!" In putting out a fire, one does not prescribe in advance the proper amount of water to be used. You use *enough!*

Remember—in treating with insulin, we are not adding a drug or a medication, but are replacing what the body does not provide!

Who Needs Insulin?

While many people, probably more than 1.5 million in the United States, use insulin, only those with *type I* (insulin-dependent diabetes) must have it to remain alive. Many others use it because in order to improve their metabolic lives, they need more insulin than they can get from their own pancreas. For them it is a means to live better. Actually, many do make quite a bit of their own insulin, but as we discussed earlier, it is made ineffective by insulin resistance of some kind or another.

Starting Insulin

So when is insulin treatment needed?
1. It is needed immediately when a youngster becomes rapidly and seriously ill with diabetes.
2. It is also required when people of any age develop the classic symptoms of diabetes and are discovered to have a high blood glucose level.
3. It is needed when someone with diabetes cannot achieve adequate control when treated with diet alone or with oral hypoglycemic agents.

In all of these people, insulin is needed. For many, insulin treatment comes as a great shock; for others, it may have been anticipated for some time. Yet, when actually faced with "taking the needle," it becomes a hurdle to overcome, a skill to master, "the unknown" to conquer. Fortunately, most people adapt to insulin therapy quite well.

A prominent sportscaster came into the clinic and discovered that he had diabetes and would have to take insulin. He appeared delighted and his face was wreathed in smiles. Quite puzzled, his physician said, "Why are you so happy?" "Oh," said this person who had just been told he had diabetes, "I felt miserable for so long. I lost weight and was so tired. I could scarcely stay awake during the game. I thought I had some hopeless condition for which there would be no help. I am so happy to have something which can be treated!"

Which Insulin?

Once it has been decided to start insulin treatment, the physician decides which insulin will be used, the starting insulin dose, and how often each day a dose should be given. Knowing the type of diabetes helps the physician make these decisions. Treatment of type I diabetes often starts with one prebreakfast injection of intermediate-acting insulin (NPH or Lente), but many times, a morning mixed dose (the intermediate insulin plus a dose of regular insulin) is needed because the intermediate may not start soon enough. If the intermediate insulin does not last long enough, a second dose late in the day is needed. In the treatment of type II diabetes, often one morning injection of intermediate insulin, alone or mixed with regular, will suffice. Either way, it is important to remember that the insulin dose may need to be changed many times over the years. That is because you change over the years. The goal is to have you as close to normal as possible both in health and in function. Remember the proper dose—"enough."

Insulin Treatment

Goals. The goal of insulin treatment is to provide enough insulin for the body to use the glucose in food as energy or store it for later use. It is therefore important not to give too much insulin so that the blood glucose levels drop too low (hypoglycemic reactions), or too little insulin so that the glucose levels become elevated. The goal of treatment is a balance, so that just enough insulin is available at any time, which can be quite difficult to achieve. Some people with type I diabetes may need several doses of insulin daily, and may need individualized testing schemes to achieve this treatment balance.

> PEOPLE OFTEN WORRY IF THEIR INSULIN DOSE INCREASES, THINKING THAT THEIR DIABETES IS WORSE! NOT NECESSARILY SO! MANY THINGS INFLUENCE THE LEVEL OF BLOOD GLUCOSE, AND THE TREATMENT MUST CHANGE WITH THE PATIENT!

There is *no* relationship between the severity of the diabetes and the number of units of insulin taken each day. For some people, an increasing insulin dose may mean that the full effects of "total" diabetes have begun, with a significant reduction in the number of insulin-producing beta cells. "Severity" of diabetes however, should be measured only in terms of the difficulty in achieving good control and the development of complications, not in insulin dose. Some people have diabetes that is easy to regulate with 40 or more units daily, while some may be difficult with only 15 or 20 units required daily. Fear of hypoglycemic (low blood sugar) reactions prevents some people from taking enough insulin. Although some of these reactions may be annoying (but rarely harmful), a proper insulin dose, properly balanced with eating and activity, reduces the chance of severe hypoglycemic reactions while allowing good, safe blood glucose control.

An insulin treatment program requires an effort by both the individual with diabetes and those responsible for diabetes care. There is no dose that works well for everyone. People are different. Can you imagine giving a size 14 dress to all women, or a size 40 suit to all men? Each person's diabetes has different requirements, too! As we pointed out previously, insulin doses change, as may the number of injections necessary and/or the type of insulin used. *Therefore, insulin treatment must be individualized* to fit the life-style and metabolism of each and every person with diabetes. The changes and modifications are made as needed throughout the life of each person.

Testing and Monitoring. Monitoring diabetes control (Chapter 8) is important in maintaining properly balanced diabetes control. Blood testing is a must for insulin-treated persons. Everyone should discuss the details of their self testing or monitoring with those responsible for their care. It is important to decide carefully which method(s) to use, how often to use them, and what to do about the test results. The results of these self tests plus the results of office blood and/or glycohemoglobin monitoring are vital in determining the course of therapy.

The Proper Dose. The physician's first concern is to be certain that the blood glucose levels are not so high that immediate danger is possible. These levels are the extremes, usually over 400 mg% or, for someone already on teratment, consistently under 60 mg%. Sometimes hospitalization or some other close supervision is needed. If the problem is not this extreme, there is time to determine how often the blood glucose levels are too high or too low and how close to the desired treatment goal the blood glucose levels already are.

Many people, especially those with type II diabetes, have stable blood glucose patterns with only occasional very high or very low values, and rarely do these changes happen suddenly. For these people with stable values, the immediate effort is to lower the glucose levels into the "normal" range. Dietary change, increased activity, and insulin dose increases are usually quite effective. However, many people with type I diabetes have unstable blood glucose patterns, with frequent highs and lows, and are prone to sudden changes in blood glucose levels. For these people, it is necessary to adjust insulin doses to smooth out the pattern, eliminating the highs, lows, and sudden shifts.

These adjustments can often be accomplished by first eliminating insulin reactions and "rebound" by temporarily accepting a stable higher level of 150 to 250 mg%. At this level, the detailed insulin adjustments can be made to establish a smooth pattern of glucose levels. Once these glucose level fluctuations are lowered, the insulin dose can be increased to bring these stabilized values down toward normal. This process may actually take a number of weeks or months, and may be done most effectively while the individual is living a normal life-style at home under usual conditions, rather than in a hospital. Unless it is an emergency situation, there is no hurry. People have diabetes for a long time and rushing changes too fast can cause imbalance as well as confusion.

Insulin Adjustment. The road to a proper insulin dose for people with type I diabetes frequently passes through many insulin dose changes before the correct dose, or range of doses, can be reached. Needless to say, a physician or teaching nurse should work with each of these people to help make adjustments. However, many physicians, including those at the Joslin Clinic, encourage patients to take an active role in this adjustment process. Frequently, with proper instruction, individuals can make dose adjustments themselves. Generally, patients do not change the insulin dose more than two units at a time and not too often, except on special instructions. This self-adjustment of insulin doses must be based on individual ability and interest. Some people can and will make many changes themselves, while others need the help of their physician or teaching nurse.

When properly taught insulin dose adjustment, many people can intelligently establish their own insulin dosing program. The basic approach is to change the dose of insulin when abnormal blood glucose or urine glucose values are noted for three days in a row.

TABLE 9–1. Insulin Adjustment Chart Based on Insulin
Action Peak Times

If the blood or urine test is poor or you have a hypoglycemic reaction:	Then you need to adjust the following insulin:	Administered at the following time:
Before lunch	Regular	Before breakfast
Before supper	NPH or Lente	Before breakfast
Before bedtime	Regular	Before supper
Before breakfast	NPH or Lente	Before supper or at bedtime

(See also Tables 9–2 A through E for detailed adjustment guidelines
for specific insulin dosing programs.)

For example, if a value is too high, it is necessary to increase the
dose of insulin that is working hardest (peaking) at the time of that
high glucose value. If the glucose is too low, the dose should be
decreased.

Adjustment Problems. It is important to remember the action times
of the various types of insulin when adjusting doses. Short-acting
("*Regular*," for example) starts acting almost immediately, is most
effective ("peaks") 2 to 4 hours after injection, and is usually gone
after 6 to 8 hours. *Intermediate insulin* (NPH and Lente) starts more
slowly and peaks at 6 to 12 hours after injection. It still may be
effective in some people 18 to 26 hours later, but in many
individuals, especially those using the newer human-like insulins,
its effects may be gone sooner (see Chapter 7, Table 7–1).

Know the Peak Activity Time of the Insulin You Are Using. This
can help you decide which insulin dose needs to be adjusted (Table
9–1). When the blood or urine glucose tests taken following the
peak activity of a specific insulin dose are not at the desired level for
three days in a row, adjustments of the dose of that particular insulin
are usually needed.

Before making any adjustments in an insulin dose, however, it is
important to be sure that there is not anything adjustable that may
be influencing the blood glucose levels. Has the diet been followed
properly? Have the timing of the eating and insulin injections been
proper? Remember, it is best to inject insulin about 20 to 30
minutes before a meal so that the insulin can arrive into the bloodstream at about the same time as the digested food arrives. Has the

insulin dose been measured out properly? (When you invert the bottle, be sure your needle has not been inserted above the surface of the insulin so that it is sucking in only air instead of insulin.) Has your exercise pattern been different than usual? Has there been any new physical stress, infection, or severe emotional stress that may affect the diabetes?

REBOUND. Finally, are there any hypoglycemic (low blood glucose) reactions? When the blood glucose level drops too low, the body usually calls on glucose stored in the liver and muscles to help return the level back up toward normal again. This rising blood glucose level is called "rebound." If the initial low glucose reaction was not detected, the resulting high blood glucose level could be confused for a high blood glucose level due to *too little* insulin, rather than *too much*. The proper adjustment for hypoglycemia and resultant rebound is a reduction in the insulin dose to eliminate the hypoglycemic reaction. In these circumstances, it is *not* appropriate to increase the insulin dose, which one might be tempted to do because of the high blood glucose values.

Once all of the possible reasons for poor control have been ruled out, an adjustment of the insulin dose is required to compensate for a high or low glucose value. This adjustment should be systematic and logical. Tables 9–2 A through E provide guidelines for insulin dose adjustments or to help you know when to go to a more complex dosing program. These should be used only after a review with your physician. It is important to remember that these apply to "well" or healthy days. The rules outlined in these guidelines indicate upward adjustments for test results that are too high. However, if your problem is hypoglycemia (low blood glucose levels) at the particular times, you should reduce the appropriate insulin dose instead.

During days of sickness, extra doses of regular insulin may be needed in addition to adjustments in the daily insulin program (see the section on sick day rules in Chapter 15). Rules for insulin adjustment are rough guidelines at best, because individuals with diabetes vary greatly. The physician who is responsible for managing your diabetes should be consulted anytime you are confused about needed changes.

TABLE 9–2. Insulin Adjustment

How to Use the Insulin Adjustment Guidelines

The rules for insulin adjustment should not be confusing if you take them one step at a time.

1. Look for the table that shows the doses **you are now taking** and follow each step. The other tables do not matter to you at present.
2. A "poor test" is one in which **the glucose in the urine is greater than 1% and the blood glucose level is above ideal** (to be determined by you and your physician).
3. Don't panic or necessarily call your physician if things do not seem to be working out. You may have to repeat the adjustments several times. Most importantly, have your physician determine **when** and **how often** he would like to be notified.
4. If two or more of the tests you do at the various times each day are poor for 3 consecutive days, adjust first the insulin dose that affects the presupper test.
5. Do not adjust more than one dose or type of insulin at a time unless directed to do so by your physician.
6. When a dose is increased, the blood glucose level at the next test time should be lower. The insulin that now begins to act over this next time period is starting off at a *lower* glucose level. *Beware!!* Because the glucose level is lower to start, this dose may now be too great and lead to a hypoglycemic reaction.
7. If there is concern, the insulin that acts over this second subsequent time period should be reduced slightly until the full effect of the increased previous dose can be assessed.
8. After making an insulin dose adjustment, wait 3 days for the tests to improve. If no improvement is noted, make the same adjustment a second time.
9. If you have any difficulty with adjustments, get help from your health care professional.

NOTE: All adjustment guidelines listed should be used *only* after they have been approved for your use by your physician.

TABLE 9–2A. Present Dose: INTERMEDIATE insulin given before breakfast

If Tests are Poor 3 Days in a Row	Do This
BEFORE SUPPER	Increase the NPH or Lente insulin by 2 units on the 4th morning.
BEFORE BREAKFAST, but good before supper	Notify your physician. You may need an evening dose of insulin.
BEFORE LUNCH, but better before supper	Notify your physician. You may need a mixed dose (NPH or Lente + Regular) in the morning.

TABLE 9–2B. Present Dose: REGULAR and INTERMEDI-ATE insulin given before breakfast

If Tests are Poor 3 Days in a Row	Do This
BEFORE SUPPER	Increase the NPH or Lente insulin by 2 units on the 4th morning.
BEFORE LUNCH	Increase the regular insulin by 2 units on the 4th morning.
BEFORE BREAKFAST but good before supper	Notify your physician. You may need an evening dose of insulin.

TABLE 9–2C. Present Dose: INTERMEDIATE insulin given before breakfast and again before supper or bedtime

If Tests are Poor 3 Days in a Row	Do This
BEFORE SUPPER	Increase the NPH or Lente insulin by 2 units on the 4th morning.
BEFORE BEDTIME	Increase the NPH or Lente insulin by 2 units on the 4th morning.
BEFORE BREAKFAST	Increase the NPH or Lente insulin by 2 units in the evening dose on the 4th day.

TABLE 9–2D. Present Dose: REGULAR and INTERMEDI-ATE insulin given before breakfast and INTERMEDI-ATE insulin given before supper or bedtime

If Tests are Poor 3 Days in a Row	Do This
BEFORE SUPPER	Increase the NPH or Lente insulin by 2 units on the 4th morning.
BEFORE LUNCH	Increase the Regular insulin by 2 units on the 4th morning.
BEFORE BEDTIME	Increase the NPH or Lente insulin by 2 units on the 4th morning.
BEFORE BREAKFAST	Increase the NPH or Lente insulin by 2 units in the evening dose on the 4th day.

TABLE 9–2E. Present Dose: REGULAR and INTERMEDI-ATE insulin given twice daily (before breakfast and before supper)

If Tests are Poor 3 Days in a Row	Do This
BEFORE SUPPER	Increase the NPH or Lente insulin by 2 units on the 4th morning.
BEFORE LUNCH	Increase the Regular insulin by 2 units on the 4th morning.
BEFORE BEDTIME	Increase the Regular insulin by 2 units before supper on the 4th day.
BEFORE BREAKFAST	Increase the NPH or Lente insulin by 2 units before supper on the 4th day.

10

Intensive Insulin Therapy
of Type I Diabetes

This is not only a chapter not found in earlier editions of this book, it is also probably not for everybody! With certain very modern developments, "intensive insulin therapy" has become both possible and necessary for many people with diabetes. In a sense, it has just been invented. Not all those with diabetes need it. Those who do, however, often need it *very* much! This is the group who must read this chapter!

What Is Intensive Insulin Therapy?

Two recent developments in the treatment of diabetes have led to the development of "intensive insulin therapy." These are the glycohemoglobin measure, which measures overall diabetes control, and self monitoring of blood glucose (SMBG), which allows daily assessment of blood glucose levels with adjustment of treatment to try to correct them.

Intensive insulin therapy uses either multiple daily injections (MDI) of insulin or the insulin infusion pumps, which provide a continuous subcutaneous (under the skin) insulin infusion (CSII). Prior to each meal, a blood test is performed. The result of this blood glucose level is used to determine the dose of short-acting insulin (regular) to be given at that time, about 20 to 30 minutes before the food is actually consumed. The goal is to achieve a better glycohemoglobin level (and thus better diabetes control) than could be achieved using a fixed insulin dose. Thus, while conventional therapy uses a dose of insulin that is essentially unchanged from day to day, intensive insulin therapy involves insulin doses (usually 3 or more per day) that are adjusted daily based on the blood glucose level at the time of injection as well as past and anticipated food consumption and activity.

The different labels—"intensive" and "conventional"—should not imply that conventional insulin therapy is somehow inferior. Conventional therapy is an important exercise in self-care. Yet there are philosophical differences in the intensive approaches to insulin therapy which differentiate it from conventional therapy. Conventional therapy is based on the assumption that the insulin dose can be fixed and that activity, eating, and the body's metabolism are similar enough from day to day that acceptable blood glucose control can be achieved. This assumption may be quite correct for many people with diabetes. Intensive therapy is based on an assumption that daily activity, eating, and metabolism are not always the same and therefore the insulin dose must vary to compensate. It is necessary to make this assumption in only a small minority of individuals.

Intensive therapy is not really a different treatment of diabetes; rather, it is a different way of using the same therapies employed in the usual treatment. As a result, there may not be a clear dividing line between conventional therapy and intensive therapy, only differences of intensity.

Why Intensive Therapy Makes Sense

Right after the discovery of insulin, the only type available was like the regular, short-acting insulin we have today, and the only treatment was several injections a day. Then longer-acting insulins were developed to decrease the number of daily injections. These insulins—PZI, NPH, Lente, and even long-acting Ultralente—were safe and eliminated the symptoms of high blood glucose levels.

There were many physicians, however, including those at the Joslin Clinic, who felt that elimination of symptoms was not enough and that the patient would be best helped by keeping blood glucose levels as close to "normal" as possible. The goals for this more "intensive" therapy were to make the patient free of symptoms and also to prevent potential longterm complications. Many physicians preferred to use more than just one daily injection of intermediate

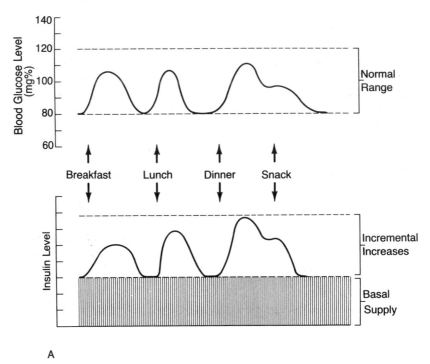

A

FIG. 10–1A. Blood glucose and insulin patterns in a person who does not have diabetes.

(NPH or Lente) insulin for patients with type I diabetes. Many used programs with regular plus intermediate insulin ("split-mix") given in the morning and in the evening.

This slightly more complicated pattern of insulins tried to imitate the action of the pancreas if it could function normally. The normal pancreas constantly secretes an amount of insulin, possibly half a unit (more or less) each hour (the basal insulin secretion), and then releases more insulin in response to meals, enabling the body to use the food for either storage or energy (Fig. 10–1A).

One injection of intermediate insulin, peaking 6 to 12 hours after injection, does not produce this natural pattern (Fig. 10–1B). For many people with type II diabetes, one daily injection may be effective. Many of these people have insulin resistance, and although their pancreases may secrete enough insulin, it is not as effective as it should be because of insulin resistance. The primary purpose of treatment with insulin in this person is to give additional insulin to overcome this resistance.

Some people with type I diabetes still are also able to secrete

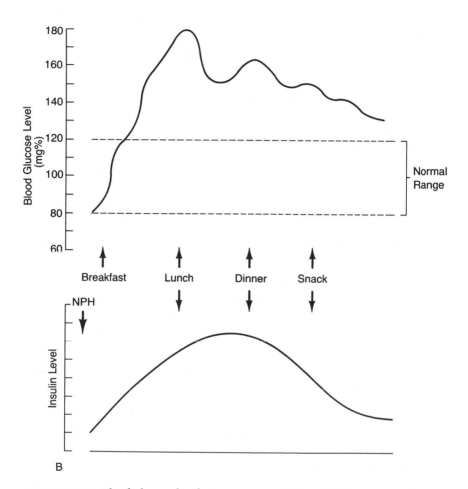

FIG. 10–1B. Blood glucose levels in a person with type I diabetes treated with one morning injection of NPH (intermediate-acting) insulin.

enough of their own insulin so that one injection of intermediate insulin may be enough. This often occurs early in the course of diabetes—during the "honeymoon" phase. Eventually, though, these individuals may lose the ability to secrete insulin altogether, and it becomes necessary to use a more complex dosing program that more closely imitates the normal insulin secretion. The split-mix schedule, for example, spreads the insulin effect out more effectively over the course of the day, with insulin peaks occurring fairly close to the times that food is eaten (Fig. 10–2). By using insulin frequently, the person always has some insulin present in the blood: the basal supply!

The goal of this conventional insulin therapy is one of *anticipation*—a dose of insulin is given in anticipation of the insulin needs over the next 6 or 12 hours. To do this, however, all of the factors that affect blood glucose level must be predictable. Hence there is a need for regular eating habits and predictable activity. Many people can live predictable enough lives for such a program to achieve good to excellent blood glucose control.

However, the standard split-mix is not, by itself, intensive therapy. Intensive therapy attempts to mimic one other characteristic of a normal pancreas—the ability to sense the blood glucose level and then adjust the output of insulin based on that glucose level. Thus the pancreas is *responsive* to present glucose levels. The pancreas of someone with diabetes obviously cannot do this.

Thus the insulin doses in intensive therapy are based on the *anticipated* need to reach a blood glucose goal, and they are *responsive* to the present glucose level.

Who Needs Intensive Insulin Therapy?

Not everyone! In fact, most carefully treated people with type I diabetes can achieve control that is good enough by today's standards. No one new to insulin or newly diagnosed with diabetes needs the intensive approach. After some years of conventional insulin treatment, however, some people may need this intensive approach.

The use of intensive therapy may be helpful to those with diabetes that is so unstable that no matter what they do—no matter how they try to control all the variables—they cannot even come close to control that is safe or adequate. This is often called "brittle" diabetes. Why some people have diabetes that is difficult to control, while others have diabetes that is easily managed, is not always clear.

Intensive therapy may also benefit people with widely variable or unpredictable life-styles, such as people who must change work shifts or travel extensively or whose activity changes hour to hour or day to day. They require a special, more adaptable program.

Finally, some people use intensive therapy in an attempt to make their blood glucose metabolism normal. Many physicians feel that a goal of normal blood glucose patterns will greatly minimize the threat of complications. The problem is deciding *how* normal it should be and how much effort should be made, since good standard therapy, when effectively used, can adequately help many people

> INTENSIVE THERAPY DIFFERS FROM CON-
> VENTIONAL TREATMENT IN THAT IT IS AN
> ATTEMPT TO MIMIC THE NORMAL PAN-
> CREAS'S RESPONSIVENESS BY ALLOWING
> THE INSULIN DOSES TO BE DETERMINED
> BASED ON PRESENT GLUCOSE LEVELS.
> THUS INTENSIVE THERAPY TARGETS A SPE-
> CIFIC, INDIVIDUALIZED BLOOD GLUCOSE
> LEVEL AS THE GOAL OF SUCH ADJUST-
> MENTS.

approach normal patterns. (See the discussion on the Diabetes Control and Complications Trial in Chapter 18.)

Insulin Dosing Schedules

The cornerstone of any intensive insulin program is the multiple daily opportunities to adjust the insulin dose, based on the results of blood glucose tests, so that a blood glucose level previously targeted by the physician and patient can be reached. Various schedules can be used. The simplest is the split-mix, with a minimum of two daily blood tests (before breakfast and supper) to determine the doses of

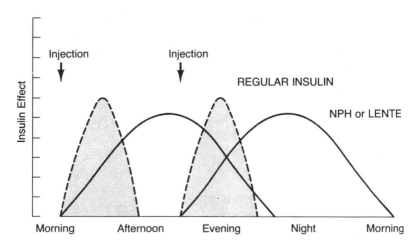

FIG. 10–2. Effect of a "split-mix" insulin program for type I diabetes: regular and intermediate insulin before breakfast and before supper.

regular insulin taken (Fig. 10–2). Of course, blood tests before lunch and the bedtime snack would also be necessary to gauge how effective the two regular insulin doses are. Variations of this program may also be used. For example, regular plus NPH or Lente insulins in the morning, regular insulin at suppertime, and NPH or Lente at bedtime may help people who need more insulin effect in the morning. People with variable life-styles may try regular insulin before each meal, mixed with NPH or Lente only at suppertime.

The use of this split-mix schedule has the advantage of simplicity. It allows accommodation for daily variations, while permitting a reduced frequency of testing and injections compared to more rigorous intensive therapy. However, the intermediate insulins (NPH, Lente) peak many hours after injection and have more variable timing than regular insulin. Therefore intensive programs using intermediate insulins are less precise than programs using multiple doses of regular insulin. Split-mix programs, even with daily adjustments, may fall short of some goals of true "intensive" therapy.

The use of Ultralente and regular insulin may be closer to the insulin secretion pattern of the normal individual (Fig. 10–3A). Ultralente is a long-acting insulin that is slowly absorbed, usually over 28 to 36 hours, but in some people may last as long as 96 hours! When given once, twice, or even three times a day, it is thought of as being essentially "peakless" and often provides a constant "basal" supply of insulin to the blood. Additional injections of regular insulin given preprandially (before meals) are based on blood testing results. The regular and Ultralente insulins can be mixed in one syringe provided the injection is given right after the insulins are mixed. Ultralente is often mixed with the prebreakfast and presupper regular insulin doses, although some physicians prefer that these insulins be given as separate injections.

A common variation of this Ultralente/regular insulin program uses regular injections, with NPH or Lente given once at bedtime (Fig. 10–3B), which provides peaking intermediate insulin during the night. This is effective with larger dinner meals or when problems with something known as the "dawn phenomenon" exist.

The Dawn Phenomenon

The dawn phenomenon is a rise in insulin requirements which occurs in many people during the latter part of the nightly sleep cycle, toward morning. Changes in certain hormone levels (probably growth hormone and possibly cortisol) change metabolism so

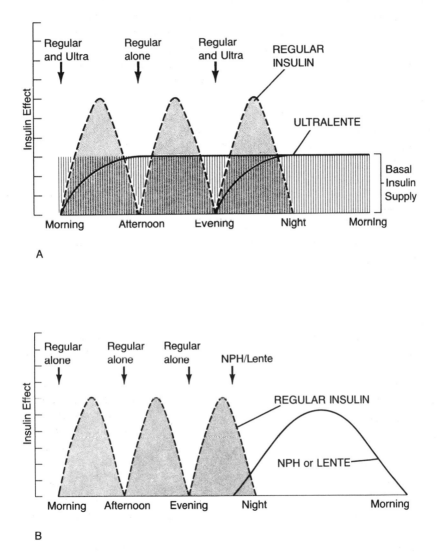

FIG. 10–3 A. Effect of an Ultralente/regular insulin program for type I diabetes: Ultralente is injected before breakfast and before supper, and regular insulin is injected before all three meals. **B.** Effect of a premeal/ regular program with one NPH or Lente injection at bedtime. Regular insulin is injected before all three meals, and NPH or Lente is injected at bedtime.

that more insulin action is needed during this time. People without diabetes can secrete this additional insulin as needed, but people using injected insulin may need to adjust their doses to compensate.

Insulin Infusion Pump

One of the great advances in diabetes therapy in recent years, which was only a dream in recent years, is the development of the insulin infusion pump. This device is intended to closely imitate the insulin actions of the pancreas. Actually the term "pump" covers a

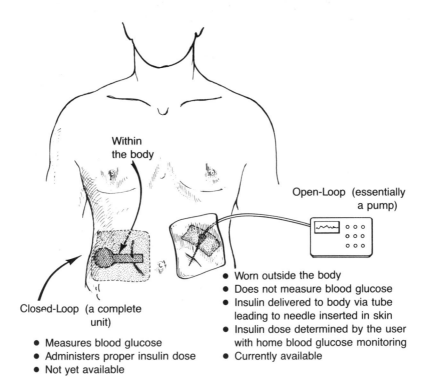

FIG. 10–4. "Closed-loop" versus "open-loop" insulin pumps. Open-loop pumps are currently available. The user must self-test blood and determine the insulin dose that the pump delivers. Closed-loop pumps would measure the glucose level and determine the insulin dose automatically. It is hoped that pumps that can be implanted within the body will be developed in the future.

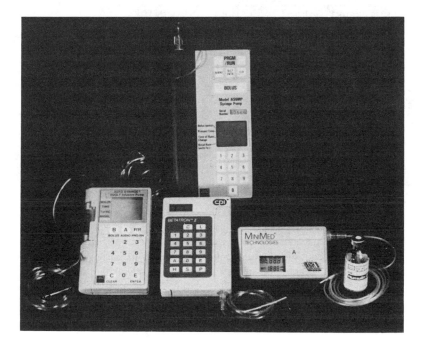

FIG. 10–5. Insulin infusion pumps that have been or are currently on the market. Top, older model of a Mill Hill. Bottom, left to right, Auto Syringe, Betatron, MiniMed.

lot of territory. What is available now is the *open-loop* pump. This is an electronic-age term that refers to the communication loop. (Fig. 10–4). The open-loop pump does not make decisions. It does not measure blood glucose levels. It is simply what it claims to be— a pump! It is on the outside of the body and releases insulin as desired via tubing and a needle into the tissues. The person using the pump has to do the thinking and the planning—thereby closing the loop. The ultimate and still experimental *closed-loop* system would probably be implanted inside the body and ideally would measure the blood glucose levels and determine how much insulin should be injected and when. Experiments with such a pump are currently under way. The closed-loop pump is the ultimate, "deluxe" model, but is not yet available.

A number of open-loop pumps are now available (Fig. 10–5). Using regular insulin only, the infusion pumps mimic the pancreas's

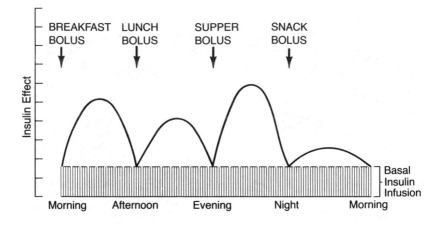

FIG. 10–6. Insulin action patterns seen with treatment using an insulin infusion pump (continuous subcutaneous insulin infusion, or CSII). The constant regular insulin infusion provides the basal insulin supply, with additional insulin boluses given before eating.

basal insulin secretion by providing a constant insulin flow through a catheter to a needle inserted into the skin, usually on the abdomen. This needle must be changed about every 2 days. The flow of regular insulin is slowly and continually absorbed into the blood stream, producing a constant, basal insulin supply. Some of the pumps can be programmed to adjust the basal insulin flow at various times of the day or night for people who need different amounts of insulin at different times. For example, more insulin during the early morning hours can be infused to treat the dawn phenomenon.

The pumps can give short bursts of additional insulin flow, called boluses, before meals and snacks. The blood glucose level at the time the bolus is to be given is used to determine the quantity of regular insulin that is needed. Figure 10–6 shows the pattern of pump insulin action.

These pumps constantly pump insulin into the body. For this reason, the safe and effective use of these devices requires a considerable amount of attention and frequent home blood testing so that proper daily dosage decisions can be made.

Preparing for an Intensive Insulin Program

A person starting an intensive insulin therapy program must be assisted by a physician who has had experience managing this type of therapy. Under *no* circumstances should anyone try to start an intensive insulin therapy program based on knowledge gained from reading material or on the advice of friends. The management of an intensive insulin program needs a skilled team of physicians and diabetes educators. While conventional insulin therapy can be properly managed by many physicians, intensive therapy programs should be managed only by those specifically trained and skilled in this approach. Improper intensive care—or unsupervised intensive care—may be more dangerous than poor conventional therapy.

Through discussions with the physician who usually cares for your diabetes you can determine whether such an intensive program is needed and who should manage it for you. Your physician can advise you whether it would be safe for you to undertake intensive therapy as well. You must also decide whether you are willing and able to perform self blood tests at least four times daily, analyze those test results and study the patterns, and decide many times daily what sort of insulin dose adjustments are necessary. The fact is that not everyone with diabetes is suited to this intense therapy.

The next step is *intensive education.* Much of the "intensity" of this therapy must come from the person using it, and therefore you must know how to routinely manage your own diabetes treatment and develop judgment to handle problems that might arise. Your education must include a thorough understanding of diabetes—why it occurs, how to control it, and its potential complications. It should also cover self-care, both in routine blood glucose control and in monitoring for other potential problems. It would be foolish to put someone on an intensive program, only to have him or her develop gangrene from an ignored foot infection or an abscess from poor hygiene.

A thorough knowledge of self monitoring of blood glucose is a must. This includes proper testing technique and understanding the results. We encourage the use of blood glucose meters because their increased accuracy over visually read strips is critical for this type of program. The function of the meter must be understood thoroughly.

Finally, through your education, you should develop a commitment to the philosophy of intensive therapy and the goals that you and your health care team set for you. Intensive therapy takes a great deal of time and effort, and it entails expense to get the program operating. It also requires a longterm determination to manage with no guarantees that the desired goals will be achieved. The immediate reward for all the effort is that it affords greater flexibility of life-style with improved diabetes control. There is possibly an even greater longterm reward for all of the effort—good health!

So if you pass the training course, you may begin!

Getting Started

The first step in starting an intensive insulin therapy program is to review with your physician all your reasons for starting intensive therapy and how it will affect your life-style. Through such a discussion you and your physician will choose the proper dosing program at the outset, although later change is certainly possible. Your physician will recommend a starting insulin dose, which may be based on your previous insulin requirements or calculated according to your body weight. Either way, this initial dose should be thought of as an educated estimate, but not a final dose by any means!

You should then discuss guidelines for daily adjustments based on self blood test results. Often physicians recommend the use of an "algorithm." Don't let this word worry you! It is defined as a mathematical rule for solving a problem. In this case, it is simply a plan that tells you what your insulin dose should be when you have a certain blood glucose level (Fig. 10–7). While much of this initial work can be done in a doctor's office, it is also common for people to be hospitalized to get the program started correctly.

The next step is experience! Go home and live it! Unless the initial estimates are way off so that glucose levels are constantly too high or too low, the initial goal is to smooth out the patterns of blood glucose measurements. Perfection is not essential at this stage—and is often quite difficult to achieve due to reactions and rebounds. Indeed, smoothing out patterns is often done more easily with blood glucose levels between 150 and 300 mg%. Staying in this range avoids both severe hyperglycemia and hypoglycemic reactions. There also may be confusion about whether high blood sugar levels are due to hypoglycemic reactions and rebounds, or not enough insulin. Pump patients are more likely to have difficulty with hypoglycemic reactions and rebounds, and it may take some time for the patterns to smooth out and for the pump user to feel better.

INTENSIVE INSULIN THERAPY ALGORITHM
(SLIDING SCALE)

Insulin Dose Schedule For:_____John Doe_____

Date: _____ Clinic Number: _____

REGULAR INSULIN:
(Your usual premeal insulin doses are:)

Blood Glucose	Breakfast	Lunch	Supper	Bedtime Snack
0-50	2	1	0	0
51-100	4	3	3	0
101-150	7	5	5	0
151-200	8	5	6	0
201-250	9	6	7	2
251-300	10	8	8	3
OVER 300	12	9	10	4

Intermediate- or Long-Acting Insulin (NPH/Lente/Ultralente):

9		9	

FIG. 10–7. Insulin adjustment algorithm for an Ultralente/regular insulin program. (Similar algorithms are used for other intensive insulin programs.) Nine units of Ultralente are given before breakfast and before supper, while the blood glucose test results at the time of the injection determine the premeal regular insulin dose.

With help from your physician or diabetes educator, the doses can be gently increased to lower the glucose levels to the desired range.

Living the Intensive Life

An intensive insulin therapy program must be a dynamic program—a program that is as dynamic as the blood glucose level changes and your life-style variations. Just how dynamic this system actually is often becomes evident during the efforts to design the program. Blood glucose levels are not like bricks, cemented in place, and changed only at the time of the next blood test. They are constantly changing, like fluid in a tank, moving up and down constantly, sometimes with more force than at other times. The direction and force of movement will be affected by the various factors that are known to influence blood glucose levels. Remember, too, that a blood glucose level is like a photograph of that water tank—it freezes the motion at one instant in time. However, the more "photographs" of your blood glucose you get—that is, the more testing you do—the better you can appreciate the ups and downs of the levels over time and the factors that cause them.

It is beyond the scope of this manual to discuss in depth the dynamics of blood glucose changes and how they relate to an intensive insulin program. While the concept is not difficult once you become familiar with the insulin adjustments and blood glucose changes, gaining a thorough understanding requires work with a diabetes educator. It is for this reason that intensive therapy requires work with a health care team and is something that cannot be started by a patient alone.

Algorithm Adjustments. The doses used in an intensive insulin program are designed to move a given range of blood glucose values toward the chosen target blood glucose level. The use of an algorithm allows for variations in the initial blood glucose range to result in variations in the insulin dose so that the target glucose level can be reached more reliably. For example, using the algorithm shown in Figure 10–7, if the morning glucose level is 137 mg%, then 7 units of regular would be taken along with the Ultralente. However, if the fasting glucose was 237 mg%, the regular insulin dose would be 9 units.

Even after you have worked with your physician to get one of these algorithms to work well, with time some of the doses may need adjustment. Needless to say, you must first be sure that nothing else—such as overeating or undereating, a change in activity, or some other factor—is causing the problems.

Adjusting an algorithm requires close contact with the health care team for guidance. It is possible that a whole scale might need to be changed. For example, for the algorithm shown in Figure 10–7, you might find that the prelunch glucose levels are *always* high and that every prebreakfast dose—from the 2 units at a glucose level of 0 to 50 mg% to the 12 units for a level over 300 mg%—would need to be increased.

Another possibility is that only part of the scale needs to be changed. Perhaps the scale worked well if you started out with a glucose level under 200 mg%. However, when starting above 200 mg%, the next glucose level may be running high, and you may need to increase only those insulin doses.

You can see that adjustments of an intensive program must take into account many more factors and possibilities than for conventional programs. It is common for it to take some weeks or months for an individual, working with the health care team, to get such a program running or to change it later on. Because an algorithm is a series of *many* doses, based on the results of numerous blood glucose tests, it can take a long time to accumulate enough data to allow analysis of these individual glucose level ranges when parts of the scale require adjustment. Hypoglycemic reactions and resultant rebounds can be most confusing and cause inconsistent responses to a given insulin dose in a particular blood glucose range.

Frequently, to sort things out, your physician may suggest that you temporarily allow the glucose levels to run a little high by reducing the "basal" insulin dose (the pump basal or the Ultralente dose) to eliminate reactions. With patterns less confused by rebounds, it becomes much easier to adjust the doses. If you are still hyperglycemic, you may need larger boluses of regular insulin. Alternatively, your physician may suggest a shift of some of the insulin from the boluses of regular insulin to an increase in the intermediate, Ultralente, or pump basal insulin doses to bring the blood glucose down closer to the targeted level of control.

Adjusting for Hyperglycemia. The basic rule to correct blood glucose levels that are too high (hyperglycemia) is to increase the insulin dose that affects that particular time period in the day.

> **THE GOAL OF INTENSIVE THERAPY IS TO SEEK NORMAL BLOOD GLUCOSE LEVELS AT *ALL* TIMES—FASTING AND PREMEALS, AS WELL AS AFTER MEALS AND UP TO THE NEXT MEALTIME.**

Despite the many factors that can affect blood glucose levels, it is the premeal insulin doses that play the key role. However, simply increasing or decreasing an insulin dose is not always the best way to correct a glucose level that has missed the target. For example, when the blood glucose level is too high immediately after eating but has reached the target level at the next meal or check time, a simple dose increase might lead to hypoglycemia. Alternatively, you could either reduce the total or concentrated carbohydrate content or increase the fiber content (to slow down food absorption) of that meal. The insulin dose should ideally be injected 20 to 30 minutes before eating, but increasing this interval might allow more of the regular insulin to be available as the carbohydrate from the meal enters the bloodstream. Of course, the insulin dose could still be increased, but a supplemental snack might be added at the insulin peak time to prevent hypoglycemia. Finally, it is important to remember that insulins don't act in compartments, unaffected by any other insulin that has ever been injected. Previous insulins may still be present when the next insulin dose arrives. Therefore, adjustment of insulins other than the one most obviously acting over that time period may be indicated. Yet adjustments can be very complex, and it is necessary for most people to work closely with their intensive insulin management team to "fine-tune" their dosing programs.

Fasting blood glucose levels are handled slightly differently. The "basal" insulin level (or overnight intermediate insulin) usually determines the level of the fasting blood glucose. If the fasting level is too high, the cause can be: (1) insufficient duration of action of the overnight insulin, (2) the dawn phenomenon—an increase in the amount of insulin required during the latter part of the sleep cycle, or (3) the "Somogyi" phenomenon—a hypoglycemic reaction during the night and resultant rebound hyperglycemia (see Chapter 15).

The actual adjustments for fasting hyperglycemia depend on which of these three common causes is the most likely explanation. Deciding which is the actual cause is the difficult part. You should work with your intensive insulin management team to find which approach is best for you.

If the duration of action of the insulin is too short, the night injection could be given later or its quantity increased. With Ultralente or pump basal infusions, the dose could also be increased, thus increasing the "basal" insulin supply. A similar approach might be used if the problem is due to the dawn phenomenon. Difficulty adjusting for the dawn phenomenon with injection therapy is one reason to switch to one of the pumps that can provide a higher basal insulin infusion during periods of the night.

Hypoglycemic reactions and resultant hyperglycemic rebounds (Somogyi) can be the most difficult cause of hyperglycemia to correct. Documented nighttime hypoglycemia can be treated by reducing the evening insulin or basal dose. However, the cause of nocturnal hypoglycemia is not always easily discovered. A careful examination of the patterns of home blood glucose tests might suggest a dip in the glucose level sometime during the night. It may also be suggested by symptoms of night-time hypoglycemia, including nightmares, restless sleep, perspiration during sleep, morning headaches, or morning urine tests that show small amounts of ketones with normal or minimally elevated glucose levels.

Adjusting for Hypoglycemia. Blood glucose levels that are too low are a common problem for people using an intensive insulin program. Every attempt should be made to document the hypoglycemic blood glucose level using home blood testing to be sure that the symptoms were not caused by something other than true low blood sugar, such as rapidly dropping blood glucose levels or anxiety. If true hypoglycemia has occurred, it should be treated immediately with rapidly absorbed carbohydrates ("quick" carbohydrates such as pure sugar, glucose tablets, orange juice, or sugar-containing tonics), and if a meal or snack is not scheduled to be eaten within one hour, a snack containing slowly absorbed carbohydrate (such as peanut butter crackers) may be recommended as well. If the individual is unconscious, either glucagon or transportation to an emergency facility is advised (Chapter 15). With intensive insulin therapy, many people become less aware of the insulin reactions, and warning signs may not be noticed. Caution and careful monitoring are advised.

After the hypoglycemia has been corrected, you should try to discover why it occurred. As discussed in detail in the chapter on acute complications (Chapter 15), there are two types of hypo glycemic reactions: "explained" reactions, the cause of which is identifiable, and "unexplained" reactions, for which no explanation is obvious. Careful notations on log sheets can help you identify the reasons for reactions and decide if insulin dose adjustments are needed.

For unexplained reactions, it is possible that an insulin dose is too high. However, unexplained reactions may also be due to a combination of factors which, on that given day, happened to all occur, resulting in a low blood glucose level. For severe hypoglycemic reactions, the responsible insulin dose should be reduced the next day. If the reaction was mild, however, and there have been no problems in the past using the same dose, then the dose should not be changed. Careful monitoring should be performed over the next few days to ensure that the hypoglycemic reaction was, indeed, just a one-time affair. If repeated hypoglycemic reactions occur, then the dose should be reduced. Some occasional, mild hypoglycemic reactions are to be expected with intensive therapies, but the risks of these mild reactions should be outweighed by the benefits of this type of program.

The insulin dose that caused a hypoglycemia reaction may not be the dose that is peaking closet to the time of the reaction. Therefore, if adjustment of the dose of insulin that is the closest peaker does not correct the problem, alternative possibilities should be considered. A "crisscross" or "piggyback" effect is one possibility. This phenomenon occurs when the apparent effect of one insulin dose is increased because there is additional insulin left over from the tail-end of a previous insulin dose or coming on at the beginning of the next. Thus when adjustment of the morning regular insulin dose, for example, dose not stop frequent late morning hypoglycemic reactions from occurring, another insulin may be the cause. It may be the leftover effect from the previous night's insulin or the oncoming morning NPH insulin beginning its effect while the morning regular insulin is still acting. Your physician or diabetes educator can help you sort out the possibilities and adjust your doses more effectively.

Diet and Weight Gain. Intensive therapy improves diabetes control, which means that calories previously lost as sugar in the urine are available for use as energy, or to be stored as fat! If weight gain is noted after intensive therapy is started, and it is not the fluid retention seen with sudden improvements of diabetes control, the eating plan may need to be reconsidered and calories reduced. With reduced calories, the insulin dose may also need to be lowered. Of course, if an improperly designed intensive insulin program was being used which prescribed too much insulin, you might be "eating to feed your insulin." This means that the insulin was lowering your glucose levels too much and you needed to eat to bring them back up. A dose reduction would help you cut down on your food consumption.

The Pump

The use of continuous subcutaneous insulin infusion (CSII) therapy with an insulin infusion pump requires even more attention than intensive insulin therapy using multiple daily injections (MDI). It is a more complex insulin delivery system than by simple syringe, and because insulin is constantly infused, the risk of pump therapy can be greater than injection therapy if proper caution is not exercised. Therefore the decision to embark on pump therapy should not be taken lightly.

The Decision to Use a Pump. You should decide whether pump therapy would really provide "better" control than other methods of intensive therapy. Remember, too, that pump use requires more intelligence, motivation, dexterity, judgment, psychological stability, self-management efforts, and finances than the other methods of intensive therapy. The $2500 to $3500 cost (present dollars) of the pumps may be covered by health insurance (as much as 80%), and the supplies, including insulin, syringes, catheters, dressings, etc., may run $20 to $30 weekly.

> The choice of pumps is like the choice of a car. There are many good ones with differing features. Your best bet is to use the pump recommended to you by your pump care team. They should know which features you will need. It is most important that you use a pump that *they* like and are familiar with.

Family and emotional support for this effort is very important. It is best that pump users not live alone, both for this support and because of the greater risks of serious hypoglycemia.

It is important to have a clear and realistic understanding of the goals of pump therapy. Many people think that the pump will prevent all complications or allow them to return to the carefree life of a person without diabetes. Not so! It usually involves more work than conventional therapy or even multiple daily injection (MDI) intensive therapy.

Pumps can be an extremely effective device for use on a daily basis to achieve normal or near normal blood glucose levels in a person with type I diabetes. The goal is improved blood glucose control. There are risks, but this is the benefit. If you are interested in using an insulin pump as part of your intensive insulin therapy, you should consult with your physician and discuss whether pump therapy would be right for you.

General Pump Care. It is important to understand the use of a pump thoroughly *before* starting treatment with it. Several sessions with a diabetes educator who knows the details of the newest pump models are recommended. Of primary importance is to know enough to avoid harmful underdosages or overdosages.

Routine maintenance is crucial to a properly functioning pump, and there are many items that need daily attention. Batteries should be changed and charged daily. Most pumps use nickel cadium rechargeable batteries, which require 10 to 16 hours to recharge. Battery life is variable. Some last up to 3 days, yet daily charging is still advised. Some pumps have self-contained batteries and must be returned to the manufacturer when the batteries wear out. Rechargeable batteries can wear out as well, especially if overcharged. All pumps come with charger devises designed for use with that particular model. We recommend having one battery in the pump, one in the charger, and one charged and ready for use. Batteries should be numbered so that it is easier to keep track of them!

Syringes also need attention and usually must be changed daily, even if the syringe size would allow more than one day's use. In preparing and using the syringe, it is very important to prevent air bubbles from getting into the system. They can take up space and lead to a reduction in the actual amount of insulin that is delivered. Air in the system has been one of the major problems in insulin pump therapy. It may actually result in ketoacidosis, especially when small doses of insulin are being used. One to two inches of air in the tubing can be a very significant amount and can cause a drastic reduction in the amount of insulin that is delivered!

Careful preparation of the syringe is therefore quite important, and everyone using a pump should be instructed "one-on-one" prior to actually starting therapy. It is important to calculate the daily insulin volume properly, being sure to include insulin that fills the tubing and needle. When disconnecting and reconnecting the pump, it is important to prevent air from getting into the system. With some of the pumps, air bubbles can get into the syringe, or insulin can seep out from around the plunger. Drawing the plunger slowly, rather than rapidly, minimizes this leakage. It is sometimes helpful to overfill the insulin bottle with air so that the increased air pressure forces insulin into the syringe rather than pulling the plunger back manually. The catheter tubing should also be prefilled ("primed") using the pump.

The catheter tubing, known as the "infusion set," can develop blockages, which can be a major cause of pump malfunction. Therefore these sets should be changed routinely, every other day. The tubing is usually 20 to 42 inches long, but the shorter the tubing, the less chance there is of occlusion. Most infusion set tubing is 27 gauge and is attached to a ⅝-inch needle, which is inserted subcutaneously.

Some infusion sets have adhesive at the site of insertion to make it easier to secure the tubing to the skin. People with sensitive skin and who are prone to rashes, dermatitis, or other skin problems are cautioned not to use these types of sets. Infusion sets without adhesive can be secured to the skin with transparent tapes (Op-site and Tegaderm are two brands), which permit the insertion site to be inspected visually. Recurrent abscesses (skin infections—usually reddened, warm, raised areas, frequently oozing blood or yellowish fluid) may form at the insertion sites. If these are noted, your physician should be contacted for treatment. The infusion sets may also need to be changed daily. In general, washing the insertion sites with antiseptic wash (Hibecleanse or Phisohex, for example) plus good general hygiene are essential.

The catheter needle should be bent at about a 45° angle prior to insertion. Once it is inserted, the extra slack in the tubing should be looped a couple of times and taped down. The tubing should not be exposed to extreme heat or cold as this may affect the potency of the insulin that is in it.

Once the pump is running, it must be attached to the body in a comfortable and safe location. Many people choose to attach it to a belt loop or the belt of a dress. Some patients have also sewn pockets into clothing, and many men can insert the pump into a shirt or coat pocket. Some women place their pumps in their bra, either on the side under the strap, or, if anatomy permits, in front. Velcro closures can be sewn into garments to allow the tubing to be run beneath them.

It is important that pump users not be "off" the pump for longer than one hour without additional insulin. This time may vary slightly if exercise is involved, and your pump management team should provide you with guidelines regarding these issues. When the pump is disconnected, the catheter needle is left inserted, but the end of the catheter is disconnected from the pump. The catheter hub and syringe tip are covered with caps when disconnected. When the pump is reconnected, the hub of the tubing is filled with insulin either manually with a syringe or with the pump itself to prevent bubble formation. (Be sure to remember this extra insulin volume that may be needed for reconnection when filling the pump and calculating the amounts of insulin that will be needed.) When manipulating the pump and tubing, catheter clamps can be used to prevent accidental bolusing of a dose of insulin. Also, the tubing should not be held up high, as the effect of gravity may draw insulin down and into the body as if a bolus of insulin were being delivered. If problems persist with air getting into the system with this method of carefully disconnecting the tubing, the whole system may need to be removed, including removing the needle from the body.

If there is concern that the pump is not working properly, there are a few things you should check to "troubleshoot" before calling for help. First, disconnect the pump and program a bolus of 3 to 5 units. Watch for the insulin coming out of the infusion needle to be sure that a blockage has not developed in the needle or tubing. Insulin can occasionally aggregate (clump up) and cause such a blockage. Also, check for leaks between the syringe and infusion set, the seal connecting the plastic tubing to the needle, or at the syringe-plunger site. Check also for air in the tubing or large bubbles in the hub of the syringe or infusion set junction. Check the needle insertion site for inflammation or leakage, especially if the infusion set has not been changed recently. Finally, be sure that the batteries are good!

Pump Dose Adjustments. General rules for adjustments of intensive insulin therapies that have been discussed earlier are applicable to pump users. The range of basal adjustments is usually 0.1 to 2 units at a time. The basal rate and the boluses should not be adjusted at the same time routinely, as it will be difficult to sort out the effect of each change. However, under supervision of the pump care team this type of adjustment allows greater flexibility. It is important for all pump users to discuss with their medical advisers the amounts to use for adjusting pump dose algorithms. Frequently, close contact is needed between the pump user and the teaching nurse to establish and maintain proper dosing programs. Therefore it is recommended that people using a pump live not more than a 2-hour driving distance from the center that is supervising their therapy.

Sick Days with Pumps. The usual sick day rules for insulin dose changes, with certain exceptions, apply for pump users as well. The usual recommendation at the Joslin Diabetes Center on clearly defined sick days is to increase the basal infusion rate by 50%. The boluses are then increased as well, using a quantity of insulin that has been predetermined in discussions with your pump care team. Often pump boluses are increased by 10 to 20% of the sum of the total daily insulin doses (basal plus boluses). The blood glucose level should be checked every 4 hours. If you get a reading over 240 mg% with urine ketones, this "catch-up" increment insulin dose should be given in addition to the usual insulin doses.

With the use of an algorithm, the bolus doses will already be higher before the catch-up is added. The nature of your algorithm— the amount of insulin given and the size of the routine dose increases for higher glucose levels as outlined by your algorithm— will determine how you should approach the sick day increases. Input from your pump care team is essential *before* you get sick, so that you will know what to do in advance. Remember that sick days require more insulin, and the syringe should be checked fre- quently.

If, after increasing both the basal and the boluses, the blood glucose level does not come into an acceptable range in a period of 2 to 3 hours, the pump should be removed and injected insulin should be used, with the alternative split-mix dose plus standard sick day rules. Sick days are not times to troubleshoot, and if there is any question whether the pump is functioning properly, injected insulin should be used. Ketoacidosis can come on quite rapidly, and any suggestive symptoms should prompt the immediate switch to injected insulin plus a trip to the physician or emergency room.

Insulin therapy is best individualized, and this is never so true as with pump therapy in general, and sick days on pumps in particular. The above guidelines are for general information. However, all people using pump therapy are well advised to be quite clear on the specific sick day instructions that their own pump management team wish them to use *before* they become ill.

Exercise Adjustments with Pumps. Exercise varies widely from person to person, and trial and error is the best way to determine what type of adjustments are needed for a given amount of exercise. Pump users are no exception. There are many ways to adjust for exercise: (1) the basal infusion rate can be reduced during exercise, (2) the pump can be taken off altogether if the exercise is strenuous, or (3) additional food may also be consumed. Needless to say, pumps should not be worn during contact or water sports. During sexual activity, the pump can be removed or worn, depending on personal preference. Most people choose to remove it.

These are general guidelines. If the exercise is to be performed within 3 hours of the last insulin bolus, hypoglycemia can occur. Additional food can help to prevent it, but if the activity is planned about 50% of the usual premeal bolus is another way. For prolonged, less strenuous exercise, such as 2 to 3 hours of bicycling or walking, reducing the basal rate by 30 to 50% may be preferable. In general, pump management teams should be consulted for guidance in determining what adjustments are needed. Careful record keeping is important so that you can later review what alterations were made, how long and how strenuous the activity was, and the ultimate effect on the blood glucose levels. With repeated adjustments you can learn what works for *you*.

Pump "Vacations." Pump vacations are times when a regular user is not using his or her pump. These may occur due to faulty equipment, other illness, travel, catheter insertion site infection or inflammation, or just simply periods of time when the pump user gets bored with the routine and wants to take a break from the intensive self-management. "Pump vacations" are usually longer than the short-term pump disconnections due to showers, exercise, or sexual activity, and are measured in terms of days off of pump therapy rather than minutes or hours.

It is essential to plan alternate insulin doses that will be given by syringe injection. It is always good to anticipate a possible emergency pump vacation due to equipment malfunction and to have a standby emergency insulin plan ready with the help of your pump care team. If you need a dose immediately and you cannot reach medical advice, here are some guidelines. The quantity of insulin given as the pump basal over a 24-hour period should be determined and given as two injections of NPH or Lente insulin, with ⅔ of the total given before breakfast, and the other ⅓ given before supper. This same pump plan for regular insulin boluses before meals can be used for injected regular insulin at those same times. Remember, however, that the prelunch regular insulin will be peaking at about the same time as the morning NPH or Lente, so alterations in either of these doses may be needed. Further dose adjustments may be necessary if the vacation is to be prolonged, if activity is different, or if the the vacation is due to a prolonged illness or severe injury.

Conclusion

Although treatment is necessary for everyone with diabetes, *not* everyone needs intensive therapies. And not everyone on intensive therapy *needs* to use a pump. Too many people mistakenly think that a pump will allow them to abandon their diabetes disciplines. This is not true. Developing a proper routine for and method of intensive insulin therapy takes time and effort. It also requires a major, longterm commitment on the part of the person undertaking this therapy and support from a skilled health care team. Results are often slow in coming, but the rewards can be great, and the feeling of success and good health can make it all worth the effort.

11

Treating Type II Diabetes

Type II diabetes, also known as non-insulin-dependent diabetes, is far more widespread than type I (insulin-dependent). It is also, strangely enough, probably more neglected and undertreated. Because people with this type of diabetes are not as dramatically in need of insulin and medical attention as those with type I diabetes, they are often taken for granted and their treatment is less than it should be. Other diseases seem to take precedence. The person with a heart problem, for example, could die rapidly, while the untreated or undertreated person with type II diabetes deteriorates more slowly—but eventually, just as surely.

What Is Type II Diabetes?

Type II diabetes is not always caused by a lack of insulin production or secretion by the pancreas. It can also result from insulin resistance, which makes the insulin that is produced much less effective at moving the glucose from the blood into the cells of the body. This insulin resistance may be related to a number of factors. It is probably an inherited trait, and, because you cannot choose your ancestors, there is nothing you can do about that once you are born! However, it can also be related both to overweight and to overeating, which contributes to overweight.

In fact, to oversimplify, you could say that you inherit *not* type II diabetes, but the ability to *get* type II diabetes. Or, to simplify further, you could say, "Heredity loads the gun, and stress pulls the trigger." Stress can be many things: infections, obesity, multiple child births, or even simply the stress of aging.

Treatment of Type II Diabetes

People with type II diabetes have a greater choice than those with type I. The latter can use diet and exercise, but must have insulin. Those with type II may have the added choice of oral hypoglycemic agents.

Diet and Weight Loss

The first treatment of people with type II is the eating plan (sometimes called "diet"). If people with type II diabetes who have been overeating and are overweight change their eating habits, they often begin to see improvements in their diabetes within a few days, and even before they have lost one ounce. This effect occurs because a proper diet may help the insulin receptors, the parts of the cell that get the message from the insulin, work more effectively. Being overweight is a major factor, however, and weight loss should be the goal.

Weight certainly contributes to insulin resistance. A person with the genetic predisposition to develop type II diabetes who would need about 40 units of insulin each day at a normal weight might need as much as 100 units daily to maintain normal blood glucose levels when overweight. This extra insulin is needed to overcome insulin resistance. Weight loss can reduce the insulin resistance and the amount of insulin needed daily. A detailed discussion of the eating plans to accomplish weight loss is found in Chapter 4, which is required reading for everyone with type II diabetes.

Exercise

Exercise is another important component of treatment. It helps reduce the blood glucose level as well and makes the insulin more effective (Chapter 5).

If a proper eating plan plus exercise do not result in acceptable regulation of diabetes, further treatments are available to many. The first choice after diet may be an oral hypoglycemic agent

(Chapter 6). If oral agent therapy plus diet and exercise are ineffective, insulin may be needed instead of oral medication.

Oral Medication

When diet and exercise are not sufficient to bring type II diabetes under acceptable control, oral therapy should be started. The oral hypoglycemic agents are discussed in detail in Chapter 6.

Is Diet Still Necessary? People sometimes wonder if diet is still needed with treatment with oral medications. The answer is a resounding *yes!* Diet is more important than ever. People using these compounds often develop a false sense of security and neglect diet, but diet is still important and may make the difference between the success or failure of oral therapy. In fact, some people with type II diabetes who have to use insulin might not really need it if they ate properly. In addition, the oral agents do not work when the eating plan is neglected. Increasing the dosage above the recommended maximum does *not* improve things. There are definite limits beyond which they are generally not more potent.

Who Might Use the Tablets

The sulfonylurea compounds are effective only in people who have a pancreas with live and effective beta cells. People with type I diabetes who cannot produce insulin may not use these medications because they will be ineffective. Insulin is the only treatment for type I diabetes.

Oral medications are most effective when the diabetes is newly discovered, in people over age 40, and in people who, when using insulin, require less than 40 units daily. There are exceptions to all rules, of course. There is an occasional youngster with adult-type diabetes (type II) who can use oral compounds, but these are rare.

At times, it is hard to determine if someone has true type I or type II diabetes. The decision is simple in many cases because the onset and symptoms are characteristic (see Chapter 1). For others, a trial-and-error system is needed. There is no simple test to differentiate between the two types. The progress of treatment must be monitored by a physician over time. If the diabetes eventually begins to act like type I diabetes—elevated blood glucose levels unresponsive to oral therapy, with weight loss and perhaps the detection of some urine acetone—then insulin treatment must start. With close observation and the change to insulin in time, there is no harm from the delay. Diabetes is for a long time. A few days or weeks may be worth a trial under medical supervision.

Oral agent therapy may also be ineffective during periods of stress, such as infection, injury, or major surgical procedures. During these periods, many physicians recommend insulin treatment, even if only temporary. At this time, many physicians prefer to use the purer human insulins to minimize the stimulation of insulin antibodies. Oral medications are not to be used during pregnancy because the effect on the fetus is not known, and at about the thirty-sixth week of pregnancy, the oral agents pass through the placenta to the fetus, thereby lowering the fetal blood glucose levels.

People with type II diabetes who are badly out of control at the onset of the diabetes may not be able to respond to the oral agents and might require insulin for a period of time. After a period of good control, the diabetes may improve to the point that oral compounds and diet—or diet alone—might be effective.

Combinations of Oral Agents

The combined use of sulfonylurea agents with biguanides (such as phenformin, sold as "DBI") was an effective treatment of type II diabetes some years ago. This approach stopped when phenformin became unavailable. Many of the people successfully treated in this manner had to start insulin therapy. The biguanides are still used in most of the world. Recently, research with newer biguanides (nonsulfonylurea) compounds has started.

Oral hypoglycemic agents combined with insulin for the treatment of type I diabetes has not proven effective. This type of combination therapy for people with type II diabetes should, in theory, have some effect. High doses of insulin are not effective in some people with type II diabetes, yet the oral compounds alone may not be effective at all. Because sulfonylurea medications can help reduce insulin resistance, some treated ineffectively with high doses of insulin may benefit from reduction of the insulin dose and the addition of the oral agent to treat the insulin resistance. In various published studies, this combined approach seems to be effective in some people with type II diabetes, but not in others. While this combination therapy is not in general use, if therapy with large doses of insulin alone is not completely effective, the addition of an oral agent under careful supervision may be worth a trial. If it does not improve control in a few months, combined therapy is stopped.

Mixing with Other Medications or Substances

Medicines used for treatment of one disease can cause problems when mixed with other drugs, medicines, or substances. These adverse effects can also occur with the oral hypoglycemic agents, although much less so with the newer "second-generation" agents. A distressing effect can be seen when alcohol is combined with some of the earlier agents, most notably chlorpropamide. A facial flush can be noted. The blood vessels of the skin surface of the face and neck become sensitized and dilate, causing a severe headache and causing the face to turn red like a neon sign. Although harmless, this reaction can be quite startling. This condition does not last long but can be alarming to the victim. Other drugs such as cortisone raise blood glucose levels and make the oral agents much less effective.

> Never take any new medication unless prescribed by your physician. WHEN IN DOUBT ABOUT THE USE OF ANY MEDICATION, including those that can be obtained without a prescription, CONSULT YOUR PHYSICIAN.

Do Oral Tablets Eventually Fail?

Eventually, many times they do. This is called "secondary failure." (Primary failure is when they are not effective originally.) Failure may be due to factors such as infection, surgery, or severe injury. Many people can resume satisfactory treatment with the tablets when these conditions have been treated adequately. Often, though, after varying periods of oral agent treatment, blood glucose levels become elevated and the physician has to increase the tablet dose or change to another agent. It is best to make these changes before the glucose levels become so high that insulin treatment is needed.

This change in tablets may fail nevertheless. Is it due to "patient failure" or "pill failure"? People may become careless with their diet. They may neglect to test for blood or urine sugar and not realize that the dose is inadequate. Other people deceive themselves by testing only the morning fasting urine (which may be the best of the day) and assume that they are well regulated. The debate over whose fault it is, really, is not productive. It may be simply that the diabetes becomes more difficult to regulate over a period of time and the pills cease to be effective. If the oral agents really are inadequate for the job, insulin is needed.

It is still difficult to predict at the time that insulin is started whether insulin treatment will be temporary or permanent. If insulin was needed because of "patient failure," it is possible that it may be stopped after restoration of good diabetes control for a period of time. However, if it was "pill failure," which should really be thought of as a progression of the diabetes, the insulin need is probably permanent. Be assured, however, that this progression is not caused by the continued use of oral agents. There is no evidence to indicate that such is the case.

Insulin Treatment of Type II Diabetes

If a proper diet, weight loss, exercise, and oral hypoglycemic agent treatment fail to achieve adequate control, then even some people with type II diabetes need insulin. Is it confusing that "non-insulin-dependent diabetes" needs insulin? It shouldn't be. While people with type II diabetes may not need insulin to remain alive as people with type I diabetes do, nevertheless, very high blood glucose levels for periods of time may be harmful—for example, promoting infections and many other complications. So for *some* people with type II diabetes, insulin is very important. Frequently, when necessary, treatment with one morning injection of intermediate, or mixed regular plus intermediate-acting insulin will suffice. Occasionally, people with type II diabetes will require two or more daily injections. The discussion (Chapter 9) of conventional insulin treatment of diabetes is important for people with type II diabetes who require insulin treatment.

12

Diabetes in the Young

Few things in the minds of parents are as devastating as the finding
of diabetes in their child. Their hopes of the child's bright future
seem to be shattered. At first, many of these parents are overwhelmed and in a state of shock with what is known as the "grief
reaction," which includes resentment, denial, anger, and guilt.
Eventually, most adapt and accept the diabetes.

While there is little to make you overjoyed about diabetes, age
9 or 90, life goes on, and the diabetes must be dealt with. The
treatment for diabetes in young people today, while demanding, is
effective and can enable the child with diabetes to live an enjoyable
and fulfilling life. While it takes time for the child and parents to
adjust, patience and support help bring understanding and acceptance. In addition to the actual management of blood glucose levels,
another important goal of diabetes therapy is this acceptance and
eventual adjustment by the young people and their parents.

You Are Not Alone!

Among adults, diabetes is very common, and most people know
at least one person with diabetes. This may not be so with children.
Frequently, the affected child may be the only person he or she
knows that has diabetes. This is especially true if the child lives in
a small town. It is estimated that diabetes mellitus affects some
100,000 children and adolescents under the age of 20 years,
accounting for about 2% of all people with diabetes in the United

States. *Prevalence* refers to the total number of people with diabetes in the population at any given moment. A study in Allegheny County (Pennsylvania) found diabetes in 140 per 100,000 people under 19 years of age, which is probably typical of the prevalence throughout the United States. The prevalence may differ in other countries.

The development of insulin-dependent diabetes (type I) occurs at any time from infancy to old age, although it is rare in infancy. The most common age for children to develop diabetes is 10 to 12 years, with boys and girls about equally affected. This group appears to be increasing in number. This increase may be because diabetes can be an inherited condition; those with diabetes are living longer and producing offspring who continue the genetic trait.

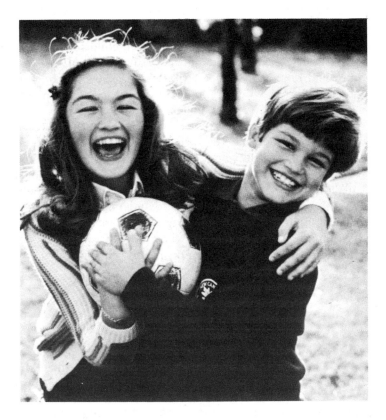

Why Do Children Develop Diabetes?

The reasons children develop diabetes are probably the same as for others (Chapter 1). In the case of insulin-dependent (type I) diabetes, the commonest form in children, the child is probably born with a genetic predisposition to diabetes. These children may also have islet cell antibodies in the blood when the diabetes is discovered. These antibodies are the signs of active destruction of the insulin-producing beta cells in the pancreas by the body's own immune system. The factors that trigger the destruction of these beta cells are not known, but may include virus infections or perhaps an environmental toxin of some sort. Specific viruses that have been blamed as a cause of diabetes include coxsackievirus B4, mumps, and Epstein-Barr virus (the cause of infectious mononucleosis). Children infected with rubella (German measles) virus before birth ("congenital rubella syndrome") have a greater risk of developing type I diabetes, usually at 15 to 20 years of age. Certainly any child in whom beta cell destruction has begun will show evidence of true diabetes when under the stress of a viral infection.

Diabetes is diagnosed more frequently during the fall and winter months than in the summer. This seasonal variation does not seem to apply to children with diabetes onset before age five. It is thought that seasonal influence in older children may be because infections unmask the pre-existing decrease in insulin production.

Types of Diabetes in Young People

Most children develop the classic form of insulin-dependent diabetes (type I). It used to be known as "juvenile diabetes" or "brittle diabetes" until it was discovered that this disease can occur at any age.

Development of type I diabetes is slow in some adults. In children, by contrast, the characteristic symptoms usually begin abruptly, especially tremendous thirst and frequent urination until medical help is sought. Recurrence of bedwetting may be a sign of diabetes in the young. The child may continue to have a good appetite and eat large amounts of food, yet lose weight. If the condition is not recognized early, dehydration may occur because of the loss of water from the body due to large volumes of urination. Vision can be blurred from temporary changes in the lens of the eye. A formerly active and robust child becomes weak, irritable, and without energy. School performance may deteriorate. The child may tire easily and complain of pains in the legs and abdomen, with difficulty breathing or chest pains.

With this abrupt beginning, the proper diagnosis can be made quickly. At times, however, the symptoms of diabetes may resemble a "flu" or stomach virus. This may be confusing for a while. Blood glucose values at the time that the diabetes is discovered are usually in the range of 300 to 1000 mg%. A child with glucose levels this high will have much sugar in the urine, as well as acetone (ketones). The diagnosis is immediately obvious. A glucose tolerance test is not necessary.

Some children will develop type II, or non-insulin dependent, diabetes (NIDDM). These children are usually extremely overweight. A rare variety of NIDDM is referred to as "maturity-onset diabetes of youth (MODY). A glucose tolerance test may be necessary to diagnose this type of diabetes.

The presence of sugar in a child's urine does not necessarily mean that the child has diabetes. Some children without diabetes can spill small amounts of glucose in the urine due to a low renal threshold. This is called "renal glycosuria" and occurs when the blood glucose is normal but there is glucose present in the urine. Nevertheless, the presence of glucose in the urine should always be taken seriously until it is checked out by the physician.

Stages of Development of Diabetes

Four distinct stages occur in the usual onset of type I diabetes in children. They are:
1. Acute onset
2. Apparently lessened diabetes (partial remission) with possible complete remission ("honeymoon phase")
3. Increasing intensity ("intensification phase")
4. Total diabetes.

Dr. Priscilla White found that 95% of children who developed diabetes before age 15 had "total diabetes" by the end of their fifth year with this condition. The number of functioning pancreatic beta cells decreases progressively so that less and less insulin is produced.

Stage I. If the diabetes is detected early, before severe dehydration, weight loss, and ketoacidosis develops, the pancreas is still able to produce some insulin but not enough to keep blood glucose levels normal. At this time, blood glucose levels may be controlled using a simple program of intermediate-acting insulin once daily in the morning.

Stage II. During this stage the diabetes seems to improve, and the patient's own insulin is more effective in keeping glucose levels close to normal. One theory is that the initial inflammation around the islet cells that produced the onset of the diabetes has subsided, and some of the ability to produce insulin returns, and, for a period, the beta cells work better. Also, with blood glucose levels returned to normal, the tissues become more sensitive to insulin's action.

Unfortunately, this improvement is short-lived. This "remission" or "honeymoon phase" varies in duration, but should not raise false hopes or be called a cure. Nor should it be thought that the diabetes diagnosis was a mistake. Ultimately the insulin dose will need to be increased, and the diabetes will again become more challenging to control. Some are tempted to eliminate the insulin dose altogether during a honeymoon. Insulin should be continued, even if only one or two units are given each day, to avoid false hopes of a diabetes cure and because discontinuing insulin may lead to sensitization to insulin so that allergies may occur when the insulin is resumed.

The remission often ends after an infection or other acute illness or with the onset of puberty and increased growth. Patients should not view this period as a vacation from the diabetes, but rather as an opportunity to learn more about it and to get used to the routines that will be needed in the future.

Stage III. When the diabetes becomes intense once again, young people with diabetes and their parents often become discouraged because blood glucose levels fluctuate so much despite conscientious efforts at regulation. While insulin is essential, there may still be some, minimal insulin secretion by the pancreas, but not enough for survival without extra outside insulin.

Stage IV. This is total diabetes resulting from the total destruction of the pancreas's beta cells. Insulin is no longer found in the blood or pancreas, and the proper use of food as a source of energy depends on the availability of injected insulin. Patients promptly develop ketoacidosis if insulin is omitted.

A common question at this time is, "Will my child always have to take insulin?" By our present-day knowledge, the answer is yes, because insulin no longer made by the pancreas must be replaced. The child cannot survive without insulin. Thus this type of diabetes is referred to as "insulin-dependent."

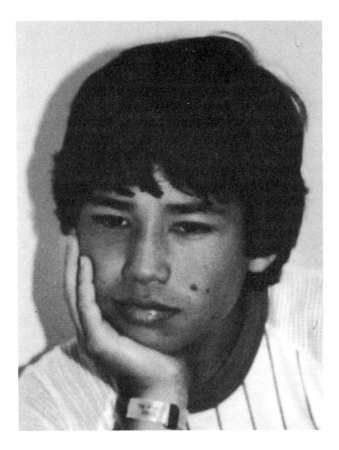

Treatment of Diabetes in the Young

Goals of Treatment. The purpose of treating type I diabetes is to relieve the symptoms caused by high blood glucose levels, prevent acute complications such as ketoacidosis and hypoglycemic coma, reduce the chances of getting the complications of diabetes, and promote a state of general well-being and physical vigor. In a child, there is also concern about maintaining normal metabolism so that the child can grow and develop normally. Current evidence strongly suggests that to achieve these goals, good control of blood glucose levels, so that they are as near normal as possible, is necessary.

To reach this goal is difficult, and at times it may seem impossible to achieve in children with total diabetes. Yet it must be the target at which one aims. In doing so, one must occasionally compromise between normal glucose levels and normal social and emotional development for the child.

The Team Approach. Children with diabetes and their families are best served by a diabetes treatment team consisting of, where available, health care professionals with special knowledge and interest in the physical and emotional development of children as well as training and experience in the management of type I diabetes. This team should include a specially trained pediatrician; a pediatric diabetes nurse specialist; a mental health professional (psychiatric social worker or clinical psychologist who understands the emotional and social problems in the family); and a dietitian who works mostly with children and adolescents to assist with nutrition education and meal planning. This is the ideal, although often it is not available. This team must work with the child's own physician and with others involved with the child such as the teacher, school nurse, school guidance counselor, or team coach.

This health care team (mentioned so many times in this volume) has a major responsibility to make sure not only that the young person and family understand and follow the initial treatment plans, but that they continue treatment into the future. This "backup" support is as important as the medical treatment itself.

Not everyone lives near a medical center that can provide primary medical care from such a diabetes team. In such a circumstance, the local physician must give routine care and emergency treatment. Nevertheless, occasional travel to centers with multidisciplinary diabetes departments may provide many of the benefits that are needed. Obviously, constant communication between all of those concerned is essential.

Education of the Young. Education is the cornerstone of all successful diabetes care. This process must start with the diagnosis and continue throughout the patient's life.

Education for a child and family consists of three stages:
1. This stage is an introduction to diabetes and to the funda-mentals of its management ("survival skills"—the basics!). These include insulin injection, self-monitoring, and recog-nition of symptoms of hypoglycemia.
2. Over the next few weeks, as the metabolism is stabilized, the family begins to acquire the skills needed for longterm care for their child at home and to enable the child to return to normal activities.
3. The final stage of education is learning the more sophisti-cated details of management to achieve near-normal blood

glucose levels. These involve coping with colds and other illnesses ("sick day rules") and other variations in the child's daily routine. This final stage of the education continues for many years and should include periodic reviews and up-dates of knowledge of diabetes self-care.

Insulin. Along with education, insulin is absolutely the major treatment of young people with diabetes at this time. Conventional insulin therapy does not replace the body's own pattern of insulin production and secretion, however. Normally insulin is secreted constantly and is present at all times in the blood. Then, in response to eating, the insulin level can increase. The use of one daily injection of intermediate insulin cannot reproduce this pattern. Therefore, most children with type I diabetes need several daily injections, usually using two types of insulin—rapid-acting (crystalline) and intermediate-acting—to achieve ideal blood glucose control.

The insulin dosing programs outlined in the chapters on insulin therapy for type I diabetes are useful for children and adolescents. Usually, once stage III (intensification) or IV (total diabetes) is reached, the standard split-mix insulin program (morning mix of rapid-acting and intermediate-acting insulins plus a second injection either before supper using a mixture of these insulins or at bedtime using only intermediate insulin) is needed. Reasons for using this program are similar to those for adults, although the more rapid progress of the diabetes in the young and their life-style variability necessitate the earlier use of this more complex program. Persistent high glucose levels at night, as shown by nocturnal urinating or bedwetting, or significant hyperglycemia before breakfast, may signify the need to start this second insulin dose. Splitting the dose is definitely preferable. If an increased morning dose of intermediate-acting insulin is used instead of two (split) doses, the risk of severe hypoglycemic reactions during the afternoon or evening is increased.

The mixtures of insulin are made in the same syringe to decrease the number of injections. The precise insulin dose must be determined based on the individual needs of each child. Children's insulin requirements are not fixed and are most likely to change during development, so periodic re-evaluation is essential. Also, children's activity is notoriously variable, and dose adjustments are often necessary throughout childhood and adolescence. For example, a child going away to camp or starting an active summer job after an inactive school year may need less insulin or more food or both. In general, dose adjustments are based on blood (and/or urine) glucose testing for a minimum of three days. Changes in the insulin dose are made when a definite pattern is observed. Changes in the dose should not be made more often than once in three days.

Whenever possible, injections should be given 30 minutes before meals, allowing the quick-acting insulin to begin work. When this is done, the blood glucose level rises less after meals than when the food is eaten right after the injection.

Preparing and injecting the insulin should be taught to the child and *both* parents. When children give their own injections, they should do so under strict parental guidance. Young children should never be pushed or hurried into full responsibility for their own injections until they are psychologically mature enough to understand fully the dangers of an inaccurate insulin dose.

Injections should be rotated, using the arms, thighs, buttocks, and belly, using new sites but not jumping from area to area. This kind of rotation prevents the development of lipohypertrophy, the puffy accumulation of fat at the sites of injections, or lipoatrophy, the crater-like depressions just under the skin at the injection sites. The newer, highly purified insulins (pure pork or human-like insulins) markedly reduce the possibility of developing these problems. The careful and purposeful rotation of injection sites not only prevents these cosmetic changes, but also makes the insulin absorption and action more predictable. Care should be taken, of course, to avoid injection in areas of the body that will shortly undergo intense exercise. This may speed up the absorption of the insulin and can change the insulin action timing.

Nutrition. Although diet and exercise are no longer the only treatment for diabetes, which was the case before insulin discovery, proper, planned nutrition is still very important. It is no longer a case of starvation.

The nutritional needs of children with diabetes are the same as for children without this condition. No special foods, vitamins, or minerals are needed. The meal plan is a basic "good" diet that provides everything needed for energy and growth. As a general rule, a child of average weight needs 1000 calories daily at age one, with 100 calories per day added each year up to the onset of puberty. All rules have exceptions, however, and each child's needs must be considered individually. For example, for obese youngsters with the rare condition of type II diabetes (MODY), the object of the diet is to reduce weight and keep it off. Generally, meal plans for youngsters should be reviewed and updated more frequently (perhaps every 6 or 12 months) than those for adults because of changing growth patterns.

It is important to coordinate food consumption with the time of action of injected insulin. Meals and snacks should be eaten at about the same times daily, and the total number of calories as well as the proportions of carbohydrate, protein, and fat should be consistent from day to day. The time of peak action is when hypoglycemia is most likely to occur. Snacks between the three main meals and at bedtime are usually needed to keep the glucose level from dropping too low. Most adolescents eliminate the mid-morning snack but should always have some rapidly absorbable carbohydrate available at that time, just in case.

THE "FREE" DIET? In theory, a free diet would permit children to eat anything they wish, as they wish. It sounds wonderful, but unfortunately it is not effective. The balance between insulin, activity, and ingested food is precarious at best, even in adults, and even more difficult in children.

Many youngsters get peer pressure regarding their eating— whether it is pressure to eat something, not to eat something, or to lose weight. Fear of low blood sugar reactions in front of their friends or being labeled "different" are powerful reasons that often cause the teenager to overeat. Also, adolescents sometimes test limits and experiment with overeating and undereating. Young people looking for their independence may try to manipulate their parents by eating improperly. The approach in dealing with these issues should be the same as in coping with such behavior in adolescents without diabetes.

Exercise. Details of the relationship of exercise and diabetes have been discussed previously. In summary, exercise in the young lowers blood glucose levels without the need for additional insulin during exertion. Regular exercise or physical training also provides a more sustained ("lag") effect. This involves an increase in the sensitivity of the body cells to the effects of insulin and persists even when the individual is not engaged in physical activity. After exercise is completed, the glycogen stores, which were used to provide energy, are replenished. As a result, further drops in blood glucose levels may occur. Additional food is usually needed to prevent these blood glucose drops. However, vigorous exercise in a person with poorly controlled type I diabetes can actually cause a further rise in blood glucose levels as well as in ketone (acetone) production. Therefore, if a child has marked hyperglycemia and ketonuria (urine ketones), strenuous physical activity should be discouraged until satisfactory control has been achieved.

Exercising an arm or leg into which insulin has been injected can increase the rate of insulin absorption into the circulation and increase the chances of hypoglycemia. If exercise is planned, it may be good to choose an injection site that will not involve vigorous muscular contraction. For example, if a child plans to do a lot of running during the day, the morning insulin injection should be given into the belly or buttocks. Unfortunately, children's activities are frequently not planned. Therefore, bursts of increased energy expenditure should be covered by providing extra snacks beforehand as well as during the exercise if it is prolonged. With a sustained increase in physical activity, such as during summer vacations, the overall insulin requirement usually decreases, and the daily dose of insulin may need to be reduced to avoid hypoglycemic reactions.

Adolescents who are responsible for their own care should be taught how to reduce their insulin dose when involved in organized sports. The exact amount of reduction has to be determined individually by frequent blood glucose self-monitoring and by trial and error. Although exercise is not a substitute for proper blood glucose control with insulin and a meal plan, it is a useful adjunct. A program of regular exercise allows young people with diabetes more choices of food, enabling them occasionally to have "forbidden" foods judiciously as sources of quickly absorbed carbohydrates to combat hypoglycemic reactions.

Monitoring Diabetes in Young People

As we discussed earlier, urine testing was, until recently, the only means to monitor diabetes control at home. Self monitoring of blood glucose has given us a more effective way to examine daily blood glucose patterns and to accommodate more interesting lifestyle variations.

Testing should not be a routine chore forced by the physician or parent. Proper use of monitoring systems requires knowing how and when to use them and what to do with the test results. Repeated daily testing is a waste of time and money unless the results are used to adjust insulin, diet, and exercise to improve control. Children are also less likely to "fake" test results if they are involved in understanding the results and the decisions made because of these results.

Although a monitoring program must be individual, it is usually recommended that young people test their blood a minimum of twice daily. They should also perform four tests a day (before meals and at bedtime) on at least one or two days each week. One or two blood glucose tests at 3:00 A.M. each month are also suggested. For the person who needs to make daily adjustments of insulin dose, activity, or food consumption, level III testing (see Chapter 8) may be necessary. Test results should be written down and this record brought to the physician or diabetes nurse educator for review so that patterns can be spotted.

Blood monitoring allows children to avoid hypoglycemia and allows adjustment of food and insulin for variations in activity. Most children tolerate blood testing well—in fact, better than their families or physicians thought they would. Most report that they prefer blood testing to urine testing because they find the data more informative. Many children and teenagers, and some adults, do not like urine testing, and, if they test at all, prefer to test blood. In infants who cannot urinate on demand (to say nothing of a double-voided specimen!) blood monitoring by heel or finger prick is advantageous.

Glycosylated Hemoglobin. In no single group of people is the glycosylated hemoglobin, discussed previously, more useful than in the child and adolescent. The constantly fluctuating blood glucose levels of young people are confusing. In addition, some adolescents do not take their diabetes seriously or may manipulate their control for various reasons. The glycohemoglobin test measures the level of control when home testing or office blood glucose levels may be confusing.

Glycosylated hemoglobin levels can be a goal of therapy, rather than only excellent office blood glucose test levels, although the exact level of blood glucose control that protects against diabetes complications is not absolutely known. While most knowledgeable physicians feel strongly that blood glucose levels as normal as possible are desirable, achieving them should be consistent with fairly normal living.

Nevertheless, individual goals can help. At the Joslin Diabetes Center, the normal hemoglobin A1 range for persons without diabetes is 5.4 to 7.4%. (Values may vary with each laboratory.) "Excellent control" (the goal) is about 8.5 to 9%. However, in young people with variable activity and eating habits, reaching a glyco-hemoglobin level under 10.5% can be difficult and may be acceptable if more strenuous efforts to improve control have failed or are not possible at a given time. Goals must be individualized for each person.

Glycohemoglobin levels may be used as a sort of "report card" to show how well the child's diabetes has fared during the past 2 months. However, it is important to avoid using the terms "good"

AVOID USING THE TERMS "GOOD" AND "BAD" WHEN DISCUSSING TEST RESULTS. TEST RESULTS ARE NOT A MORAL ISSUE. THEY SHOULD BE "HIGH" OR "LOW." YOUNGSTERS HAVE SOMETIMES BEEN PUSHED INTO FALSIFYING TEST RESULTS IN ORDER TO BE "GOOD"!

and "bad" to describe the glycohemoglobin or the blood glucose test results. Young people often interpret these terms to be judgmental. This can cause resentment and anger and may decrease the youngster's interest in any control of the diabetes. Children have been known to give false test results in order to please their parents. "High" and "low" are better terms. The glycohemoglobin indicates the degree of success at achieving optimal control or the need for more effort.

What Every Parent Should Know

The parents of a child newly diagnosed with diabetes are understandably overwhelmed. In addition to sorrow and possible resentment at their child's diabetes, they may be thoroughly confused. The complexity of diet overwhelms them; the prospect of insulin reactions frightens them, and, if the child is small, they are terrified at the thought of giving injections to what they think will be a squirming, screaming loved one. Most parents become overwhelmed because they try to learn everything there is to know about diabetes at once. This is neither possible nor necessary.

Learning "survival skills" should be the first undertaking. Parents should learn the general plan and goals of treatment and how to achieve them. The more important early tasks requiring mastery are: (1) the technique of insulin injection and simple dose adjusting; (2) prevention and treatment of insulin reactions; (3) self monitoring of blood glucose and its relationship to the insulin dose; (4) fundamentals of diet and how to provide the proper balance of interesting foods; (5) how to handle the child's diabetes during the generally short but frantic illnesses that occur during childhood (sick day rules). This is not the time to worry about possible foot problems of adulthood, eye problems, neuropathy, and other

> IN THEIR INITIAL FEAR AND FRUSTRATION
> ABOUT DIABETES, PARENTS SOMETIMES
> BLAME EACH OTHER'S FAMILIES FOR
> "CAUSING" THE DIABETES. "THERE IS NONE
> ON *OUR* SIDE OF THE FAMILY!" THE FACT IS
> THAT NO ONE KNOWS, AND IT DOES NOT
> MATTER. WHAT IS NEEDED IS A UNITED
> FRONT TO HELP THE CHILD!

complications that might be possible in the longer term picture, if ever.

What the Child Must Know

It is important that young people with diabetes develop the proper attitudes toward the condition. Diabetes will not go away— it will be with them *forever*, but it can be lived with. Once this is accepted, they will be much more receptive in learning what they need to master. They will also begin to pay attention to their bodies and learn to recognize the subtle clues that will help them succeed.

The actual facts and skills to be learned depend on the child's age and stage of maturity. Most children can learn to inject their own insulin by the time they are about 12 years old. Accurate measurement of insulin is a serious matter, and most children are not mature enough to take this responsibility until that time. Some should be older. Complete responsibility for managing insulin treatment requires experience and maturity. The potential for problems when mistakes are made is great. It is best not to impose these responsibilities on young people until they are mature enough to handle them.

Children should learn to understand the reasons for self blood glucose testing, whether or not they can do these tests alone. Most important is for young children to recognize the symptoms of a low blood glucose reaction and how to treat it (detailed in Chapter 15). Later, children will begin to appreciate the general goals and purposes of treatment and will become motivated to accept self-care. Children often learn at an early age that the care needed to maintain good health will allow them to participate in the normal activities of youth.

The Emotional Response

Diabetes is not simply a matter of mechanical treatment. It also involves a child's emotional and social development, which are very much influenced by their parents' reactions to the diabetes. Diabetes in a child involves the whole family and often imposes a considerable strain. When parents, perhaps already struggling with other problems, give up and leave the child alone with diabetes, the consequences can be disastrous in terms of dreadful glycemic control and many bouts of ketoacidosis.

Diabetes challenges the young person and the entire family to gain and use complex knowledge about physiology and nutrition, and to acquire technical skills such as measuring and injecting insulin. They must perform testing procedures which in previous years were done in the laboratory. This knowledge and these skills are usually associated with trained medical professionals. On top of all of this, they live with the anticipation of potential future complications.

> DON'T UNDERESTIMATE THE YOUNG AND THEIR ABILITY TO UNDERSTAND AND TREAT THEIR DIABETES. YOU OUGHT TO SEE WHAT THEY ARE DOING WITH COMPUTERS!

Although research always continues, it is now widely accepted that maintaining near-normal metabolic control may prevent or delay future complications. However, because conventional therapy cannot achieve truly normal blood glucose levels throughout the day and night in most young people with total insulin deficiency, they are haunted by the anxiety-provoking uncertainty about whether the level of control achieved will be sufficient to prevent complications.

The Onset of Diabetes. For parents and for older children and adolescents, the diagnosis of a probable lifetime condition usually stirs emotions that are much like those experienced by the bereaved: shock, disbelief, denial, anger, and depression. The initial emotional upheaval that follows diagnosis may temporarily limit a family's ability to comprehend, to say nothing of learning. Therefore, the educational goals should initially focus on the immediate necessities of care.

The burden of care for the young child rests with the parents who must plan, execute, and monitor the plan. Normally, the gradual transfer of responsibility from parent to child is the goal of all child-rearing. In dealing with diabetes, however, the delicate balance between dependency and independence is most difficult, and parents find it difficult to "let go."

The worry about daily care may foster the parents' belief that they alone can satisfactorily meet their child's special needs. Parents should transfer some responsibility to others, such as relatives, school personnel, athletic coaches, and even friends. All can be taught not only to be observant, but also how to manage emergency situations.

Parents must not hurry the child into taking responsibility for injecting insulin. The administration of correct insulin doses at the appropriate times is a life-sustaining matter for the child with total diabetes. Many times, the child who is forced too soon to accept full self-management calls for more parental help by purposely omitting insulin injections, with disastrous results. While many school-aged children can master the mechanics of diabetes care, their tasks will be easier when parents continue to lovingly oversee all aspects of care, even occasionally assisting with injections. The school-aged child can be involved in care by helping in meal planning, recognizing low blood sugar symptoms, and helping with urine or blood testing, as well as drawing up and occasionally injecting insulin with parental supervision. The concern that not making the child take full responsibility early will result in a dependent young adult is not true. No one has been seriously harmed by too much real love. Older children are usually eager to take over injections when it is important to them to do so. It is amazing how well they do when making an overnight visit to a friend's house or going on a camping trip or class outing.

> Caring for the young patient with diabetes is not solely a medical problem. Emotional and behavioral issues inevitably arise, must be identified, and must be dealt with.

The Adolescent. A major problem for any growing youngster is to develop responsibility with some independence. This is often difficult, but not as difficult as some adults make it. Growth toward independence is, of course, complicated by diabetes. The need for closer medical care occurs at just the time when the teenager is trying to be less dependent on others and wants to "do his own thing." Another problem in this struggle for teenage self-identity is their temporary rejections of the values of parents or other figures of authority. Diabetes often becomes the battleground for this struggle. Many adolescents want to find out whether they *really* have diabetes and want to know what happens if they do not follow instructions. This may mean overeating, omitting insulin injections, or refusing to do any testing. Adolescence is a period of rapid physical growth and sexual maturation. Both physical and mental factors lead to more erratic diabetes control during the adolescent years than occur during childhood or in later life.

The peer group is all important during adolescence as well. The

> **Youth is a strange period. Young people deplore being "different." They want to be one of the group. Later in life adults can make a scene trying to be "different," whether by driving sportier cars, wearing outlandish clothes, or bragging at parties.**

teen with diabetes, already sensitive to "being different," has extra need for peer support. They may omit insulin injections, eat haphazardly, and omit monitoring in order to prove "nothing is wrong." Occasional omission of insulin, lapses in following diet plans, and periodic refusal to test should be expected and watchfully tolerated. However, this is different from severe self-destructive behavior which results in repeated episodes of ketoacidosis. Numerous emergency room visits often signal the need for intensive psychological intervention and support. In this regard, the nurse-educator, psychiatric social worker, or clinical psychologist is a very important member of the diabetes treatment team.

Growth and Development

The records of Dr. Priscilla White, the pioneer in treating youngsters with diabetes, collected over many decades, provide an interesting historical footnote on how diabetes affected growth and development. Between the years 1922 and 1940, 1 boy in 4 with diabetes and 1 girl in 10 fell below the standard average growth for their age by as much as 4 to 13 inches. These people were called "diabetic dwarfs." The picture has changed! Today, with modern insulin and monitoring methods, most children treated with usual insulin therapy who achieve "fair to good" metabolic control grow at a normal rate, despite some abnormal metabolism.

The goal of treatment should certainly be better than "fair to good" control. It should be fairly easy to achieve control that is good enough to maintain proper growth and development. Therefore, if normal growth and development are not proceeding as expected, closer attention to diabetes control is essential. Of course, there may be reasons for poor growth and development which are unrelated to diabetes, and these causes should be ruled out and treated.

The onset of puberty usually proceeds normally in people with diabetes, but poor control can delay it. One of the problems sometimes found at puberty among girls with diabetes is delayed menstruation. If the thyroid function and other hormones are normal, this delay is frequently self-correcting with a bit more time and good diabetes control. Such delays cause great anxiety and distress among both parents and youngsters.

Infants with Diabetes

Babies with diabetes are very rare, but increasingly diabetes is being found under age five. Home blood testing allows accurate insulin doses. Because infants need relatively tiny amounts of insulin, the insulin concentration should be diluted down from the usual U-100 strength to U-50 or even U-25, although U-40 may still be used. Insulin manufacturers provide the fluid to make this dilution, and your physician or teaching nurse can tell you how to make a proper mixture with as low a dilution as you need. The amounts of insulin needed will increase as the child grows.

> Parents often are upset because their children need increasing amounts of insulin as they grow from babyhood. They think that the "diabetes is becoming worse." Not so! As children grow toward adulthood, they need adult-sized doses.

Because they start receiving insulin injections from infancy and only know life with insulin injections and testing, infants and young children adapt to diabetes quite well and manage self-care, when older, without difficulty.

The Effect of Menstruation

During menstruation the kidney threshold may be reduced, so that more sugar is found in the urine. This may confuse those using urine testing. Also, many women notice a rise in blood glucose levels for a few days just before the beginning of the monthly flow. Temporary increases in the insulin dose may be needed.

School

It is important that children going to school keep their diabetes well regulated for normal growth and development as well as for freedom from high and low blood glucose levels that may be distressing as well as calling attention to them as "different." The teacher should be told of the diabetes, but must not shelter or overprotect the youngster. Teachers should not make obvious special allowances for the diabetes. The child should be allowed to participate fully in all school activities. Parents should meet with the child's teacher at the beginning of the year to explain the nature of diabetes and to indicate the need for snacks and for eating meals on time. Most important is information about hypoglycemic reactions—their prevention and treatment. School nurses and others will be helpful in informing the teachers so that they feel secure with the child with diabetes. It is useful to prepare written instructions for the teachers, just in case.

Leaving the Child with a Babysitter

It is important for parents to get away, even if just for an evening out. Parents also have lives! This will take a little extra thought and planning, with a responsible person at home.

The choice of the person to care for the child is crucial, and finding such a person may be difficult. Many thousands of parents have found such people, however, and so can you! Nurses, students, other people with diabetes or who have relatives with diabetes, or even your relatives are possible sitters. Social service or other local agencies may be able to find appropriate personnel to provide a change for parents of children with diabetes. Time should be set aside to teach the babysitter the simplest basics of diabetes care and what to do in emergencies, which may never occur. Most important, review the recognition and treatment of insulin reactions. If the parents are to be away for longer than an evening, have the person come a day or two earlier while the parents are home to see the normal day-to-day routine for handling the child with diabetes. Of course, parents must leave the phone number of the family physician and the phone number and address where they can be reached while they are away. A phone call can solve many problems. The care of older children usually poses no great problem, but with the very young, it is important that the parents' fears not ruin what should be a happy time for the whole family.

Camps

Since they started in the 1920s, camping programs for young people with diabetes have been recognized as beneficial physically and emotionally and are good sources of diabetes education. Camps may be either regular camps with special facilities or special staff to supervise and care for children with diabetes, or camps devoted primarily to children with diabetes. Two such camps are the Elliott P. Joslin Camp for Boys in Charlton, Massachusetts, and the Clara Barton Birthplace Camp for Girls, 3 miles away in North Oxford, Massachusetts. Both are 50 miles west of Boston, in central Massachusetts. Older teenagers and young adults are employed as counselors, program directors, and other members of the camp staff. The American Diabetes Association also has lists of camps. There are also camps in many other countries. The primary purpose of these camps is to provide an enjoyable recreational experience for the youngster while also insuring good treatment of diabetes. The camp staff is responsible for assisting the campers to gain mastery over their diabetes by acquiring the necessary knowledge and technical skills.

Diabetes education is a vital part of the total program and is ideally carried out in a manner that is enjoyable and effective. A successful camp experience should leave the child with a feeling of greater independence and self-esteem, due to his or her increased competence in self-care as well as seeing many other youngsters cope with their problems. Camp also relieves the anxiety and depression that some children experience at being different. Staff members who have mastered some of the difficulties of diabetes management that each young person must face can be positive role models. An added dividend of such camps is that they also provide

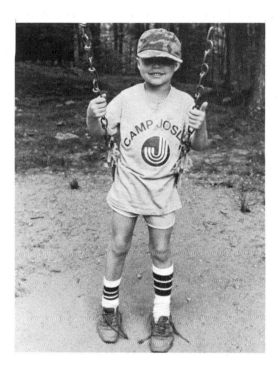

parents with several carefree weeks away from their children, knowing that they can safely postpone their direct responsibilities for a while. Everyone ends up healthier!

A feature writer once asked some youngsters *why* they attended a camp for those with diabetes. "Wouldn't it be more fun to go to a camp that doesn't focus on diabetes?" The unanimous response was quite startling to the questioner. "No, we love it. It is the only time in our lives when *we* are the normals and those without diabetes are the outsiders!"

Sports of all types are encouraged for youngsters with diabetes. The coaches and teammates should know of the possibility of insulin reactions, but with simple precautions and increased food on the days of strenuous activity, virtually no sport should be an impossibility to a physically capable youngster with diabetes.

All Our Goals

The goal of treatment of diabetes in young people is the same as that for all people with diabetes: to achieve blood glucose levels as close to normal as possible, safely and practically, while allowing a life-style that is as free of restrictions as possible. A child must grow, both physically and emotionally, and it is important that diabetes not prove too great an obstacle. There are challenges that need to be met, but they *can* be overcome, and many young people with diabetes enter adulthood with bright futures and great potential.

In summary, the child has the diabetes and will have to live with it the rest of his or her life. Let your child learn how to do it. Help with love and understanding. Don't do all the thinking for your child. Parents and youngsters and all the family must work together. This is one place where group function is vital.

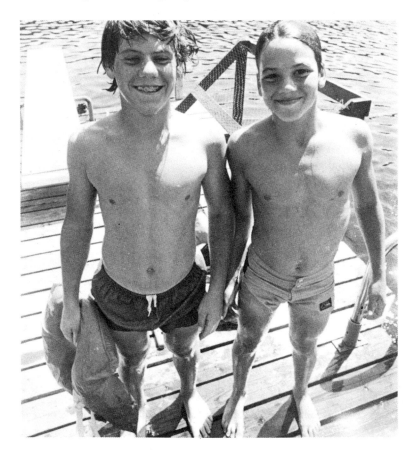

An important thing to keep in mind is that there is an increasing number, probably in the thousands, who have had diabetes for more than 50 years since they first got it. Almost all have type I, the so-called juvenile-onset diabetes, and require insulin. The outlook is better than it has ever been before . . . and research and education are improving.

13

Pregnancy and Diabetes

The tremendous progress made over the last 30 years in treating pregnant women with diabetes is one of the great success stories in the history of diabetes! Nevertheless, diabetes does make pregnancy more difficult, and one should start planning before conception. Certainly, throughout the pregnancy, careful attention to both the diabetes of the pregnant mother and the health of the growing child is crucial.

Pregnancy for women with diabetes was once a great threat to health and well-being. In the preinsulin era the experience of pregnant women with diabetes at the Joslin Clinic was considered "modestly successful," with a survival of 65% of the mothers and 40% of the infants. When insulin became available in the early 1920s, a dramatic improvement was seen in the survival of the mothers (Table 13–1). Today, with ideal care, the maternal death rate is the same as that of the general population. Although maternal death does occur, it is very rare, and infant mortality has also declined. Infant survival in experienced diabetes pregnancy centers is almost 98%. The sudden tragedy of the "unexplained" stillbirth is now infrequent, although, as in the general population, it does occur.

Nevertheless, problems do still exist and every woman with diabetes planning pregnancy must be aware of the potential difficulties. Infants of diabetic mothers can still have serious difficulties at the time of birth and often require specialized management by an obstetrician who deals with high-risk cases and by a neonatologist (a specialist in the care of newborns) in a newborn intensive care unit of a medical center. It is the special equipment and the highly experienced team of personnel that make the difference between life and death for these infants. There are also increased risks of birth defects ("anomalies") in infants of mothers with diabetes as well. Defects can affect many different organs, but those affecting the heart and skeletal systems are the most frequent. With proper diabetes control, however, the frequency of these defects is not much greater than among the general population. It is obvious, therefore, that pregnancy in women with diabetes still requires special care and attention, and successful outcomes cannot be taken for granted.

It is the very careful treatment of diabetes in preparation for conception and through the first 12 weeks that lowers the number of major birth defects. The glycosylated hemoglobin (Chapter 8) determines the adequacy of diabetes treatment. This measure of control has helped centers such as the Joslin Diabetes Center and the Brigham and Women's Hospital in Boston, Massachusetts, and others achieve control good enough to reduce these birth defects.

Many of the needs of good diabetes care as discussed in other chapters apply to women before and during pregnancy. Other chapters in this book that are relevant to an expectant mother's diabetes should be reviewed in addition to this chapter. This chapter focuses on the changes that occur in the body during pregnancy and on how diabetes can affect these changes. There is a lot going on during pregnancy—and a lot that can go wrong. Despite the complexity of pregnancy, though, it is truly a miracle that all of the things necessary for pregnancy usually proceed properly. You are a very important person in helping this miracle take place!

TABLE 13–1. Improvements over the Years in the Survival of Mothers with Diabetes and Their Infants at the Joslin Clinic

Dates	Viable Pregnancies*	Percent of Babies That Survived*	Percent of Mothers That Survived
1898–1915	10	40%	67%
1924–1938	128	54%	>99%
1939–1958	900	86%	>99%
1959–1974	1119	90%	>99%
1975–1976	147	97%	100%
1977–1979	201	98%	100%
1980–	Data being collected: survival still improving!		

*All pregnancies that reached 28 weeks for the years up to 1974, and 24 weeks since 1974.

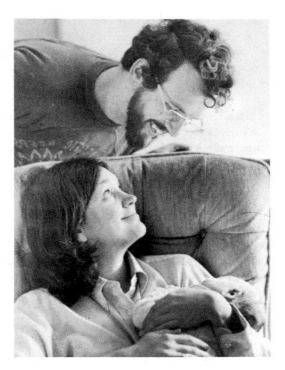

How Is Pregnancy with Diabetes Different?

Glucose provides most of the energy that the body needs to function. This is true for everyone. If nonpregnant people do not have enough glucose available to meet their needs—either because they have not eaten or because they have diabetes and have not taken enough insulin—their bodies utilize alternative sources of energy. Fat is the major alternative source of energy. Protein can also provide energy. While nonpregnant people can use either of these fuels, pregnant women are more likely to burn fat as an alternative fuel when the glucose supply is insufficient or unavailable due to poor diabetes control. Protein is conserved to be used for the growth of the fetus.

The presence of ideal amounts of insulin allows the body to use glucose as efficiently as possible, minimizes the amount of fat that is used as fuel, and helps replace the fat when it is used. This is important to prevent ketoacidosis. With insufficient insulin supplies, this balance cannot be maintained. A key difference between pregnancy in women with and without diabetes, is the increased chance of developing ketoacidosis in the woman with diabetes. The biochemical and hormonal changes of pregnancy predispose the pregnant woman with diabetes to a much more rapid onset of more severe ketoacidosis, even when the symptoms may seem to be mild.

All pregnant women require more insulin than nonpregnant women. People without diabetes can usually produce this additional insulin without any difficulty. However, some women with no previous evidence of diabetes may have higher blood glucose levels during pregnancy. The insulin-producing beta cells in their pancreases, which formerly had been able to supply enough insulin, cannot maintain the increasing insulin needs of pregnancy. This condition is called "gestational diabetes."

Women who require insulin before pregnancy will usually need much more insulin (often 1½ to 3 times as much) by the time they are close to delivery. In addition, the diet must contain more calories, including increased carbohydrate and protein to provide for the needs of both mother and fetus. The balance of insulin, food, and activity may need many readjustments during pregnancy!

Gestational Diabetes

Elevated blood glucose levels are found in 1 to 2% of pregnant women, but of these, only 1 in 10 are known to have diabetes before pregnancy. Thus most patients with diabetes during pregnancy discovered it during the course of the pregnancy itself.

Gestational diabetes is more likely to occur in women with other diabetic family members and who themselves are overweight, over age 30, occasionally show urine glucose, or have had some previous, even slightly, elevated blood glucose levels. A previous pregnancy with complications suggestive of maternal diabetes is associated with an increased likelihood of developing diabetes during the current pregnancy.

If any of the factors associated with maternal diabetes is present, a glucose tolerance test (GTT) (discussed in Chapter 1) may establish the diagnosis of "gestational diabetes." (Specific criteria for the GTT in pregnancy are given in Table 13–2.) The tendency of pregnancy to make diabetes appear increases from the first trimester (the first three months of pregnancy) to the second and third trimesters. Therefore, if diabetes is suspected early in pregnancy but the GTT is normal, it may be necessary to repeat this test later. Recently it has been recommended that all pregnant women without diabetes be screened at about 24 to 28 weeks gestation with a shorter form of the glucose tolerance test known as the glucose load test (GLT), to be followed by a full GTT if needed.

It is increasingly evident that precise control of blood glucose levels during pregnancy reduces the chances that the infant will show signs of diabetic complications. For this reason even the mildest gestational diabetes is treated aggressively. Insulin treatment is often recommended, although most women who develop gestational diabetes do not require it after delivery. For those who need continued treatment, it is likely that they had been in early stages of diabetes anyway, and the pregnancy just made it obvious. Testing before pregnancy might have shown early diabetes in these women. Women with gestational diabetes not needing treatment after delivery may develop diabetes later. It is important for them to inform their physicians about the gestational diabetes so that they can be correctly followed.

Effects of Pregnancy on Diabetes

Young women with diabetes planning pregnancy ask whether pregnancy will worsen their diabetes or its complications. To answer this question, any complications that are already present must be carefully evaluated, before conception. A thorough review with appropriate physicians is needed.

Before retirement, Dr. Priscilla White was a pioneer in the care of women with diabetes, both generally and during their pregnancies. Early in her career, Dr. White recognized certain factors that increased the risk to the pregnancy. If diabetes had been diagnosed many years before the pregnancy, if it was diagnosed when the woman was very young, or if vascular (circulatory) complications

TABLE 13–2. Glucose Tolerance Test in Pregnancy (upper limits of the normal range)

Time	Venous Whole Blood (mg%)	Venous Plasma (mg%)
Fasting	90	105
1 hour after eating	165	190
2 hours after eating	145	165
3 hours after eating	125	145

were already present at the time of pregnancy, there was a greater likelihood of a complicated pregnancy and of having a baby born with problems. The risks were less if the diabetes had been diagnosed recently, at a more mature age, and without evidence of vascular disease.

To help other physicians and their patients recognize the importance of these predictive factors of the outcome of these pregnancies, she developed risk categories, now known worldwide as the White classification (Appendix 6). This classification was first formally used in about 1948. It was later modified by Dr. White and more recently in association with Dr. John Hare to include gestational diabetes.

With better care, this classification of patients has been less necessary, but a general awareness of these risk factors is helpful in planning the course of your next pregnancy with your health care team.

The insulin doses and food required to control diabetes will change during pregnancy, but after the pregnancy, the treatment program becomes similar to that used before pregnancy. The overall health of the mother usually returns to about what it was before she became pregnant. Any increase in complications usually return to a level that might have been expected had the complication progressed anyway, without pregnancy. However, there are a few conditions requiring special attention because even temporary worsening may be dangerous.

Retinopathy, the changes in the inside of the eyes, is one of these conditions. If this complication has reached the stage known as "neovascularization" (formation of new, undesired blood vessels on the retina), rapid deterioration in eyesight may occur. Because pregnancy may speed up the eye changes in diabetes and because these changes can result in permanent vision loss, pregnancy should be postponed if these changes are present. Neovascularization that has been successfully treated with laser therapy and has stabilized is much less likely to worsen during pregnancy. "Background" retinopathy, an earlier form of retinopathy with less risk of visual loss, may progress somewhat during pregnancy, but not usually to a threatening stage.

Because it is so important to know what the condition of the retina of the eye is at the beginning of pregnancy, the woman with diabetes who is considering pregnancy should be evaluated by an ophthalmologist (particularly one experienced in diagnosing and treating diseases of the retina), preferably before conception. This physician can determine if the diabetic retinopathy is in a particularly vulnerable stage and may advise postponement of pregnancy to avoid more severe damage. While even the most skilled physicians are unable to predict with certainty what will happen to each individual, close attention to these details can reduce the chance of problems. We also recommend that consultations with the ophthalmologist should continue during pregnancy. If the condition of the eyes worsens, the close observation will allow these changes to be found early and treated without delay. As with other complications, the eye changes during pregnancy may improve gradually after delivery.

Kidney function needs to be considered in preparation for, and during, pregnancy. If the kidneys function well before pregnancy, then it is likely that they will continue to do so. If, however, protein is being lost in the urine (over 400 mg of protein in a 24-hour urine collection) before conception, even with normal filtering ability, pregnancy may cause this protein loss to increase, accompanied by symptoms such as high blood pressure (hypertension) and fluid retention (edema). If this occurs, prolonged bed rest at home or in a hospital may be necessary. If kidney function is more seriously affected by the diabetes before pregnancy, with an actual reduction in filtering capacity, it may become worse during the pregnancy, and great caution and care must be taken. Your physician can give you a good idea how well your kidneys are working by performing simple examinations of collected urine.

Even with good diabetes control, *neuropathy* (nerve damage or irritation due to diabetes) may worsen during pregnancy, perhaps causing some foot and leg tingling, numbness, or discomfort. Diabetic neuropathy frequently occurs unpredictably, but does not usually occur just because of pregnancy itself.

Managing Diabetes and Pregnancy

The Joslin Clinic has, for a long period, believed in this team approach to care of pregnancy. The team is made up of a diabetes specialist, an obstetrician expert in high-risk pregnancies (called a perinatologist), a diabetes nurse-educator, a nutritionist, and a social worker. Another person who should be available is a neonatologist, a specialist in the care of newborn infants, to minimize difficulties that the child may have around the time of delivery.

You, the pregnant woman with diabetes, are the center of this health care. Your participation is the key to success. When a health care team is not available, active coordination between an internist, obstetrician, and pediatrician can be arranged.

Preparing for Pregnancy. The best way to insure the proper health and development of the fetus is to make certain that the diabetes control is as good as humanly possible, even before conception. You should plan for pregnancy with your diabetes health care team by getting your diabetes into the best control possible before contraception is discontinued. This control should be documented monthly by favorable glycohemoglobin results.

The decision whether to become pregnant is yours. However, to make an intelligent decision, you need all the facts so that you can increase the chances of good health for you and your baby. You should also be aware of the early warning signals of problems so that you will know when to seek help.

Managing Your Pregnancy. It cannot be emphasized enough that management during pregnancy requires coordination between the people caring for your diabetes and the people caring for your pregnancy. The better this coordination is between all concerned persons, the less likely it is that there will be difficulty.

The first three months (the first trimester) are critical to the fetus. It is during this time that the basic body structures begin to form. Uncontrolled diabetes at this time is associated with major structural abnormalities in the fetus. Careful monitoring of both diabetes and obstetrical progress are most vital during this period.

Amniocentesis is a test in which a small amount of the amniotic fluid—the fluid that surrounds the fetus within the uterus—is obtained via a syringe and needle. This may be performed early in the second trimester to look for evidence of any chromosomal abnormalities that might affect the health of the child if the pregnancy is continued. This is usually called a "genetic amniocentesis," and it allows the examination of the baby's chromosomes. Amniocentesis is more likely to be recommended if the mother will be 35 years old by the time the baby is born. The frequency of babies born with Down's syndrome (mongolism) increases with the age of the mother. By the age of 35, the chances of this happening due to a detectable change in chromosomes is high enough to warrant the risks of this test. The risk, although slight, is that the test could start a spontaneous abortion.

Of course, you should notify your obstetrician of any inherited abnormalities that may run in the family of either parent. Some, but not all, of these conditions can be detected by an amniocentesis. In addition, this test may be recommended if evidence of other problems is discovered by other screening tests performed during pregnancy. You should review the reasons for having amniocentesis, including your family history, with your obstetrician so that you can make an informed choice about whether to have the test done.

The Course of Pregnancy. During the first trimester, a full assessment of diabetes and its complications must be completed if it was not done prior to conception. Diet should be adjusted for pregnancy requirements. Iron and vitamin supplements are often started. Close and frequent monitoring of blood pressure, weight, and the eyes (retina) is important. Diabetes management must be as perfect as possible. Frequently, insulin doses will be decreased a little at first because of nausea and vomiting ("morning sickness"), which may make the treatment of diabetes more difficult. Weekly visits to the diabetes/obstetrical team often begin as soon as the diagnosis of pregnancy is made.

The monitoring and intensive care continue in the second trimester. For many women, the diabetes tends to become more stable than in the first trimester, although the insulin dose may increase. It is necessary to watch closely for increases in blood pressure, edema (fluid retention), or decreases in kidney function. These symptoms and signs can be worrisome and may need to be treated with prolonged bed rest. Obstetrical observation continues during this second trimester. An ultrasound examination of the fetus may be performed between week 16 and week 20 and other tests of fetal health may be performed as well.

Weekly monitoring continues through the third trimester. For many women, the diabetes remains relatively stable, although the insulin dose often increases more rapidly until weeks 34 to 36. Although some women will remain at the insulin dose that they used prior to pregnancy, many will need two to three times as much insulin as before. For some, the proportion of (ratio between) regular and NPH or Lente insulins will change. Insulin adjustments vary from person to person; the goal is good control, regardless of the insulin dose that is needed. Often, toward the last few weeks of pregnancy, the amount of insulin needed begins to decline.

During the third trimester, any sign of edema, hypertension, or declining kidney function would be of concern. Ultrasound examinations are performed periodically, and fetal heart monitoring is done with increasing frequency. Additional testing will be performed during your pregnancy in accordance with usual prenatal practices as well as special individual needs. For example, testing for blood type is routine. In your particular case, your doctor may want to measure your thyroid function or check on other measurements if it is important to you and your baby. Your hemoglobin level may be checked regularly to make sure that you are not anemic.

Anemia is a common problem during pregnancy, and treatment with iron supplements may become necessary.

Urine cultures are frequently performed to make certain there is no urinary tract infection. These infections occur commonly and may not produce noticeable symptoms in some women. Approximately 5% of pregnant women have bacteria growing in their urine at the time of their first visit for pregnancy care, and antibiotic treatment is often needed. Some studies suggest that infections occur more frequently in women with diabetes. Urinary tract infections can affect diabetes control, and therefore the urine must be checked frequently. Certainly if you develop fever or urinary burning or urgency, you should contact the doctor at once. Sometimes it is difficult to tell the symptoms of urinary infection from the simple pressure of the fetus on the bladder.

Monitoring Diabetes during Pregnancy. Throughout pregnancy, the goal of diabetes treatment is to achieve blood glucose control as close to normal as possible. Of course, "close to normal" may vary from person to person, but ideally the goal of treatment is a fasting capillary (finger-stick) blood glucose level of 60 to 100 mg% and a level 2 hours after eating of 100 to 150 mg%. To achieve this, it may be necessary to test the blood at home at least four times daily: fasting (before breakfast), and 2 hours after breakfast, lunch, and dinner. Urine testing is not good enough, as the renal threshold tends to be lower in pregnancy, and urine test results can be confusing. Before adjusting insulin doses, consider all other possible explanations for the changes in blood glucose levels—for example, eating, timing of the insulin dose in relation to meals, or variation in physical activity.

Guidelines for adjusting insulin doses (discussed in Chapters 9 and 10) are generally useful for pregnant women, but changes adjusting for postmeal glucose values are listed in Tables 13–3 A through D. Usually the same insulin types as used before pregnancy can be used during pregnancy.

With growing evidence that precise control is especially important just before and during pregnancy, many women decide to use more intensive therapy during this period. Some choose to use one of the insulin infusion pumps (Chapter 10). The same reasons and criteria that other people with diabetes have for using an insulin pump apply to pregnant women. At one time it was more common to start pump therapy at the beginning of pregnancy to achieve the tightest possible control. However, it took too long to establish excellent control with these devices during the first trimester—the most critical for the development of the fetus. Control, measured by

TABLES 13-3. A through *E.* Insulin Adjustment in Pregnant Women

HOW TO USE THESE INSULIN ADJUSTMENT GUIDELINES FOR PREGNANT WOMEN

Daily insulin doses are determined by various factors and can vary for many reasons. The use of insulin, as outlined in Chapters 9 and 10, is relevant to women who are pregnant as well. The adjustment rules listed here are designed specifically for the pregnant woman. However, as with any set of general guidelines, you should discuss them with your physicians to determine how they might apply to you. A careful review of Chapters 7 through 10 is advised.

The goals of insulin therapy of pregnant women with diabetes are outlined in the text. However, actual goals for a given individual should be determined after discussion with your physician about the use of these adjustment rules. For the purposes of these tables, therefore, we refer to glucose levels above the determined goals as being "high" rather than giving specific glucose levels.

The insulins most commonly used, and for which these guidelines apply, are regular (clear) insulin (short-acting) and NPH and Lente (cloudy) insulins (intermediate-acting).

The use of these tables is similar to the use of Tables 9-2 A through *E*:

1. If two or more of the tests you do at the various times each day are high for two consecutive days, adjust first the insulin dose that affects the presupper test.
2. Do not adjust more than one dose or type of insulin at a time unless directed to do so by your physician.
3. When a dose is increased, the blood glucose level at the next test time should be lower. The insulin that now begins to act over this next time period is starting off at a *lower* glucose level. *Beware!* Because the glucose level is lower to start, this dose may now be too great and lead to a hypoglycemic reaction. Therefore . . .
4. If there is concern, the insulin that acts over this second subsequent time period should be reduced slightly until the full effect of the increased previous dose can be assessed.
5. After making an insulin dose adjustment, wait two days for the tests to improve. If no improvement is noted, make the same adjustment a second time.
6. If you have any difficulty with adjustments, get help from your health care professional.

TABLE 13-3A. Present Dose: INTERMEDIATE insulin given before breakfast.

If Tests are Poor 2 Days in a Row	Do This:
BEFORE BREAKFAST OR BEFORE TAKING INSULIN	Notify your physician. You may need some evening intermediate insulin.
TWO HOURS AFTER BREAKFAST	Notify your physician. You may need short-acting insulin with the intermediate insulin.
TWO HOURS AFTER LUNCH	Increase the intermediate insulin by 2 units the next morning.
TWO HOURS AFTER SUPPER	Increase the intermediate insulin by 2 units the next morning.

**TABLE 13–3B. Present Dose: REGULAR and INTERME-
DIATE insulin given before breakfast.**

If Tests are Poor 2 Days in a Row	Do This:
BEFORE TAKING INSULIN OR EATING IN THE MORNING	Notify your physician. You may need an evening dose of intermediate-acting insulin.
TWO HOURS AFTER BREAKFAST	Increase the amount of short-acting insulin by 1 to 2 units the next morning.
TWO HOURS AFTER LUNCH	Increase the amount of intermediate-acting insulin by 2 units the next morning.
TWO HOURS AFTER SUPPER	Increase the amount of intermediate-acting insulin by 2 units the next morning.

**TABLE 13–3C. Present Dose: INTERMEDIATE insulin
given before breakfast and in the evening.**

If Tests are Poor 2 Days in a Row	Do This:
TWO HOURS AFTER LUNCH	Increase the amount of intermediate-acting insulin by 2 units the next morning.
TWO HOURS AFTER SUPPER	Increase the amount of intermediate-acting insulin by 2 units the next morning.
BEFORE TAKING INSULIN OR EATING IN THE MORNING	Increase the amount of intermediate-acting insulin by 2 units in the next evening dose.
AFTER BREAKFAST	Notify your physician. You may need some short-acting insulin.

TABLE 13–3D. Present Dose: REGULAR and INTERME-DIATE insulin given before breakfast and INTERMEDIATE insulin given before supper or bedtime.

If Tests are Poor 2 Days in a Row	Do This:
BEFORE TAKING INSULIN OR EATING IN THE MORNING	Increase the amount of intermediate-acting insulin by 2 units in the evening.
TWO HOURS AFTER BREAKFAST	Increase the amount of short-acting insulin by 1 to 2 units the next morning.
TWO HOURS AFTER LUNCH	Increase the amount of intermediate-acting insulin by 2 units the next morning.
TWO HOURS AFTER SUPPER	Notify your physician. You may need an evening dose of short-acting insulin.

TABLE 13–3E. Present Dose: REGULAR and INTERME-DIATE insulin given before breakfast and before supper.

If Tests are Poor 2 Days in a Row	Do This:
BEFORE TAKING INSULIN OR EATING IN THE MORNING	Increase the amount of intermediate-acting insulin by 2 units in the evening.
TWO HOURS AFTER BREAKFAST	Increase the amount of short-acting insulin by 1 to 2 units the next morning.
TWO HOURS AFTER LUNCH	Increase the amount of intermediate-acting insulin by 2 units the next morning.
TWO HOURS AFTER SUPPER	Increase the amount of short-acting insulin by 1 to 2 units the next evening before supper.

glycohemoglobin, did not improve substantially more with pump therapy than with multiple injection therapy, and therefore pump use has decreased somewhat in favor of multiple injection programs.

Monitoring urine ketones is also important because the risk of getting ketoacidosis is greater during pregnancy. Ketoacidosis can be dangerous to a fetus. You should check for ketones each morning before taking insulin or eating. If ketones are present for two days in a row, but with normal or close to normal blood glucose levels, you should call your physician or other health care team members. The cause could be low blood glucose reactions during the night, and an additional or a larger nighttime snack may be needed. You must monitor for ketones on days that you feel well if your blood glucose level is above 240 mg%, and call your physician if ketones are greater than "trace." Of course, it is even more important to monitor for ketones on days when you are ill, even if the illness is minor, such as a common cold, upset stomach, flu, or diarrhea. Chapter 8, Monitoring Your Diabetes, should be reviewed carefully by any pregnant woman with diabetes.

Monitoring Fetal Development. Certain tests are performed during pregnancy to make sure that the baby is developing properly.

The *alpha-fetoprotein blood test*, performed at about the sixteenth week of pregnancy, tests for possible defects in the covering of the baby's brain or spinal cord. An *ultrasound* test may also be advised on occasion. This test uses sound waves which pass through the mother and fetus and are bounced back to a microphone-type pickup device or sound probe, which then translates these returning impulses into a picture image on a screen. With this device it is possible to see images of your baby and the surrounding organs and structures. This instrument works as sonar works on ships, whereby an image of an underwater object can be pictured quite accurately. This test does not use x-rays, which may be harmful to a developing fetus. At the Joslin Diabetes Center, the ultrasound is usually first performed at week 16 or 18 and is used to estimate the expected delivery date. It is usually repeated between weeks 26 and 28 and again near the time of delivery to be sure that the baby is growing properly and to determine the baby's weight and size. The size is important in determining whether the baby can be delivered normally or if a cesarean delivery might be necessary.

A *nonstress test*, done weekly from week 32 and twice weekly after week 36, measures the heart rate of the baby as it changes with movement. This test also uses a sound pickup device, but it is different from the one used for the ultrasound. This is often the first opportunity for the new child to exhibit contrariness, as many a fetus has decided to take a nap just as you get the equipment ready and want movement! Of course, these babies can hear, even while in the uterus. Although it may not sound very scientific, banging on pots and pans is sometimes used to wake up the sleeping fetus. Some babies still do not respond to this "alarm clock" and keep right on sleeping. On such occasions, a small amount of medication (oxytocin) can be given to the mother to cause a small uterine contraction, and observations can then be made on how the baby responds to this change in the environment. This is called the *oxytocin challenge test* or *stress test.*

Fetal monitoring tests have been one of the great advances in the last decade. Along with other data, these tests have made it possible to gauge accurately when the delivery time will arrive. An amniocentesis may again be performed as the pregnancy nears term, this time to check the maturity of the baby's lungs. The higher the "test scores," the more mature the lungs are and the less likely the baby will have breathing difficulty at birth. As your pregnancy approaches the delivery date, the obstetrical team watches your progress closely and determines which of these tests need to be done and how often to do them.

Obstetrical Complications. Pregnancy and childbearing are exciting—parents-to-be are filled with expectations of the arrival of a new family member. The dedication and extra work by the pregnant woman and her family enhances the joy of a happy outcome. However, there are potential complications of pregnancy that cause some anxiety. These can occur in any pregnant woman, but they are more common in pregnant women with diabetes. Some are serious, others not. For women with diabetes, the goal is to reduce the chances of serious complications. Pregnancy is *not* the time to ignore anything or to play ostrich, with your head in the sand. Pay attention to anything that does not seem to be correct. Seek help early, rather than delaying it until serious problems have developed.

Diabetic ketoacidosis (DKA) is a serious complication for anyone with diabetes, but it is even more dangerous for a pregnant woman and the fetus. Careful self monitoring of blood glucose is a must! *Spontaneous abortions* are no more common with diabetes than in the overall population, but they do occur. If a spontaneous abortion does occur, there is usually no reason why a later pregnancy should not be successful.

Urinary tract infections are more common during pregnancy

because urinary tract drainage is slowed by the enlarging uterus. These infections may be symptomless, so the urine should be checked frequently. Certainly, if you do have symptoms of discomfort with urination, seek care at once.

Preeclampsia is a condition of elevated blood pressure, protein in the urine, and edema (fluid retention) formation during pregnancy. It can progress to *eclampsia,* which involves seizures. Preeclampsia differs from the edema and hypertension seen in patients with diabetic kidney damage (nephropathy). However, preeclampsia can occur in someone with preexisting kidney damage, and the effects of these factors may be difficult to differentiate. Preeclampsia and eclampsia still occur more often in women with diabetes than in the general population. Treatment is aimed at preventing eclampsia by diagnosing preeclampsia early and instituting treatment, which includes bed rest at home, or hospitalization if the blood pressure remains high.

Polyhydramnios is the accumulation of an excess amount of the amniotic fluid that normally surrounds the fetus during pregnancy. This can increase the pressure in the uterus and on the fetus and can cause premature labor and early delivery. This complication occurs in about one-third of pregnancies in women with diabetes. It also can occur with twins.

One of the most painful tragedies, which is now very rare, is that of *stillbirth.* Just when everything seems to be going well, an examination fails to find the heartbeat and no fetal motion is detected. Further examination will show that the fetus is no longer alive. What can be most stunning is that, when such a tragedy occurs, the baby is often found to be perfectly formed. The parents, of course, are crushed. "How could this happen? What went wrong? Why? Why didn't any of the tests pick up a problem? I did everything they told me to do no matter how difficult it was, and nobody can explain to me what happened."

Unfortunately, despite many theories, there is no good explanation for a stillbirth when it does happen. We can just be grateful that modern medical/obstetrical practices have reduced the frequency of this so-called classical accident of the diabetic pregnancy. Stillbirth is not related to the severity or duration of diabetes because it can also occur in women with gestational diabetes or even those without diabetes. The nonstress testing of the fetal heart rate is one of the main tools that has allowed better assessment of fetal health during the last weeks of pregnancy and has reduced the frequency of this complication.

Diet

"You are what you eat!" "You are eating for two!" Old, trite phrases, but as true today as ever, and especially for women with diabetes. During pregnancy, as with all diabetes treatment, diet cannot be overemphasized.

Weight. It is expected that an average-sized woman will gain 24 to 28 pounds during pregnancy. Overweight women are advised to gain less weight during this time (15 to 24 pounds), while underweight women may gain more (28 to 32 pounds). The weight gain is needed to ensure that there is enough food to provide sufficient nutrients for the developing fetus. In addition, it is important to supply enough carbohydrate so that fat is not used up for energy, resulting in ketone production.

About half of the weight gain during pregnancy is due to changes in the mother's body and the growth of tissues which support the growth of the baby. This includes an increase in the blood volume, breast size, and fat stores. The other half of the weight gain is the baby, the placenta, and the amniotic fluid.

The rate of weight gain varies over the course of pregnancy. It is expected that only about 3 pounds will be gained over the first trimester (up to week 13). During the second and third trimesters, one-half to one pound per week is expected. While some variation in this pattern may occur, gradual weight gain is ideal, with no dramatic increases or plateaus. Weight loss during pregnancy needs to be evaluated and treated energetically. Your weight gain is monitored frequently during pregnancy.

The Eating Plan. Regardless of the eating plan followed before pregnancy, you should meet early during the pregnancy with a dietitian skilled in nutrition for pregnant women with diabetes. Together you will develop the eating plan for the first trimester of pregnancy. At the beginning of the second trimester, this plan may need changes to meet the increasing needs of the growing baby.

These eating plans are based on the same principles as for anyone with diabetes (Chapter 4), except that during pregnancy, calories, minerals such as calcium and iron, and sufficient vitamins must be provided. Supplements (especially iron, folic acid, and calcium) are often recommended.

In addition, between-meal snacks are especially important during pregnancy. In all pregnant women, there is an increased rate of metabolism and some insulin resistance. The result of these changes

> **TABLE 13-4. When to Contact Your Dietitian during Pregnancy**
>
> YOU SHOULD CONTACT YOUR DIETITIAN (OR PHYSICIAN) FOR A REVIEW OF YOUR EATING PROGRAM IF YOU NOTICE ANY OF THE FOLLOWING:
> 1. KETONES are present in your urine when your blood glucose level is within or near the normal range. This may indicate you are not eating enough food and particularly that you may need a larger evening snack.
> 2. WEIGHT LOSS. This may indicate that you are not eating enough food.
> 3. INADEQUATE WEIGHT GAIN (2 pounds or less per month during the second and third trimester or no weight gain in 3 weeks). This may indicate that you are not eating enough food.
> 4. EXCESSIVE WEIGHT GAIN (more than 1 pound per month in the first trimester and thereafter 7 pounds or more per month or more than 2 pounds per week). This may indicate that you are eating too much food or that your body is retaining fluid.
> 5. WIDELY FLUCTUATING BLOOD GLUCOSE LEVELS. This may indicate that you are eating too much food during certain times of the day. (You should be sure to contact your physician for this problem in particular.)

is that the blood glucose levels rise more rapidly after eating, reach a higher peak, and then drop more rapidly to lower blood glucose levels before the next meal. As a result, a larger proportion of insulin tends to be given as premeal regular (rapid-acting) insulin and proportionately less insulin is given as intermediate insulin (NPH or Lente). This heavier emphasis on regular insulin helps to keep the glucose levels down between meals. However, snacks may become more important to prevent the low blood glucose levels that can occur as the regular insulin peaks later after the meal.

Proper nutrition is so important that problems with eating should be dealt with at once. Notify your physician or dietitian if any of the conditions shown in Table 13-4 are noted.

Delivery

For many years, the babies of women with diabetes used to be delivered as early as 4 to 6 weeks ahead of their due date. As stillbirth was a major complication of pregnancy in women with diabetes, early delivery was induced to lower the risk to the fetus during the last weeks of pregnancy. With modern techniques of care and monitoring, the risk is small enough that now hospitalization for uncomplicated pregnancies can be delayed until between the thirty-sixth and thirty-eighth weeks. Delivery often occurs at the thirty-eighth or thirty-ninth week, or even at full term (40 weeks).

By the thirty-eighth week most babies are mature enough to deliver, and preparations can be made. To confirm proper maturity, an amniocentesis may be performed, which helps determine the maturity of the baby's lungs. The size of the baby is determined with ultrasound. The size determines in part whether the baby will be delivered vaginally or by cesarean section. Infants of diabetic mothers traditionally have been larger than those born to women without diabetes. This large size is called *macrosomia*, and it carries with it health problems for the child, including an increased need for a cesarean delivery and a greater chance of birth trauma. Cesarean deliveries are needed in about half of all pregnant women with diabetes. They are also recommended in women with certain stages of diabetic retinopathy, since "bearing down" during delivery can increase pressure on the eye vessels, which may cause them to rupture.

After the baby is born, it is often cared for in the newborn intensive care unit of the hospital to monitor for any lurking problems. If an infant is delivered too early and the lungs are not mature, breathing difficulties ("respiratory distress") can develop. A respirator may be used until the lungs improve enough for the baby to breathe alone. Infants of mothers with diabetes can also develop hypoglycemia (low blood glucose) at or shortly after birth. If the baby has been exposed to high blood glucose levels from the mother's blood while in the uterus, these stimulate insulin production by the infant's pancreas. After birth, this insulin is still being released by the baby's pancreas and may cause a drop in the blood glucose levels. Prompt treatment with glucose corrects this, but treatment may need to be repeated during the first 12 to 24 hours of life. Sometimes even longer treatment is needed.

Other unusual metabolic abnormalities occasionally occur. These include low calcium (which can cause the baby to be jittery) and a high bilirubin level. Bilirubin is a chemical substance that is produced in the liver and, when present in increased amounts, can cause a yellow appearance (jaundice). These metabolic abnormalities are most often self-limited and can be treated in most instances.

As soon as the baby is born, the mother's insulin requirements drop significantly. The dose of insulin required is often less than it was before pregnancy for anywhere from a day to about a week. However, as the mother readjusts and returns to normal, insulin requirements usually return to prepregnancy ranges.

Breast-Feeding (Nursing)

Breast-feeding (nursing) or bottle feeding is a choice the mother makes after considering the advice of her obstetrician and pediatrician. Breast-feeding does not cause significant problems in treating the mother's diabetes. Most pediatricians recommend breast-feeding, and diabetes does not interfere with this normal maternal function.

Women with diabetes who are planning to breast-feed their child should remember that doing so may cause their insulin requirements to be reduced. If you decide to nurse, you should watch out for low blood glucose levels and discuss insulin adjustments with your physician in advance. Frequently, an increase in diet (about 300 more calories per day) is suggested, but this varies from person to person. Snacks before nursing may be needed to prevent hypoglycemia. An adequate calcium intake is also important. In addition, some women with diabetes have a greater chance of developing mastitis (breast infection) than those without diabetes. If any inflammation or soreness is noted, the physician should be contacted.

Pregnancy, Diabetes, and Life

As recently as the 1960s, it was assumed that if you were pregnant, you were in your early to mid-twenties and married. In this modern age, people begin or add to a family under many possible circumstances. Whatever the situation, your stability is important. Perhaps you are a single parent. Or perhaps your new baby will be joining children of a previous marriage. There are teenage mothers on the one hand and mothers in their late thirties or even early forties on the other. The possibilities are many, and each brings specific worries and problems to deal with. Whichever group you are in, no one of them is free from worry during the 9 months of pregnancy, although oftentimes women in one group think they might be better off if they were in one of the other situations. A married woman who is having trouble with her husband might wish she were on her own. The single parent might tend to be jealous of the seemingly easy path of the married couple. Each group has its strengths—and its hurdles.

In addition to the specific kind of relationship (or lack of one) with the father of the baby, you and every other woman come to a pregnancy with your own particular history. Your story has its own unique particulars: just completing high school or finishing your Ph.D., supportive family or no support at all, three children already or pregnant with your first, diabetes for 1 month or diabetes for 20 years, obstetrical problems in the past, or smooth sailing with past pregnancies, a history of psychological upheavals or a history of handling stress well in the past. **You are unique,** and you come to pregnancy with a varied background and approach it from a slightly different direction than anyone else. It is therefore unlikely that you will experience the emotional aspects of pregnancy in exactly the same way as any other woman.

Yet what is common to you and to all women experiencing pregnancy is the anxiety or apprehension that you face during certain times within this exciting period. The reason is that all of you have the same goal: being a healthy mother with a healthy baby. These intensely powerful wishes have many ramifications. The amount of work and flexibility that go into a pregnancy can be astounding. Most women convince employers to permit time off to attend clinic appointments. Most work hard to keep their diabetes in the best possible control. Most actively participate in and become knowledgeable about caring for themselves in ways that women without diabetes do not need to do. If they are hospitalized during or toward the end of pregnancy, they permit the upheaval to occur, knowing that it is not easy to leave a family at a time when they are most necessary.

The particular sacrifices required often result in strong friendships with other pregnant women in the diabetes clinic. Moreover, with frequent visits, strong relationships may develop with one or more of the physicians. These relationships, and other relationships that developed outside of the health care environment, are ones that can be relied on during particularly stressful times.

You should be encouraged to ask any questions you may have about yourself or the pregnancy. The various members of the team—the internist, the obstetrician, the dietitian, the nurse-educator—all have their various areas of expertise and all will be able to help in answering your many questions.

If your support system is not working quite the way you want it to, or if you are finding it difficult to talk about vague or specific worries, you may also want to speak with a mental health professional (psychiatrist, psychologist, or social worker). At the Joslin Diabetes Center, for example, it is common for a social worker to work with the pregnant woman and her family to help smooth out the rough edges. Do not hesitate to ask your physician to refer you to a mental health professional who is knowledgeable in the psychological aspects of pregnancy complicated by diabetes. Having

physically and emotionally healthy mothers and babies is a goal
shared by you and the health care team members.

Conclusion

We have come a long way from the days when pregnancy in a
woman with diabetes was fraught with danger and despair. What
has allowed this progress, in addition to modern treatment techniques, is intensive monitoring and care of both diabetes and fetal
development, as well as education of the mother so that she knows
what to expect and watch for in her role as the center of the
pregnancy care team.

If you are contemplating pregnancy, this chapter is just the
beginning. There is no substitute for direct care and instruction
from your diabetes/obstetrical team. All details of your care should
be reviewed with them.

Further reading may also be helpful. You may want to obtain a
copy of the Joslin Diabetes Center pregnancy guide, "A Guide for
Women with Diabetes Who Are Pregnant . . . Or Plan to Be"
(revised, 1986). It is available through the Joslin Diabetes Center,
One Joslin Place, Boston, Massachusetts 02215.

14

Diabetes and Aging

Everybody Is Doing It

Aging is something which everyone does but which most people
are not happy about. It is true that Robert Browning said, "Grow old
along with me! The best is yet to be, the last of life for which the first
was made," but almost no one believed him. A number of alleged
wits have remarked that while aging is not fun, it is better than the
alternative. There is one interesting facet about aging—the definition changes as you do! It is safe to say that "old age" is 10 years
older than you are at any age.

It is not that people are so worried about their chronological age
as they are about the infirmities, lack of adequate funds, and most
of all, a type of ill health that will cause them to be dependent on
others. But there is also good news! While everyone is aging, people
are living longer and healthier lives, and those with diabetes are no
exception. About 11% of the population is now over age 65, and by
the year 2020, that figure may be as high as 17%. In addition, the
age group that is growing the most is people over 85 years!
However, while 5% of the total population may have diabetes, it has
been estimated that as much as 20% of the population over 65 years
of age may have reduced glucose tolerance. Diabetes is indeed a
prominent disease among people in this mature (not "old") age
group. At times the effects of diabetes and the effects of the aging
process itself become difficult to sort out.

More good news for older people with diabetes is that since
May, 1970, the Joslin Diabetes Center has awarded the 50-year
medal (for living at least 50 years since the onset of diabetes) to more
than 700 people. There is good reason to believe that there must be
thousands of these!

For the older individual who is otherwise reasonably healthy both physically and mentally, the management of diabetes is essentially the same as for a younger person, and possibly simpler. When other diseases complicate the picture or when infirmities make self-care more difficult, however, the basic tasks become more difficult, and care becomes a challenge.

Effects of Aging on Glucose Tolerance

Blood glucose levels gradually increase in everyone after about age 50. This rise is more striking in the blood glucose levels measured 1 and 2 hours after a meal than in the fasting level. There is no difference in this change between men and women. If this increase in blood glucose level is too great, it may be true diabetes. Several studies have shown that people with even relatively mild elevations of blood glucose levels have increased risk for heart disease. These mild abnormalities must be taken seriously. It is false to assume that in aging, good control is not important because "someone is old and probably won't live very long." Healthy individuals 70 or 75 years old may live long enough to develop some of the complications of diabetes. Furthermore, people over age 80 or 85 can better themselves and be less of a "burden" to others if they haven't lost their limbs or sight! Diabetes must be taken seriously, at any age.

There are a number of reasons why there may be decreased glucose tolerance in older individuals. The insulin may not be as effective because of so-called insulin resistance, which is more common in those who are overweight. Aging also causes changes in body composition—a decreased muscle mass and increased adipose (fat) tissue (also increasing insulin resistance). Physical activity, so important to improve glucose tolerance, may be reduced in older people.

Dietary changes may also be a factor. Older people may overeat. Cicero, the ancient Roman politician, said, "I am grateful to old age because it has increased my desire for conversation and lessened my desire for food." But then he was an exception and relatively lean!

At the other extreme, starvation or reduced food intake can lead to a false impression of glucose tolerance (a "false positive") when a person is given a glucose tolerance test.

Diabetes is said to accelerate the aging process. Collagen ("connective tissue"), which helps maintain the smoothness and youthful appearance of the skin, has been shown to age more rapidly in people with diabetes. Blood vessels also age rapidly, becoming narrow or leaking. This can result in poor circulation to the heart, brain, legs, and feet.

Diabetes Treatment in Mature Individuals

Although older people may have either type I or type II diabetes, more often they have type II. The treatment for type II can be an adequate diet alone, oral medications, or sometimes insulin injections. For people with type I diabetes, the treatment is an eating plan plus insulin. This type of diabetes can develop after age 40, but it may have developed earlier in life, as many people now aging had type I diabetes diagnosed as children or young adults.

The treatment goals for the older person with diabetes are the same as the treatment goals for anyone else, with some modification. The goal is to bring blood glucose levels and glycohemoglobin measurements as close to normal as is *reasonably and safely possible*. The actual target for control varies with each person. However, for some older persons, "reasonable and safe" may need some compromise. Although still possible, some complications such as ketoacidosis are less likely. Some aging persons have decreased circulation to many areas, including the brain, and it would do them no favor to impose severe hypoglycemic insulin reactions on top of generally decreased circulation. This does not mean *not* watching or monitoring these senior citizens. It means *a bit* less restriction, but *never* decreased care and observation.

To treat the older person with diabetes, it is necessary first to evaluate the individual's abilities and interests and to find out what resources are available. For example, an 80-year-old person with poor vision and failing memory who requires insulin for diabetes would have difficulty self-monitoring, preparing syringes, and adjusting insulin. He or she would need modified goals of therapy if it were not possible for family, friends, or visiting nurses to provide needed help. There are many active 80-year-olds who still work and play golf or take daily walks. "Control" for this person may be easy to achieve. For many of these active people, age is not an issue.

When age brings infirmity, however, the treatment approach does need to be modified. Frequently there is a need for the help of others.

Eating

An eating plan can be difficult for anyone, but some age-related problems can make eating properly even more difficult. For those with less sharp memories, remembering or understanding the instructions may be nearly impossible. Also many people are reluctant to change a lifetime of habits. Eating may be one of the few pleasures remaining. When restrictions are made in fat, salt, fiber, or dairy products, "proper eating" becomes dull indeed.

A successful eating program should start with a dietary session. The presence of another family member or friend is helpful. The dietitian can plan a program that fits the person's interests, abilities, and resources. It can also be simplified or given some flexibility to make it more acceptable. Meal and other instructions should be printed with large type to help those with poor eyesight. Family and friends can help by making certain that proper foods are obtained and prepared as well as giving encouragement and support. Social agencies ("Meals on Wheels," for example) can be called upon if necessary.

Exercise

The benefits of exercise (Chapter 5) are applicable to nearly everyone with diabetes, but some older people may not be able to undertake a formal exercise program on a daily basis. Nevertheless, activities such as walking three times per week can be helpful and should be encouraged. Even this amount of activity helps maintain general health and better diabetes control. It helps one's mental state as well! People living in areas with poor climate can get exercise by walking in enclosed shopping malls. But leave the extra cash or credit cards at home, as frequent stopping to shop reduces the benefit of continued walking, to say nothing of making the trip expensive! In general, the physician should be consulted to determine how much and what type of exercise is safe and effective.

Pills or Insulin

The choice of medical therapy of diabetes is based on individual need. For some older people, however, it may be almost impossible to use prescribed treatments such as insulin. For those with reduced vision, magnifiers are available to assist with syringe filling. Frequently, others must prepare the syringes in advance when an older individual cannot see or has unsteady hands. Refrigeration of these prefilled syringes is not necessary, and a week's supply can be prepared at once. Even mixed insulin can be prefilled in the syringe (NPH is probably better than Lente for this). If two daily injections are needed, one should put the morning syringes in one place, and the afternoon or evening syringes in another place, to prevent confusion. Relatives, visiting nurses, or even some pharmacies can prepare these syringes. For those who cannot self-inject, daily visits by someone (relative, friend, visiting nurse) may be needed. Of course, attention to detail is important.

Even the proper use of tablets is not simple. Supervision by others may become necessary to ensure that these medications are taken on time and in the proper dose. Also, other medical problems may mean that the person needs other medications. It is important that there are no interactions between such medicines and the treatment for diabetes. The physician in charge should be aware of these potential interactions.

Monitoring

It is useless to test glucose levels at home without knowing what to do with the results. For some, self blood testing can be confusing or difficult to perform or interpret. Therefore, for some older people, urine testing may be more practical than blood testing, as it may be easier to perform and interpret. This approach can be used as a safety monitor, and patients can be told when to call for help if the tests show too much sugar spilling. Beware of some pitfalls! The renal threshold often increases as we age, making urine testing less useful because many times the glucose does not appear in the urine until *blood* glucose levels are very high. In this case, urine testing may have little value, except for acetone. Therefore, even if the patient has a high threshold or cannot perform self blood glucose tests, it is important to have a family member or friend learn to perform blood testing so that in the case of illness or other emergency, a blood glucose level can be done and the information phoned to the doctor. Physicians often use the glycohemoglobin measurement to get a more accurate picture of overall control levels in those people whose self testing is limited.

Preventing Complications

Prevention is the goal of diabetes care, and this is most important for older individuals. It is important to watch for signs of problems before they become serious. Regular visits to ophthalmologists (eye doctors) and podiatrists (foot doctors) are recommended. Treatment of high blood pressure and high blood fat (cholesterol) levels is also important. Smoking is always discouraged. The excuse that "I've been smoking so long, what difference does it make?" is not valid! Regular checkups to monitor for heart, circulation, or kidney problems are also advised. In general, good self-care permits an older person to live and enjoy life more fully.

Summary

For the many healthy active people who are over 65 taking care of their own diabetes can be no more difficult than it would be for a younger person. For those less able to care for themselves, however, physicians, other health care professionals, relatives, and friends must work together to overcome some of the inabilities that age has created and to help those with diabetes take better care of themselves. It is a true team effort.

To simply live *long* is not enough. It is more important to be well enough to enjoy this living. Increasingly in our society, living beyond the biblical "three score and ten" can have its rewards, but to enjoy these, one must have good health. Plato put it nicely: "Aging has a great sense of calm and freedom . . . You have escaped, not from one master, but from many." While one may not escape from diabetes, knowledge can give the freedom to master *that* master.

Appendix 7 lists associations that offer assistance to the elderly.

15

The Acute Complications of Diabetes

Every person's experience with diabetes is different. Just as there is no "typical" person, there is no "typical" diabetes. It is difficult to make predictions for any given person or situation. This difficulty also applies to the complications of diabetes—both the "acute" complications (those coming on rapidly) and the "chronic" complications (the results of a number of years of diabetes). No one can say exactly what the chances are of developing complications, although those with better care and control seem to have far fewer problems. Actually, acute and chronic are not really good classifications. One could use "early" and "late," but these are not much better. The fact is that the acute or early complications such as insulin reactions, ketoacidosis, and infections can happen at any time. They are also called acute complications to bring them to the attention of all people with diabetes, even those just diagnosed. These complications can and should be prevented with early discovery of the diabetes and vigorous and prompt treatment.

Acute versus Chronic Complications

Acute (or early) complications are those that can occur at any time during the life of a person with diabetes. While they can be dangerous, they are almost always preventable and usually remediable. The commonest are hypoglycemic ("insulin") reactions and diabetic ketoacidosis or coma. Infections are another such complication.

The chronic (or late) complications are discussed elsewhere. These are usually more serious. While they can be treated or managed, they often do not go away as the acute problems do. Research is now under way on how to prevent these complications, or at least treat them better.

Hypoglycemia (Low Blood Sugar)

The commonest acute complication is hypoglycemia, which is low blood glucose. Anyone can develop hypoglycemia, but it is most common when associated with treatment of diabetes. Low blood glucose levels can result from overtreatment with insulin or oral hypoglycemic agents, from insufficient food intake, or from too much exercise without enough food intake. Few people with well-controlled diabetes who have used insulin for any length of time can say that they have never had an "insulin reaction." In fact, those most tightly regulated may have very minor ones frequently.

The Symptoms of Hypoglycemia. If the blood glucose level drops too low, symptoms of hypoglycemia may occur. The level of symptoms varies with each person. Even in a given individual, the level below which symptoms are produced may change from time to time. While often the symptoms occur at a glucose level of about 50 mg%, this threshold can be higher, especially if the person's average blood glucose levels have been higher. Conversely, those using intensive therapy may be used to fairly low glucose levels and may not feel symptoms until the glucose level reaches about 40 or even 30 mg%. In addition, rapidly falling glucose levels can produce some of the symptoms of hypoglycemia without the glucose level actually being "too low."

In the clinic it is not unusual for a physician to find a blood glucose level of 20 or 30 mg% without the patient being aware of it, although admittedly, at that time, he or she may not be thinking too clearly! Some people may have reaction symptoms at a level of 150 mg%, especially if they had been at about 250 or 300 mg% and had dropped rapidly.

The early symptoms of a low or falling blood glucose level may include hunger, trembling, weakness, sweating, confusion, irritability, acute nervousness, tingling of the mouth and fingers, or many other symptoms. What actually happens is that the body senses the dropping glucose level and tries to bring it back up by releasing hormones such as glucagon (from the pancreas) and epinephrine (adrenaline) to trigger the release of glucose from glucagon (the glucose storage form) in the liver and muscles. Adrenaline is secreted as part of the "flight or fight" mechanism, which prepares the body to take emergency measures. If you are crossing a busy street and notice a truck bearing down on you, you jump quickly to get out of the way. Once you reach the safety of the sidewalk, you notice that you are shaking, sweaty, and nervous. These symptoms are due to the secreted adrenaline and are the same as those noted when the adrenaline secretion is due to low or dropping glucose levels. The symptoms are not produced directly by the glucose levels alone.

Severe Reactions. However, if the glucose levels continue to fall, different symptoms can occur. These symptoms include headache, confusion, drowsiness, or unconsciousness. With very severe hypoglycemia, seizures may even occur. In rare cases, the symptoms may also resemble a stroke, including weakness of one side of the body. Unlike the earlier symptoms caused by adrenaline, all of these symptoms are a direct result of blood glucose levels being too low for too long, with insufficient glucose available to the brain. These severe symptoms, while fairly rare, can be dangerous. Therefore the early symptoms of hypoglycemia should be taken seriously and treated at once to prevent more serious consequences.

> **WHEN IN DOUBT, BUT SUSPICIOUS OF HYPOGLYCEMIA, DON'T HESITATE. IMMEDIATELY TAKE SOMETHING SWEET, PREFERABLY LIQUID. IF YOU ARE CONTINUALLY IN DOUBT ABOUT YOUR SYMPTOMS, LEARN TO TEST YOUR BLOOD SO YOU CAN TELL FOR SURE!**

In treating a reaction, it is important to remember that once a person has taken insulin or an oral hypoglycemia agent, the glucose-lowering effect continues until the medication runs its course, regardless of what else happens. Thus if there is not enough glucose supplied to provide fuel for the action of these medications throughout the time they are working, glucose levels can fall too low. Even for severe reactions, a "quick fix" with orange juice may not be enough. Even if the orange juice has made you symptom-free for the moment, the insulin (or pills) may still be working. Take the next meal or a snack with some additional protein and fat, which will help hold the glucose levels up until the insulin or oral agent has run its course.

Although a few hypoglycemic reactions can be severe, most are so mild that they may not be easily recognized. Studies have demonstrated that when people have had diabetes for a period of years, they may lose the ability to judge truly what their blood glucose level is by how they feel. Of course, prolonged low blood glucose levels may cause impaired judgment, emotional upset, or a loss of physical control. One of the earlier signs of insulin reaction is difficulty expressing oneself.

Reaction Denial. A most confusing thing about insulin reactions is how differently they affect people. Some people, while unable to do involved work or think deeply, can perform automatic, habitual tasks quite well during an insulin reaction. People sometimes deny that anything unusual has occurred or that they have a reaction until someone has persuaded them to drink some orange juice or ginger ale. An insulin reaction can be dangerous to others as well if it occurs while the person is driving an automobile.

> **SOMETIMES THE PEOPLE *MOST* IN NEED OF SOMETHING SWEET FOR TREATING REACTIONS BECOME MOST STUBBORN AND NEGATIVE. THIS IS BECAUSE THE BRAIN LACKS ENOUGH GLUCOSE TO LET THEM THINK CLEARLY. IT TAKES CLEVERNESS TO TREAT REACTIONS!**

In some people, hypoglycemia can cause a Jekyll-and-Hyde effect. The quiet person may become belligerent, or the lively person somber. Mothers often recognize a low blood glucose level when a usually peaceful child becomes hyperactive or, sometimes, irrational. Experienced physicians can be caught unawares. One day, a child was rambunctious, crying, and refusing to permit his blood to be drawn for testing at the Joslin Clinic. Cajoling, threatening, and reasoning with him were equally ineffective. Dr. Elliott P. Joslin noticed this and tried unsuccessfully to convince the child to permit the test. He then asked whether the child usually behaved that way. The mother replied that this was most unusual. Dr. Joslin gave the youngster a small glass of ginger ale, after which the mood change was striking. The child cooperated, and it was obvious that his low blood glucose level had changed the usual behavior pattern.

Hypoglycemia causes some people to behave as though they are intoxicated. They are confused, unstable, and erratic in their behavior. One reason for people with diabetes to abstain from drinking even a small amount of alcohol and then driving is that alcohol may be blamed for erratic driving when the problem is actually due to hypoglycemia. More than one person has been arrested (or threatened with arrest) for drunken driving. The police officer cannot be expected to have clinical judgment, although with education, more and more of them are aware of diabetes and its problems.

> One reason to carry diabetes identification with you: It may help persuade the police officer that you have diabetes and need help, rather than a trip to the "drunk tank"!

Rebound: The "Somogyi Effect." Rebound, or the Somogyi effect (named after the physician who first described it), refers to hyperglycemia (high blood glucose level) that follows a severe hypoglycemia reaction. It usually occurs when the blood glucose falls to below normal levels. The body tries to compensate by releasing too much glucose that has been stored as glycogen into the bloodstream. Sometimes the liver overdoes it and releases too much, producing elevated blood glucose levels. A rebound is more common in some people than in others. It is harmless, unless not understood, in which case someone may give you *more* insulin, rather than less.

There is no usual pattern to "rebounds," but they may last 12 to 24 hours after the severe hypoglycemic reaction has occurred. The resulting upward swing of blood glucose levels may last even longer. This condition usually corrects itself if left alone. Extra insulin should not be used to lower the blood glucose unless the high levels continue for several days. Normal amounts of food should be eaten during rebounds. The danger comes from giving still more insulin or eating less. Doing so may drop the blood glucose level and start the same cycle over again. If the symptoms of hypoglycemia have not been obvious, self monitoring of blood glucose to observe the blood glucose patterns can be helpful.

Diagnosing Hypoglycemic Reactions. Diagnosing insulin reactions is easier if there are classic symptoms and if the low blood glucose level is proven by testing. If they occur during sleep or exercise without the usual symptoms, diagnosis can be more difficult. In fact, insulin reactions may not be obvious unless you look for them.

Self blood glucose testing has made the diagnosis of hypoglycemic reactions much easier. When only urine testing was available, a negative urine test might represent a blood glucose level of anywhere from 40 to 180 mg%. Now self blood glucose testing tells you the real story. A low blood glucose level at the time one is feeling the symptoms early hypoglycemia makes the diagnosis easy. Even if the glucose level is not very low when the symptoms occur—perhaps over 60 mg%—it is still possible that hypoglycemia is present. The blood glucose level when the test was done could have been dropping or going up from a lower value. It is here that watching blood glucose patterns becomes so important.

PATTERN HUNTING. Tests of the blood at least four times daily for several days can reveal patterns that might tell you when a hypoglycemic drop has taken place. For example, blood glucose levels of 350 mg% before breakfast, 240 mg% before lunch, 70 mg% before supper, and 340 mg% at bedtime could represent subtle hypoglycemia in the late afternoon, which may require treatment adjustment.

It helps to determine why each hypoglycemic reaction occurs. There are two types of reactions: explained and unexplained. Some reactions can be explained easily—lunch was delayed, breakfast was missed, dinner was too small, exercise was too intense, or too much insulin was given. Other causes should be considered. For example, alcohol prevents the body from being able to use its glycogen stores, thus making hypoglycemia more likely and possibly more severe. Injection of insulin into an area that is in use during exercise may speed up insulin absorption. Change of injection sites from "lipohypertrophy areas" (fatty buildup at injection sites) to normal areas may also speed up insulin absorption and make hypoglycemia more likely. If repeated explained reactions occur, you can adjust the factor that caused them to occur—the meal time or quantity, etc.—if possible.

Unexplained reactions are reactions that you cannot find reasons for. When these take place, it may mean that the insulin dose needs adjustment or some other part of the treatment plan needs changing. Unless you understand how to adjust for these, they should be reported to your physician so that the treatment program can be changed.

WHEN IN DOUBT ABOUT A REACTION, TREAT IT ANYWAY!

Prevention. The best treatment of hypoglycemic reactions is to prevent them. People with diabetes should avoid sudden changes in diet, insulin, or exercise unless their diabetes is well controlled and they know how to make changes to maintain proper glucose levels. For example, before exercising vigorously for an hour or more, more slow-acting carbohydrate should be eaten. Rapid-acting car-

---

TABLE 15–1. Products and Foods That Can Be Used to Treat Hypoglycemic (Low Blood Sugar) Reactions

PRODUCTS
3 B-D glucose tablets
½ tube Glutose (80 gram container)
½ tube Insta-Glucose (31 gram container)
1½ packages of Monojel

FOODS
4 ounces of orange juice
6 ounces of regular (nondiet) soft drinks (ginger ale) or 5 ounces of Coke or Pepsi
3–4 teaspoons of sugar dissolved in water
8 Life Savers
1 tablespoon of concentrated syrup such as Karo, Coke, or honey
1 small tube of cake icing
3 large or 25 miniature marshmallows
1 tablespoon of marshmallow creme
4 teaspoons of maple syrup
6 jelly beans
9 small gumdrops
2 tablespoons of raisins
1½ portions of dried fruit (see Appendix 1 for portion sizes of various fruits)
3 ounces of cranberry juice, regular
3 ounces of grape juice, sweetened
4 ounces of sweetened orange drink (for example, Tang or Hi-C

If the dose recommended above does not effectively treat the symptoms of hypoglycemia, increased amounts of food or products should be tried.

After symptoms of low blood sugar have subsided with treatment, you should have something else to eat if a meal or snack is not scheduled within the next hour. This should consist of longer-acting foods such as crackers with cheese or peanut butter, or milk and crackers.

REMEMBER: Do not try to feed food by mouth to a person who is unconscious, nearly unconscious, or delirious. A person with these conditions due to low blood glucose levels should be treated with glucagon injections or brought to an emergency facility.

IF IN DOUBT, OR IF THE BLOOD GLUCOSE LEVEL DOES NOT RISE WITH TREATMENT, CONTACT A PHYSICIAN OR EMERGENCY FACILITY AT ONCE.

bohydrate is used quickly and should be used if short (20 to 30 minutes), sudden, intense exertion is planned. Exercise is the most common cause of low blood sugar reactions. Chapter 5 discusses adjustment of the treatment program to prevent this problem.

Treatment. People who are able to swallow during a hypoglycemic reaction should use the simplest, fastest-acting, sweet drink or food available. Allow about 10 minutes for the sugar to be effective and repeat the same treatment if no improvement is seen.

Commonly available drinks are orange juice and regular (nondiet) sodas—in fact, any sweetened liquid. Table 15–1 lists other effective choices of foods and products available to treat hypoglycemic reactions. The instant glucose tablets or jells are alternative treatments and have the advantage that they are not tasty snack foods that people may nibble at times other than with hypoglycemia. Once the reaction is treated and the symptoms subside, a meal or an extra snack of longer-acting carbohydrate, perhaps with protein, should be eaten to prevent the blood glucose level from dropping too low later on. This might include one meat and one bread exchange. This extra food is not counted in the diet.

The longer people wait before treating a reaction, the more likely they are to become confused. Once they are confused,

> Do not use the low-calorie diet drinks in your refrigerator to treat reactions. If you are having an insulin reaction, you might confuse them. Diet drinks are useless for treating hypoglycemia!

treating the reaction becomes even more difficult, and the chance of injury increases. Always carry something with you and treat the reaction right away! In a pinch, almost any gasoline station has sugar-containing drinks or candy for sale in vending machines. You can carry sweets in your car, purse, or pocket. A supply can also be kept in a desk at work. Supplies should be checked from time to

> An easy antireaction treatment to carry around is a low-cost, simple tube of confectioners' sugar icing— the kind you use to spell "Happy Birthday" on top of a cake. Squirt some in the mouth and replace the top so that it can be used another time.

time. One person who suffered a severe reaction was asked by his physician why he did not carry some fast candy in the glove compartment of his car. He replied that he did have some, but a night or two before the reaction, his young child had found the candy and eaten it.

Severe hypoglycemia does sometimes result in unconsciousness, although fortunately not very often. Treatment of unconsciousness presents special problems because liquids should not be force-fed.

LOW BLOOD GLUCOSE LEVELS CAN RESULT FROM:
1 too LITTLE (or no) food
2. too MUCH exercise, without extra food
3. too MUCH insulin

YOU MAY FEEL:
1. shaky
2. sweaty
3. hungry
4. weak
5. dizzy
6. confused

YOU CAN CONFIRM THAT THIS IS A LOW BLOOD GLUCOSE LEVEL BY:
1. testing your BLOOD glucose level and seeing a low value
2. testing your URINE sugar level and finding it negative, but this does not actually confirm that it *is* true hypoglycemia

YOU SHOULD TREAT THIS CONDITION BY TAKING:
1. Commercially prepared glucose preparations (see Table 15–1)
2. 4 ounces of orange juice or 6 ounces of regular ginger ale
3. 3–4 teaspoons of sugar dissolved in water
4. 8 Life Savers or similar product. Chew if possible
5. 1 tablespoon of concentrated syrup such as Karo, Coke, or honey
6. Any additional foods listed in Table 15–1

When unconscious, the person may aspirate (inhale) liquid into the trachea (windpipe), causing lung complications. Unconscious patients should be treated with injections of glucagon or taken immediately to the hospital emergency room for intravenous glucose.

Glucagon. Like insulin, glucagon is a hormone produced by the alpha cells of the pancreas. It is also a protein chain and, like insulin, must be injected because if taken orally it would be destroyed by the stomach's digestive juices. If a person with diabetes is unconscious, glucagon can be given easily by a family member or friend. It is effective in the treatment of severe hypoglycemia because it releases stored glycogen from the liver and helps to convert it into glucose in the blood. This temporarily raises the blood glucose level enough so that the unconscious patient will usually awaken and be able to take liquid nourishment by mouth.

> **You may never need glucagon, just as you may never have to use your fire extinguisher, but it should be there—in case. . . .**

Most people who use insulin should keep glucagon available for the emergency that may never come. This is particularly important for those who have had, or have come close to, severe or unconscious reactions. A family member or friend should know how to use glucagon, which is injected in the same way as insulin. An infrequent side effect of glucagon is nausea and vomiting, so individuals receiving glucagon injections should be on their side to avoid vomiting and aspirating the stomach contents into the lungs. Usually the person can be aroused in 5 to 10 minutes and then can be given additional nourishment by mouth to prevent another reaction. If there is no response, a second injection may be given. If the response is still insufficient, more intensive treatment may be needed in a hospital emergency room. If no one knows how to use glucagon, it is best to get the person to the emergency facility rather than try to learn the use of glucagon for the first time with the person lying unconscious. Actually, glucagon is much simpler to use than insulin. The dose need not be as exact because you inject a vial-full (or more) rather than worry about units.

Glucagon is available by prescription from Eli Lilly & Company in a kit that contains two vials. One vial contains 1 mg of glucagon as a white powder; the other, 1 cc of sterile solution for preparing the injection. Wipe tops of both vials with alcohol—the same way as for the top of an insulin bottle. Using the U-100 insulin syringe and needle, withdraw all of the diluting solution and inject it into the vial of glucagon. Then shake the vial, dissolving the powder, and withdraw all of the resulting solution into the syringe. This solution is injected anywhere under the person's skin, exactly as insulin is injected. Recently, premixed glucagon syringe kits have become available.

The person who does not respond to glucagon and is rushed to an emergency facility will likely be treated with an intravenous glucose mixture. This treatment usually brings about rapid and complete recovery, even if the insulin reaction is severe. When the person recovers, try to determine the reasons for the reaction. Often this will turn out to be quite simple, like a delayed or skipped meal. Steps must be taken to prevent a recurrence.

Are Insulin Reactions Harmful? Reactions are frightening far beyond their potential harm because they make the person feel uncomfortable and out of control. Mild hypoglycemic reactions may be an indication of good regulation, not because they are desired, but because occasional mild reactions appear to be unavoidable with present-day methods of tight control. Many patients have an exaggerated and unnecessary fear of insulin reactions, not just because they are uncomfortable, but also because they fear that repeated bouts of hypoglycemia may result in permanent brain damage. The possibility of lasting damage from the minor hypoglycemia that occurs with good, thoughtful diabetes control is almost nil.

By contrast, a very severe, prolonged reaction with unconsciousness for several days can be quite threatening. Such a reaction may be due to neglect, some catastrophe in insulin dose, or even a series of mishaps. Fortunately, these kinds of reactions are very rare. There is no reason anyone with diabetes should have severe reactions, as monitoring and attention to the daily routine should prevent them. Predisposing factors such as not eating or excessive alcohol intake make a severe reaction more likely.

> Many older people living alone, especially those who use insulin, have a "buddy system" with a friendly neighbor, or even someone else with similar problems. They make certain to phone each other daily or to check in some other way. A great idea!

Almost all insulin reactions can be prevented, and most are readily treated. However, they can cause difficulty indirectly, as with an automobile accident caused by a driver's hypoglycemia. People with diabetes must be careful to risk neither their own lives and property nor those of others. Increasingly, regulations for driving privileges are becoming stricter, and the loss of the license to drive is a real threat. Physicians and educators can instruct a person on proper self-care and how to avoid hypoglycemia, but it is the responsibility of each person with diabetes to follow these instructions.

Other Causes of Hypoglycemia. "Reactive Hypoglycemia" is a condition that is receiving a lot of attention. It results from the stimulation by glucose in the blood of an excessive release of insulin in people who do not have diabetes and do not take insulin. The resulting symptoms are just like those that occur with an insulin-induced hypoglycemic reaction with diabetes. Reactive hypoglycemia is quite rare, and it is frequently overdiagnosed because it seems to explain a lot of symptoms and complaints. Even if present, many physicians do not consider it a "disease." Treatment is with diet adjustment so that large amounts of carbohydrate are not present to stimulate insulin release. A few of these individuals may go on to develop true diabetes in the future.

Tumors made up of pancreatic beta cells may cause hypoglycemia because they may secrete excessive amounts of insulin. This condition has no relationship to diabetes and not only is very rare but is diagnosable and treatable.

The Hyperglycemic "Comas" of Diabetes (High Blood Sugar)

At the opposite pole from hypoglycemia is an acute complication that can be most dangerous for those with diabetes—very high blood glucose levels that result in diabetic *ketoacidosis* or "diabetic coma." Ketoacidosis can occur any time during the life of someone with type I diabetes and even, in unusual circumstances, someone with type II. Usually, however, people with type II do not get ketoacidosis. More likely, they can develop something called *hyperosmolar, nonketotic* coma. There is a vast difference between the two comas, but both of these conditions are very serious and can be life-threatening.

Before the discovery of insulin in 1921, nearly half of the deaths of people with diabetes at the New England Deaconess Hospital in Boston were due to diabetic coma. At present, the death rate is only about 1% of those admitted with this diagnosis. The sad fact is that all of these comas are completely preventable with knowledge and proper monitoring and use of insulin. Even after it starts, if treated early and vigorously enough, it is almost curable!

Ketoacidosis. People with type I diabetes lack insulin. In these people markedly elevated blood glucose levels are usually due to not enough effective insulin. Insulin, of course, enables glucose to enter the cells to be used for energy. It also helps deposit fats in the fat (adipose) cells for storage. When the blood insulin level is *low*, the glucose cannot get into the cells to be used as an energy source; however, the body cleverly can use fat cells as another source of energy. When fat cells are used for energy, the blood glucose level is quite high, which results in large amounts of sugar in the urine. High urine sugar levels cause the urine volume to increase, and a tremendous amount of fluid can be lost from the body. This state of reduced body fluid levels is known as dehydration, and is the cause of symptoms such as increased thirst and dry mouth that are characteristic of high glucose levels. Meanwhile, as the body, in desperation, turns to fat for energy, ketone bodies are produced because the fats are not completely used. These ketones accumulate in the blood and also spill over into the urine. The presence of ketones in the urine is called "ketonuria." With further dehydration and ketone buildup, the blood becomes more acid. This is now ketoacidosis. In extreme cases or when enough insulin and fluids are not given in time, coma and unconsciousness occur. This is as serious an emergency as any that a person with diabetes can face. It is every bit as much of an emergency as acute appendicitis and much more complicated to cure.

Hyperosmotic Coma (The Other Coma). People develop type II diabetes not because of insulin lack, but because of insulin resistance. Many with this condition produce insulin of their own; some, indeed, produce more than a normal amount. As with type I diabetes, if some stress, infection, or serious illness increases the insulin required to overcome insulin resistance beyond what is available, the blood glucose levels can climb markedly.

However, unlike people with type I diabetes, these people have some insulin present. While a lack of insulin would allow the metabolism of fat as an alternative energy source and the production of ketones, in these people the presence of insulin prevents fat from being used. Very high blood glucose levels can develop. The body reacts by trying to lower these levels through the kidneys. The glucose-containing urine may result in a high urine volume. In fact, a tremendous amount is lost, causing dehydration. This fluid loss can be even more severe than that of ketoacidosis. With massive fluid loss, the blood becomes more concentrated. This blood concentration is due to dehydration called "hyperosmolar" (increased concentration of the blood).

Why These Happen. Both of these comas result from definite causes. With *ketoacidosis*, all of these causes are related to a deficit of needed insulin. With the *hyperosmolar coma* the insulin is present but is not effective. The pattern of both these problems often starts with neglect of diet, neglect of *blood* or *urine testing*, infections, or some other very definite reason. Poor diet alone is not likely to cause either of these, but it does give the comas a start. With a chronically poor diet setting the stage, it is not difficult for an infection with fever, for example, to make insulin even less effective. At this time increased insulin is needed. The situation is like inflation. What used to be 5 or 10 units of insulin is now worth much less. If more insulin is not given, the blood glucose level will rise and rise, and the usual insulin dose is not enough. If the demand for more insulin is not met, the situation rapidly deteriorates. At this point, the problem can be worsened if the person erroneously does not even take the usual insulin dose because of illness or reduced eating, and ketoacidosis becomes almost a certainty.

Symptoms. The onset of diabetic acidosis leading to coma is usually more gradual than the onset of a hypoglycemic reaction. Blood glucose or urine tests are poor and urine acetone tests may be positive for days before the coma develops. In a young person developing diabetes or in someone with unstable diabetes, this onset may be more rapid. Although the treatment is different, you should treat the onset of hyperglycemic comas with the same urgency as you treat an oncoming hypoglycemic reaction. Even if the blood glucose climbs quite rapidly over 12 to 24 hours, there is still enough time to avoid coma.

At first, the symptoms are often those of untreated diabetes—dry mouth, thirst, and excessive urination. Nausea and vomiting are usually present, and abdominal pain is often felt. Later symptoms may be deep, labored breathing (Kussmaul respirations), flushed features, dryness, and a generalized feeling of acute illness that gives way to drowsiness and finally coma. The breath has a sweetish acetone odor. Although the word "coma" implies total loss of consciousness, the patient may not be completely unconscious, but

---

HIGH BLOOD GLUCOSE LEVELS CAN RESULT FROM:
1. too MUCH food
2. too LITTLE exercise
3. too LITTLE insulin
4. illness

YOU MAY:
1. be THIRSTY
2. URINATE frequently
3. LOSE weight
4. be very TIRED, DROWSY, OR WEAK
5. have BLURRED VISION

YOU CAN CONFIRM THAT THIS IS A HIGH BLOOD GLUCOSE LEVEL BY:
1. TESTING YOUR BLOOD GLUCOSE LEVEL and finding that it is HIGH
2. testing your urine and getting a POSITIVE result.

YOU SHOULD:
1. test urine for ACETONE
2. CALL YOUR DOCTOR
3. TAKE MORE INSULIN

---

rather disoriented and increasingly stuporous. The hyperosmolar type of coma can develop in similar ways, although the urine ketone test is usually negative. Symptoms of dehydration and general illness are obvious.

One of the most common mistakes made by people with diabetes is neglecting to take insulin on days when they are ill. Although they may be eating less, insulin may be less effective. They might need *more* insulin, not less!

Treatment. Real diabetic acidosis or coma requires emergency medical care in a hospital as fast as possible. The urgent treatment includes insulin and replacement of body fluids. Insulin can be given in various ways. Some physicians give a large dose and then smaller ones. Many physicians now give frequent, even hourly, insulin, while in many major hospitals automatic infusion pumps

TABLE 15–2. Habits That Will Help Prevent Diabetic Comas

1. Develop a routine monitoring plan (Chapter 8) and follow it.
2. Be sure you understand how the balance between insulin, food, and activity affects *your* diabetes.
3. Test for acetone (ketones) if the blood glucose level is above 240 mg%, or if your urine glucose levels have been 1% or higher for 2 consecutive tests.
4. During an infection, increase the dose of insulin if the blood or urine tests are strongly positive (see Table 15–3, Sick Day Rules).
5. Take additional insulin as your doctor may order.
6. Treat all illnesses as possible impending coma and follow sick day rules.

replace the needed insulin injections. By monitoring blood glucose and other blood chemicals such as acetone, the insulin dose is adjusted to bring the glucose level steadily and safely toward the normal range.

IN EVERY URGENT EMERGENCY SITUATION, REGULAR, CLEAR, FAST-ACTING INSULIN IS ALWAYS USED!

As mentioned, the other vital treatment is to replace body fluid to correct the intense dehydration that accompanies both these comas. Potassium (denoted by the letter K) that is lost because of excessive urination must be replaced, and shock must be treated. Later, liquids can be given by mouth, starting at first in tiny amounts as tolerated. By the second day, the person is usually able to take small amounts of food, and when the blood chemistry is almost normal, the person returns to the usual program of insulin and diet. Often several more days of careful diabetes regulation are needed to help the return to normal.

Prevention. Although diabetic coma is not the dreaded catastrophe that it was in the past, it is still very serious and can be fatal. With these complications, prevention is the key. At this time, with the possible exception of comas occurring at the onset of diabetes (when the diabetes is not known), ketoacidosis can nearly always be avoided. It is here that the education of people with diabetes and their families is most important. ALWAYS TAKE YOUR USUAL DAILY DOSE OF INSULIN. DO NOT OMIT IT WHEN FEELING ILL. Remember that during illness the liver is releasing

---

TABLE 15–3. SICK DAY RULES

1. Always take your usual daily dose of insulin. NEVER OMIT IT, EVEN IF YOU ARE UNABLE TO EAT.
2. Test your urine or blood glucose level every 4 hours. A minimum of 4 times a day (before each meal and at bedtime) is absolutely essential. It is usually preferable to test every 4 hours around the clock, setting an alarm during the night. If you use urine testing, use *freshly made samples* of urine. If you are feeling too sick to test, ask someone to do it for you.
3. If the urine glucose levels are 1% or higher, or the blood glucose levels are above 240 mg%, you should also test for urine ketones. DO THIS WHEN ILL FROM ANY CAUSE. If ketones are present along with high glucose levels, you ALWAYS need extra insulin. Regular (short-acting) insulin should be used. Guidelines for how much regular insulin you should use and how often to take it appear in Table 15-4. Do not use extra insulin if only ketones are present, or if blood tests are less than 240 mg% or urine glucose tests are less than 1%.
4. Take liquids every hour (see Table 15-5). Refer to the food suggestions for sick days in Table 15-5. If you are unable to take liquids because of nausea or vomiting, contact your physician immediately. He or she may prescribe a medication to stop the nausea or vomiting.
5. If you are too ill to follow your usual meal plan, refer to the food suggestions for sick days in Table 15-5.
6. Rest and keep warm. Do not exercise. Have someone take care of you.
7. If you are vomiting and cannot hold down food or liquid, if you have persistent severe diarrhea, if you cannot bring your blood glucose levels down (Table 15-4), or if you are in pain, contact your physician immediately.

---

glucose *even when one cannot eat,* so insulin is still needed. Prevention of diabetic comas involves good habits at all times, (Table 15–2). These habits are even more important during sick days, when special rules must be followed (Table 15–3). Guidelines for increased insulin doses (Table 15–4) and how to eat during and after illness (Table 15–5) are important parts of the sick day routine as well.

High and Low

Because ketoacidosis and insulin reaction are so serious, you must be able to tell them apart and start proper treatment as early as possible. Table 15–6 lists the different signs for each. It is usually easy to tell high blood glucose from low. The nature of the onset of

---

TABLE 15–4. GUIDELINES FOR USING EXTRA INSULIN ON SICK DAYS

---

1. Extra insulin is needed when glucose levels are high and ketones are present in the urine. Use regular (clear) insulin for your extra doses. Keep a bottle of regular insulin on hand for sick days even though you may not use it on a daily basis.

2. If you are sick with high glucose levels, the amount of regular insulin you should take for a sick day "catch-up increment" dose is based on the number of units of all the insulin you take on a day when you are well. The sick day catch-up increment dose should be 20%, or ⅕, of this usual daily dose total. To find out the number of units of regular to use, divide the number of units of all the insulin you take in your usual daily dose by 5.

3. This catch-up increment dose of insulin should be taken every 3 or 4 hours for as long as tests for glucose and ketones remain high. Your physician may direct you to take it even more frequently.

4. The extra units of regular insulin that are the catch-up increment dose may be combined with your usual dose if you are taking them at the same time. If you do not know how to mix 2 insulins together, you can take each insulin separately.

5. If you are sick, and your blood glucose level is 240 or greater with negative ketones, use a 10% booster instead of a 20% booster (i.e., divide the total number of daily units taken by 10). However, if you have taken two 10% boosters in less than 24 hours and the blood glucose level is still 240 or more with or without ketones, use the 20% catch-up increment dose.

6. Taking additional regular insulin will eventually lower your glucose, and ketones will no longer be present in the urine. The decline of the glucose levels will be more rapid than the elimination of ketones. Once glucose levels are less than approximately 240 mg%, discontinue using the extra catch-up increment dose even though ketones may still be present in the urine.

7. Call your doctor for help if:
   a. You have taken 2 boosters every 24 hours for 3 days and the blood glucose level is still 240 to 400 mg%
   b. You need more than 2 20% boosters in 24 hours
   c. The blood glucose level remains over 400 mg% for 12 straight hours.
   d. You cannot hold down food or fluids for 2 hours or have a fever of 101° or above

8. Sometimes people hesitate to take what seem like large doses of insulin. When you are sick and have high glucose and ketone levels, you need more insulin. DO NOT HESITATE TO TAKE EXTRA INSULIN.

---

symptoms is important. A fast change from normal is usually a sign of low blood glucose levels. With the availability of home blood glucose testing, there is no excuse for not knowing the difference between high and low!

TABLE 15-5. Food Suggestions for Sick Days

Following are suggestions on how to eat if you do not feel like following your usual eating plan due to illness. Eat and drink whatever your body can tolerate, but you must consume at least 6 to 8 glasses of fluid a day. Take some each hour, alternating fluids with sugar one hour, without sugar the next. Fluids that may be used include:

water	fruit juices
tea	regular (nondietetic) soft drinks
consommé	broth made from bouillon cubes

If you cannot drink liquids because of nausea and vomiting, call your physician.

Upon recovery from an illness, food sources of carbohydrate that may be more easily digested include (each portion provides 15 grams of carbohydrate, or about 1 bread exchange):

apple sauce (sweetened)	½ cup
apple juice	½ cup
baked custard	½ cup
Coke syrup	1½ tablespoons
cooked cereal	½ cup
cream soups	1 cup
eggnog	½ cup
fruit yogurt	⅓ cup
frozen yogurt	
on a stick	1 bar
from container	⅓ cup
grape juice	3 ounces
honey	3 teaspoons
Hershey's syrup	2 tablespoons
Life Savers	7
Popsicle (twin-pop)	1
pudding (sweetened)	¼ cup
regular ice cream	½ cup
regular Jello	⅓
regular soft drinks	¾ cup (6 ounces)
saltine crackers	6
sherbet	¼ cup
toast	1 slice

While nothing is "always" in medicine, in general, if it happens rapidly, it is probably an insulin reaction. If it happens gradually, it is more likely to be ketoacidosis.

THE ACUTE COMPLICATIONS OF DIABETES   265

TABLE 15–6. Differentiating between Hypoglycemia (Insulin Reaction) and Hyperglycemia (High Blood Glucose Levels) with Possible Ketoacidosis

CHARACTERISTIC	HYPOGLYCEMIA (INSULIN REACTION)	HYPERGLYCEMIA AND IMPENDING COMA
Onset	Sudden	Slow
Appearance	Moist Skin	Dry Skin
Actions	Nervous, sometimes confused	Drowsy, sometimes stuporous
Symptoms	Sweating Shakiness Hunger Weakness	Nausea Vomiting Dehydration Sweetish breath (acetone)
Blood glucose	Low	High to very high
Urine sugar	None, but possibly present if bladder not emptied for a long period	Very high (+ + + +)
Urine Acetone	None	Very high (+ + + +)

Blurred Vision (Presbyopia)

Early in the insulin treatment of new or uncontrolled diabetes, many people have a frightening occurrence. As their diabetes becomes controlled, their vision starts to blur. This blurring (presbyopia) is not continuous, but things appear to be out of focus, as if one is looking through a camera with the wrong distance setting. Those already worried about diabetes and eye problems can be very frightened. Be reassured! This experience is usually short-lived, lasting several days to weeks, and is not related to eye damage. With longterm poor control of the diabetes, much body fluid, including that contained in the eyeball, may be lost. This happens so gradually that the eyes adjust to it and visual changes are not noticed. With rapid good regulation, fluid shifts in all areas of the body, and fluid may enter or leave the eyeballs. This changes the eyeball shape, and there is edema (swelling) of the lens due to the fluid shifts. It takes time to adjust to this, and the vision is temporarily blurred. The condition is not permanent. It is one reason eye doctors do not fit glasses for people with poor diabetes control. Actually they prefer to wait for several weeks after the diabetes has been under control; otherwise a new set of glasses would be required every few days.

Insulin Edema

Another condition sometimes found in people who have had a marked improvement in blood glucose control is "insulin edema" (swelling). This is seen more often in younger individuals and is more common in females. It is characterized by puffiness, due to fluid accumulation, most commonly around the ankles, but elsewhere as well. Although the fluid amounts are often minimal, the swelling can be frightening. It is rarely severe enough to require more than reassurance, although sometimes a diuretic (fluid-removing) drug may be used temporarily.

Diabetes Better, Neuritis Worse?

Neuropathy is a fairly common complication of diabetes (Chapter 16). It can affect almost any nerve. Sometimes when diabetes control improves fairly rapidly, there is a temporary worsening of this neuropathic discomfort. It is important to remember that this worsening is, indeed, usually temporary. Usually time will bring relief. Fortunately, most people experience only mild discomfort from this temporary form of neuropathy which lasts only a few weeks to a month or so. Rarely is any treatment necessary.

Insulin Allergy

Although generalized allergy to the protein insulin is rare, when it does occur it may be serious. It usually occurs in people who had been treated with insulin in the past, discontinued insulin, and then later restarted. Insulin allergies may be due to impurities in the insulin or an insulin of a different species than human. The new human-like insulins are less likely to cause insulin allergies, although allergies are possible with any type of medication.

People can be desensitized from allergy by repeated tiny injections of insulin. The individual is usually hospitalized for this treatment. The injections are started with very minute doses of insulin, such as *1/1,000 of a unit or less*. The amount is doubled until signs of allergy disappear and the person is desensitized. Much more common are minor allergic reactions with itching and some redness at the site of injection. This generally disappears, although medication to relieve itching can be helpful.

Atrophy and Hypertrophy

Atrophy is a complication that may be caused by insulin injections. It may be a type of immunologic response (a response caused by antibodies to a substance) to some of the impurities in the insulin. Although use of the purer insulins has made this problem much less common, it can happen, most often in girls and young women. It consists of a loss of fatty tissue just beneath the skin at the sites of injections, resulting in unsightly hollows located unfortunately, in thighs and arms—a highly visible location. Parents fear that these hollows will continue to spread and that all of the body fat will waste away. This is not true. These hollows are usually localized and self-limited. The only significance is cosmetic. However, insulin injected into these sites may be absorbed at a different rate than elsewhere, which affects its action.

Sometimes these hollows will improve spontaneously over a period of years. One way to avoid them is to rotate the insulin injection sites and especially to avoid injections into the same area. Some people have reported improvement using the new purer insulins, and injecting them into the normal skin areas at the edge of the hollows. In some cases, this practice has led to the hollows filling in somewhat.

Hypertrophy is another complication of insulin injection—just the opposite of atrophy. Hypertrophy refers to buildup in the areas of injection, usually on the thighs or arms. It is harmless but unattractive, although these areas are not usually as unsightly as the craters of atrophy. In fact, they may look like "Popeye" muscles, which, of course, they are not. New purer insulins are much less likely to cause this problem. One should avoid injecting in these areas because the absorption of insulin from them can be erratic.

Insulin Abscess and Infection

Abscesses and infections at the injection site can develop because of careless injection technique. These are preventable with careful cleanliness and sterile technique. Some abscesses may be small and treatable with antibiotics; others may develop into large areas that may require surgical treatment. Abscesses and infections at the sites of self blood test punctures are also possible, but they are unusual.

Insulin Resistance

Insulin resistance means that the insulin is unable to signal the cells of the body to allow glucose to enter so that it can be used for energy. Nearly everyone with diabetes has had some degree of insulin resistance at one time or another. It is commonest with type II diabetes. There are other types of insulin resistance as well. Most often, this resistance is mild and is caused by an illness, too generous a diet, or some other reason that can be corrected easily.

There are other conditions in which severe insulin resistance can occur, and these can be difficult to treat. In these cases, insulin resistance is defined as requiring 200 units of insulin or more daily. Some people may need as many as 500 to 2000 units daily for a period of time. Several years ago, a person receiving treatment at the Joslin Diabetes Center required 16,000 units daily before the period of resistance ended. U-500 insulin (500 units in 1 cc) is available if necessary. Such cases are rare. They can be caused by a large number of antibodies to insulin. Although resistance to human insulins is possible as well, it is very rare, and insulin resistance is often reduced by changing to a purer, or human-like insulin. Resistance will occasionally subside spontaneously. In very stubborn cases, it may be necessary to use large doses of insulin or other measures to break the resistance.

Genital Infections

People with diabetes get genital infections more often than people without diabetes. The infecting organisms are often a type of fungus ("yeast") and include vaginal infections and balanitis, or infection of the tip of the penis. These can be very annoying. They are usually related to poor diabetes control, which reduces the body's ability to resist infection as well as causing a high sugar content in the urine, which encourages the growth of these organisms. There are medicated creams and ointments that can be used to treat these conditions. However, the infections are often resistant to any treatment until diabetes control is improved.

16

The Longterm
Complications of Diabetes

By now you know that some of the things that may go wrong with
diabetes can happen in a hurry. The acute problems can actually
happen anytime, often early in the course of diabetes.
Hypoglycemia (low blood sugar reactions), for example, can occur
with the first doses of insulin, or after many years. Infections can
also happen anytime. The complications discussed in this chapter
usually occur only after many years of diabetes, especially if the
condition has not been well taken care of. These are generally the
dreaded complications that, although serious, really take place
much less often than is generally thought. Considering that there
are about 100 million people with diabetes in the world, perhaps
more than 12 million in the United States alone, it is amazing how
many patients *do not get* serious forms of these complications. The
problem lies in the fact that some of these disastrous problems are
highly visible. The patient with a limb loss or a marked visual defect
is noticed by everyone, yet the many, many others who have none
of these problems go unnoticed. Having 50 or more years of
diabetes *without* any of the stigma of this condition is becoming
more and more common.

Can really good control prevent all of the longterm problems? It
is difficult to make a bold statement of that kind. Studies are now
under way to help find answers, but there is gradually increasing
evidence that many of the microvascular (small blood vessel)
changes can indeed be helped or possibly prevented. For now we

will look more closely at the various chronic complications and see what can be done.

The Eyes

Eye problems are probably the most terrifying of all the well-known complications of diabetes. The fear often starts shortly after diagnosis. Upon starting insulin treatment for the first time, some people get blurred vision called "presbyopia" (see Chapter 15). This is not uncommon. A panic sets in, with thoughts of "diabetes blindness." In reality, this blurring is caused by fluid changes in the eye which accompany better diabetes control. The condition usually clears up within a matter of days or weeks!

Anatomy of the Eye. The eye is a strange and wonderful instrument. Essentially it is like a hollow Ping-Pong ball separated into two segments by the lens (Fig. 16–1). All of the structures of the eye that are in front of the lens are bathed in a watery bath called the aqueous humor, while structures behind the lens in the main cavity or "ocular cavity") of the eyeball are bathed in a concentrated fluid called the vitreous humor. Next to the vitreous humor is the retina, which is the delicate nervous membrane that responds to light stimuli. The retina transforms these stimuli from appropriately focused light to nerve impulses. These nerve impulses travel along nerve fibers that line a layer of the retina and then extend out of the eyeball at the optic nerve. The human optic nerve has about 1.2 million individual nerve fibers. These are most densely packed in the center of the nerve that carries images from the middle of the retina. The optic nerve at the back of the eye goes directly to the brain, which interprets what the eye pictures.

As the physician looks into the pupil of the eye, he or she sees a pale, yellow, flat object, much like a pancake, on the back of the eyeball. That is the flat side of the optic nerve facing toward the observer. Coming out of all the sides of this optic disc are blood vessels, like the spokes of a wheel (Fig. 16–2). These blood vessels are important because they nourish the eye. The arteries and veins are called retinal vessels. The physician also sees another area close to the optic disc, called the macula, which controls central vision.

While the macula measures only about 1.5 millimeters in diameter (about the size of a small letter "o" in this text), it is responsible for our ability to see colors and fine detail. It is the macula that enables us to read and see clearly and distinctly, while

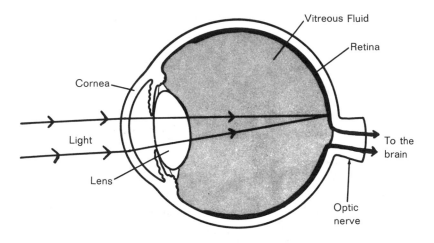

FIG. 16–1. Basic structure of the eye (profile views). Light passes through the cornea and the lens and is focused on the rear of the eyeball at the layer of the retina. The optic nerve carries the image from the retina to the brain, where it is interpreted. The vitreous humor is a clear fluid that keeps the eyeball in constant shape. Four areas of potential trouble are (1) clouding of the lens, which is known as *cataract;* (2) increased pressure of the aqueous, which can damage the optic nerve, a condition known as *glaucoma;* (3) rupture or hemorrhage of the blood vessels in the retina, a condition called *retinitis* or *diabetic retinopathy;* (4) accumulation of fluid in the macula area which has leaked from retinal blood vessels, a condition called *macular edema.*

the rest of the retina enables us to see motion, shades of gray, and peripheral vision.

Although the eye has often been described as "like a camera," it is much more complicated than anything a photographer might use. It chooses the proper amount of light needed and adjusts its own focus better than the most perfect camera made. It even protects itself with a lid when necessary. It has a lens in front, very much like the lens in a camera. Clouding in the lens itself is called a *cataract,* which can prevent sharp vision. The lens with a cataract is like a windshield that is dirty so that it is difficult to see through. The fluid going in and out of the front (anterior) of the eyeball is constantly changing. If something stops the proper drainage of fluid from the eyeball so that the pressure increases, this condition is called *glaucoma.* Inflammation of the outer front covering of the eye, so that it looks red or hemorrhagic, is known as *conjunctivitis.* Damage to the retinal blood vessels so that they break, leak, or bleed in the interior of the eye is known as *hemorrhagic retinitis* or *diabetic*

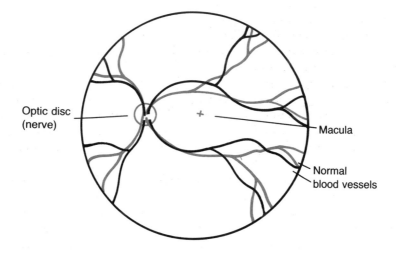

FIG. 16–2. The fundus of the normal eye. The optic nerve and blood vessels pass into the back of the eye (the retina) through the optic disc. The blood vessels radiate from the center like spokes in a wheel. The ones depicted in red are arteries, the ones in black are veins. The macula is an oval depression in the retina and is the point of clearest vision in the center of the retina. The + shows the center of the viewed field. (Sketch by Dr. Sabera T. Shah, of the William P. Beetham Eye Research and Treatment Unit of the Joslin Diabetes Center.)

retinopathy (Fig. 16–3). It is this condition that most threatens vision for many people with diabetes. Vascular (blood vessel) changes in the eye are fairly common in people with long-standing diabetes, but complete blindness is not nearly as common as supposed. Although about 90% of those who have had diabetes for more than 25 years have some vascular changes, sometimes these changes are not obvious to the person with diabetes, who is surprised when told about them by the doctor.

Subconjunctival Hemorrhage. Occasionally a person looks into the mirror and sees a bright red, pie-shaped wedge in the white of the eye. This is frightening but quite harmless. It represents a tiny blood vessel that somehow broke and bled beneath the clear outside covering of the eyeball. It is not exclusive to people with diabetes; anyone can have it. It is not caused by diabetes. If left alone, it usually improves and disappears within a few days.

Glaucoma. Many people over age 40 may have glaucoma, and people in that age group should be tested for glaucoma every year

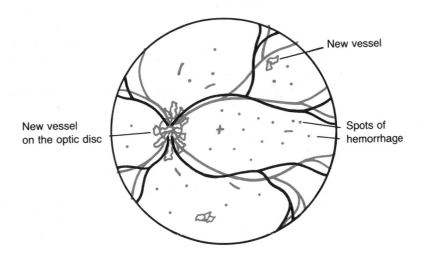

New vessel

New vessel
on the optic disc

Spots of
hemorrhage

FIG. 16–3. Fundus of an eye affected by diabetic retinopathy. Characteristic changes of retinopathy include small spots where small blood vessels
have bulged (aneurysms) or hemorrhaged and new blood vessels (proliferative retinopathy), which can form on the optic disc and elsewhere on the
retina. (Sketch by Dr. Sabera T. Shah.)

or two. The test is a simple, quick, and painless measurement of
eyeball pressure. Increased pressure is due to too much fluid in the
eye. At first the condition usually causes no symptoms. As the
pressure increases, the symptoms may include visual loss and bright
flashes or rings of lights around the eyes. Later there may be eye
pain. If left untreated too long, the pressure damage is irreversible.
Early on, the condition is treated with drops that permit the fluid
exchange to continue. Sometimes surgery is needed. The usual
forms of glaucoma (increased pressure without hemorrhage) can
occur with or without diabetes. Glaucoma resulting from hemorrhage in the eyeball is, fortunately, unusual. Special forms of laser
treatment are now used instead of or in conjunction with eye drops
to control glaucoma.

Cataract. A cataract (clouding of the lens) is one of the commonest
eye problems in older people. As we said earlier, the lens must
remain transparent if vision is to be normal. If the lens becomes
clouded, the transmission of light is blocked. There are two types of
cataract. One type is the metabolic cataract, which develops

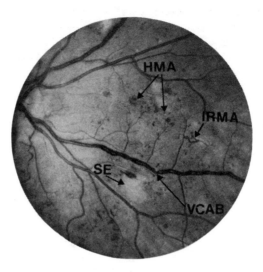

FIG. 16–4. A fundus from someone with diabetes showing changes that are characteristic of diabetic retinopathy. These include microaneurysms (bulges in the blood vessel) and small hemorrhages of the blood vessels (**HMA**); soft exudates (**SE**), or small diffuse areas where fluid has leaked out of the blood vessels; and damage to the blood vessels such as narrowing or weakening of the walls (**VCAB** and **IRMA**).

because of the accumulation of the by-products of abnormal metabolism in the lens of the eye. This type of cataract is sometimes found in younger people. Before insulin, metabolic cataracts were quite common in people with diabetes. The most common type of cataract is the age-related cataract, frequently found in older people with or without diabetes. Cataracts seem to occur as part of the normal aging process, although there is some evidence that poor diabetes control may speed up the process. Either of these two types of cataracts can be treated surgically by removing the lens. Traditionally, new eyeglasses were used to replace the lens and help the eye focus light after cataract surgery. In recent years, ophthalmologists have also used contact lenses as well as artificial lenses that are surgically implanted in the eyeball.

Diseases of the Retina. Damage or disease of the retina (retinopathy) is the most serious of all the diabetic complications of the eye. The early changes of diabetic retinopathy start subtly (Fig. 16–4). The small retinal vessels weaken and their supporting basement membranes (the lining of the vessels) become thickened and develop leaks. The vessels themselves become fragile. Recent research has shown that the chemical makeup of this basement membrane is changed in diabetes.

A more obvious change is the microaneurysm, a dilated bulge on the wall of a small vessel, which is something like the bulge on the side of a weakened automobile tire in the days when they had inner tubes. Such little bulges may leak serum from the blood. A more dangerous type of retinopathy is the formation of many new and very fragile vessels. This process of new vessel formation is called neovascularization (Fig. 16–5). When new vessels form in the retina, the individual is said to have proliferative retinopathy (the new vessels proliferate). Major hemorrhages of these fragile vessels can result in the formation of small, dark streaks. If the hemorrhages are large enough or cover a sensitive area, they interfere with vision. They may rupture through the retinal lining into the vitreous humor, discoloring this fluid so that vision is blocked. This is known as vitreous hemorrhage. With the potential to hemorrhage that proliferative retinopathy has, it is, indeed, the stage of diabetic retinopathy that is the most threatening and thus the one that requires the most immediate attention.

Some of the small hemorrhages may be absorbed, and within days or weeks even the vitreous hemorrhage may clear up because the eye fluid is continually being changed. If the new vessels shrink and scar, the visual loss may not become worse. It has been estimated that in about 30% of patients with proliferative retinopathy, the visual loss does not necessarily progress but remains static or even improves spontaneously sometimes for many years. In one large study of patients whose eyes were observed from the time they first showed some evidence of retinal damage, 18% had an increased visual loss after 15 years, but twice as many (36%) were either no worse or actually had improved.

Nevertheless, treatment of proliferative retinopathy is frequently needed. A technique of injecting a dye (fluorescein) into the eye circulation through arm blood vessels so that the vessels can be studied gives the physician a precise view of the damage. This, in turn, helps to pinpoint areas suitable for treatment.

Treating the Damaged Retina. The treatment of diseased retina has improved recently. In the past there have been many attempts to treat retinal disease, and most have been useless.

Good control of diabetes has always been considered helpful in preventing retinopathy. People who have lived 20 to 50 years with diabetes without severe forms of eye damage have usually taken better care of their diabetes than those who have severe eye damage

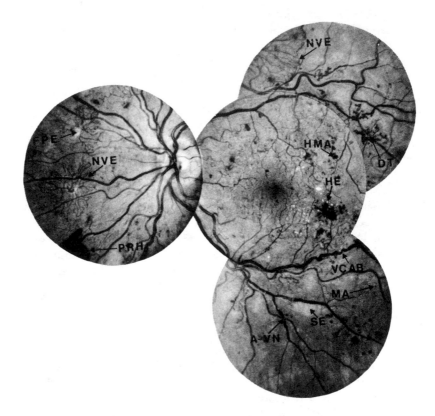

FIG. 16–5. Photos showing more advanced retinal disease. Many of the characteristics seen in Figure 16–4 are present, but in addition hard exudates (**HE**) signify leaking capillaries (very small blood vessels). Neovascularization—the haphazard formation of new blood vessels—is the hallmark of the "proliferative" type of retinopathy, and is indicated by **NVE** in the figure. (**HMA** = hemorrhages and microaneurysms; **VCAB** and **IRMA** = vessel narrowing or abnormalities)

after this length of time; however, the effect of control is difficult to relate directly to the development of retinopathy. Some people with diabetes are found to have retinal changes as early as ten years after the onset of their condition; others escape for many years. The development of retinal changes is one of the primary factors being followed in the Diabetes Control and Complications Trial (described in Chapter 18), and so we hope soon to have a better idea about the relationship between diabetes control and the development of retinopathy.

In sheer desperation many treatments were tried over the years.

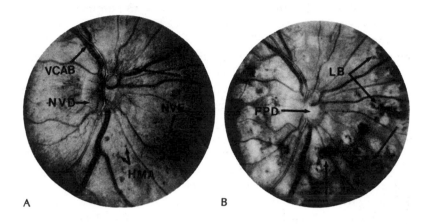

FIG. 16–6. Retina of a 20-year-old person with diabetes of 10 years' duration. Figure 16-6A, taken prior to laser treatment, shows new vessels on the disc (**NVD**) and elsewhere (**NVE**), in addition to other signs of advanced retinopathy. Figure 16–6B shows the same fundus after laser treatment. New vessels on the disc have cleared; laser burns (**LB**) are present. (**HMA** = hemorrhages and microaneurysms; **VCAB** = blood vessel narrowing; **FPD** = small fibrous membrane)

Almost every type of medication available was tried, including snake venom, which was also useless.

Because the hormone from the anterior pituitary was known to worsen diabetes, removal of the pituitary by surgery, freezing, or x-ray was tried. Removing the pituitary did help preserve vision in some but caused so many other complications that this procedure was generally abandoned in favor of the newer, safer, and more effective laser beam treatments.

Photocoagulation by Laser. A new and exciting era in the treatment of retinopathy dawned with the development of retinal photo-coagulation (treatment with light) techniques, commonly referred to as laser treatment. "Laser" itself is an acronym (artificial word) derived from the first letters of the words "Light Amplification by Stimulated Emission of Radiation." Laser photocoagulation has proven the most effective treatment to date of diabetic retinopathy. This procedure uses a bright, powerful beam of light intensely focused on the retina. This light "burns" areas of the retina that are affected by diabetic retinopathy and prevents its spread (Fig. 16–6). Research over the last few years has clearly demonstrated that this treatment is, indeed, effective in stopping the progression of diabetic retinopathy, the process that can lead to blindness.

Some 30 years ago, a xenon-arc photocoagulator was used for photocoagulation therapy of diabetic eye disease. While this proved effective in many cases, it caused greater vision loss than present lasers because the retinal damage necessary with this older technique was more extensive. It also produced more scar tissue on the retina than today's lasers, yet patients were happy to sacrifice some vision throughout this treatment in order to prevent greater vision loss from retinopathy itself.

Today's lasers are more convenient and safer than these older types. The most widely used lasers today are the blue-green argon and the green-only argon lasers, which were developed relatively recently. It was an earlier laser, the ruby, that Drs Beetham, Aiello, and co-workers used to demonstrate the technique of *pan-retinal photocoagulation*. This technique, with the newer lasers, is now used to treat proliferative eye disease. This pan-retinal technique provides focused, precise destruction of damaged or unneeded blood vessels without major side effects. By systematically placing hundreds of tiny burns on the retina with the laser, the skillful ophthalmologist is often able to achieve a dramatic reduction in proliferative retinal disease.

The efficacy of pan-retinal laser photocoagulation was definitively demonstrated in a nationwide clinical trial called the Diabetic Retinopathy Study (DRS), which began in 1971 and was sponsored by the National Eye Institute. The study was quite remarkable because it involved 1758 people who had either severe proliferative retinal disease in one eye (the other eye having less severe proliferative or nonproliferative retinopathy), or severe nonproliferative retinopathy in both eyes. One eye was treated using one of the photocoagulation techniques, while the other eye (the control) was untreated. The early reports showed that the incidence of severe loss of vision in the eye treated with pan-retinal photocoagulation was 61% less than the incidence of severe vision loss in the nontreated eye. This was remarkable for something for which there was previously no really good treatment. Now there was really hope for significant prevention of blindness if severe loss of vision could be decreased by 61% in eyes that already had advanced stages of retinopathy. What would be the result if the eyes were treated much earlier in the course of the disease? A subsequent study, the Early Treatment Diabetic Retinopathy Study (ETDRS), was started by the National Eye Institute in 1980 to determine if *earlier* laser treatment for retinopathy, a small daily dose of aspirin, and laser treatment for macular edema would further reduce visual loss from diabetes. This study, with 3,925 patients, is projected to continue for several more years, but it has already shown that proper laser treatment for macular edema may reduce the risk of moderate visual loss by 50%.

Specific treatment of the macula reduces the risk of moderate visual loss (visual acuity between 20/40—driving vision—and 20/200—legal blindness) by 50%. The overall loss of vision associated with diabetic retinopathy, therefore, can be reduced by 50% if treatment is started early enough in expert hands. This exciting news is the reason people with diabetes must have frequent eye examinations to find developing problems at an earlier stage and treat them.

> Many people can have severe eye damage without knowing it. The damage can be in areas that do not affect vision, and there is often no pain. Only a careful examination at regular intervals will find it.

Vitrectomy. A remarkable surgical procedure called vitrectomy has been used recently to treat vitreous hemorrhages. A problem with leaking retinal vessels in the eye is that when there is a large hemorrhage into the vitreous humor, the eyeball fluid becomes mixed with blood, preventing light from passing through the eye and thus causing blindness. Remember in the old-fashioned pharmacies (now few and far between) there were large jars of colored fluid hanging in the window. The fluid was mostly water with just a bit of chemical added to make the color. This color kept light from going through, just as hemorrhage into the eyeballs colors the fluid and prevents clear vision. Until recently, little could be done because even lasers could not be used if the doctor could not see into the eye. Vitrectomy uses an instrument containing a drill and suction. Under anesthesia, this instrument enters the eyeball, sucks out the vitreous hemorrhage, and replaces it with normal saline. The instrument is removed and the hole is sealed. The ophthalmologist can then see into the eye and determine whether lasers might be helpful. Some remarkable results have been obtained, and some who were absolutely blind now have vision.

Vitrectomy surgery is an attempt to restore vision after diabetic retinopathy has already caused serious eye damage. The procedure is not without risks, but in the hands of a skilled and experienced ophthalmologist, vitrectomies have restored vision for many who otherwise would have lived with blindness. While blindness is probably the most feared complication it is amazing how well many blind people can do with considerable eye damage yet with enough vision to get around. It was a wise man who once said, "In the kingdom of the blind, the one-eyed man is king," and with these new techniques many more people retain significant vision.

Eye Examinations for People with Diabetes. With the remarkable advances in diagnosing and treating eye problems, regular eye examinations become a great personal responsibility for anyone with diabetes. As we mentioned above, many retinal changes cause no change in sight until they have reached an advanced state. Because frequently there are no symptoms associated with even severe retinopathy, it is advisable for people with type I (insulin-dependent) diabetes mellitus to have their eyes examined by an ophthalmologist within five years of the onset of diabetes and *at least* yearly thereafter. For those with type II (non-insulin-dependent) diabetes mellitus, a preliminary examination looking for any possible early changes of retinopathy should be made *on diagnosis* and *at least* once yearly afterwards. In no field of diabetes complications have the treatment changes over the past dozen or so years been as dramatic and hopeful.

The Kidneys and Urinary Tract

The kidneys are among the least appreciated and most abused organs of the body. The urinary tract consists of two kidneys, one on each side of the backbone. Long slender tubes called ureters carry the urine from the kidneys to the bladder, which is a storage reservoir for the urine until it is released.

The kidneys have a most important function. They screen any waste products from the blood, reclaiming useful things for further use. This is "recycling" at its very best. The end products of protein metabolism are nitrogen substances, which are removed by the kidneys and eliminated. The proteins themselves are saved and reused. The urinary tract often becomes infected in people (especially women) with diabetes, particularly in those with poor diabetes regulation. In the presence of elevated blood glucose levels, the phagocytes (cells that are part of the body's defenses) are less effective in destroying bacteria. Thus these people are more likely to develop infections of the urinary tract which can spread up into the kidneys and damage them. Figure 16–7 shows common urinary tract complications in diabetes. In addition to infections, other

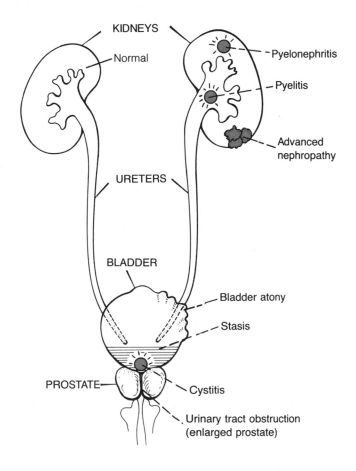

FIG.   16–7. Common   urinary   tract   complications   in   diabetes.
Nephropathy means pathology of the kidney (see text). *Pyelitis* is infection
of the pelvis, the area where urine is collected before going down the
ureters to the bladder. *Pyelonephritis* is infection of the tubules (which
collect the urine), the glomeruli (the little structures that filter the urine
from the blood), and the blood vessels. *Cystitis* means inflammation of the
bladder, usually as a result of infection. *Urine stasis* means the retention of
urine in the bladder owing to obstruction of free urine drainage or bladder
atony (see text). The longer urine remains in the bladder, the greater the
risk of infection.

common conditions that can result in damage to the kidneys are elevated blood pressure, inflammation of the connective tissues, and changes in tissues caused by diabetes.

Urinary Tract Infections. As with many other complications, the best solution to urinary tract infection is early diagnosis and treatment. Infections can be suspected from symptoms such as burning or painful urination, frequency of urination, or cloudy or bloody urine. Early mild urinary infections may produce no symptoms and are found by periodic microscopic examination of the urinary sediment by a physician at routine diabetes checkups, with cultures of urine specimens when needed.

Many antibiotics are available to treat urinary tract infections. This treatment must be medically supervised to be certain that the proper and specific antibiotics are chosen. This often requires culture of the urine to determine which bacterium is responsible for the infection and a sensitivity test to determine which antibiotic is most effective. Treatment must continue until the infection has been removed from the bladder and urine; otherwise it will recur and become chronic. This may mean taking an antibiotic for many days and often after the symptoms have disappeared.

Nonfunctioning Bladder (Atony). A less common problem is diabetic bladder atony. The bladder becomes insensitive and overdistended and loses much of its muscle power because of damage to the nerves that control urinary function. This condition usually is caused by diabetic neuropathy and is often associated with

---

The ending-"PATHY" means bad news in the language of medicine. It is short for "pathology," or disease. RETINOPATHY is disease of the eye retina. NEUROPATHY is pathology of the nerves, and NEPHROPATHY is disease of the kidney (nephros). These are the commonest severe complications of diabetes and are often lumped together as "TRIOPATHY" because of the organs involved.

---

other types of neuritis as well. It results in incomplete emptying of the bladder and stagnation of urine. Stagnation builds a sort of cesspool which favors the growth of bacteria and the development of infection. Bladder atony is difficult to treat. Sometimes medicine can be helpful. At other times, surgery is necessary to improve the drainage. Now you know why your physician tells you to drink lots of water with or without treatment. It is important to keep drainage flowing and urine from stagnating.

Kidney Disorders. Nephropathy is the most serious kidney disorder of diabetes. The word "nephropathy" refers to a combination of changes often found in the kidneys of people with diabetes of long duration. These changes are infection, sclerosis (hardening of the small kidney arteries), and damage to the glomeruli (filtering apparatus of the kidney). These often progress with long duration of diabetes so that kidney function slowly deteriorates. At first, protein, which is usually saved by the thrifty kidneys, starts to appear in the urine in increasing amounts. This means that the kidney is not screening properly. This protein (albumin) is wasted in the urine in increasing amounts. Meanwhile, more of the body's waste products are retained in the blood (uremia). In time, water is also retained, which causes swelling (edema). Blood pressure becomes elevated, and the classic signs of uremia become obvious.

The earliest changes of diabetic kidney disease involve a thickening of the basement membranes (part of the inner lining of the filtering mechanism) of the kidney. This basement membrane thickening may begin quite early. However, recent evidence suggests that this type of kidney disease is related to poor diabetes control. Repeated urinary tract infections also damage the kidneys. Thus early recognition and treatment of these infections is very important.

Treating Kidney Disease. In the past, little could be done for people with advanced diabetic nephropathy. Now much more is possible. Newer diets and medications (some still experimental) for early nephropathy are being studied. Some may decrease the accumulation of body wastes. In advanced cases, it is now quite common to rid the body of wastes normally excreted by the kidneys by using dialysis, either peritoneal or with the artificial kidney machine. When dialysis is performed with a machine, the blood is taken from the patient, and the machine removes the impurities and then returns the blood to the patient. With peritoneal dialysis, dialysis fluid is put into the abdominal cavity through a catheter. The membranes that attach the intestines to the inner walls of the body are rich in blood vessels. The wastes filter out from these vessels into this dialysis fluid, which is then removed from the body through the catheter. This method of dialysis can be done at home on some people and is referred to as continuous ambulatory peritoneal dialysis (CAPD).

Another means of treating chronic renal failure is *renal trans-*

plantation. This involves the removal of a healthy kidney, preferably from a near relative of a person with diabetes, or, if such is not available, from some other acceptable donor, and placing it into the person whose kidneys have failed because of diabetes. Kidney transplantation is a complex and difficult procedure, which is becoming increasingly successful in growing numbers of people. People with diabetes who undergo kidney transplants are living longer and enjoying a better quality of life thanks to this procedure. Transplantation has the advantage of freeing the individual from the burden of dialysis sessions and allows many people to return to a life-style closely resembling "normal." One drawback, of course, is the need to use drugs regularly to suppress the immunity factors that might cause rejection of the kidney.

In general, an important part of the care of someone with diabetes is monitoring kidney function and watching for evidence of infection. Microscopic urine testing can tell a physician a great deal about what may be happening within the kidney and bladder, and allows the doctor to advise treatment when necessary. Recent advances have allowed longer survival and a better quality of life for those with failing kidneys.

Recently, researchers at the Joslin Clinic have reviewed records of people treated at the clinic over the years since Elliott P. Joslin began his practice, looking at the development of complications. The results of the review of people who developed type I (insulin-dependent) diabetes mellitus before the age of 21 are quite encouraging. Researchers found that those whose diabetes was diagnosed between 1949 and 1959 had only half of the incidence of diabetic renal disease of those whose diabetes was diagnosed in the year 1939. The reasons for this decline are not known but may be because of newer treatments for high blood pressure and antibiotics to treat infections. The most exciting thing about these studies is that only about one-third of the people diagnosed at this very young age developed renal disease. For whatever reason, hopes are improving that modern methods will uncover ways to predict who will develop kidney disease before it progresses to a dangerous stage so that measures to stop its advance can be started.

Neuropathy

Numerous nerve-related problems are lumped under the term "diabetic neuritis" or "neuropathy." These are among the most puzzling complications of diabetes and are often difficult to diagnose with certainty. Almost any nerve pathway in any part of the body can be affected by diabetic neuropathy, and while most neuropathies are mild and annoying, they can also be very disabling and painful. Yet despite the severe disability that some neuropathies may cause, they almost never cause death without other complications being present.

Neuropathies are often thought of in two categories. One category is the sensory ("peripheral") neuropathies, which affect nerves controlling sensation in the feet, hands, or joints, and the other category is the autonomic neuropathies, which affect the nerve function controlling various organs such as the digestive or urinary tracts.

Symptoms of Sensory Neuropathies. Numbness, coldness, tingling, a feeling of walking upon wool, and pain are the most frequent symptoms described by people who have painful diabetic neuropathies. The extremities (arms and more often legs) are most often affected, but occasionally bands across the chest or abdomen can be affected. These sensations are often most obvious at night, on cold, wet, rainy days, and in winter. The skin of the feet, legs, and thighs may be so sensitive that the weight of bedclothes can be intolerable. The discomfort can range from mild to severe, from occasional to constant. In fact, the symptoms can range from almost complete sensation loss to severe pain. These symptoms do not respect age or sex; anyone with diabetes can have these manifestations.

A period of uncontrolled diabetes often, but not always, precedes the appearance of symptoms. In some adults, these symptoms lead to the diagnosis of diabetes. Sometimes the first severe symptoms start after treatment begins, but more often they occur after long duration of diabetes. On occasion they will worsen for a while, perhaps a few weeks or months, just after the control of the diabetes has been improved, almost as if the nerves were being further irritated as they "healed." Fortunately, the pain often abates with careful, prolonged treatment of the diabetes.

Although peripheral neuropathy can occur in nearly any nerve, certain nerves are affected more frequently than others. Sensory neuropathies are most common, but the nerves controlling muscles may be affected as well. It is more common to have sensory neuropathies in the feet than in the hands. Of additional concern is that when the symptoms include loss of sensation, further foot problems may result. Unfortunately, people often fail to recognize minor injuries, blisters, and trauma. Immediate medical treatment of even the most innocent-looking lesion of the foot is most important.

Amyotrophy (muscle wasting) is a special form of diabetic neuropathy. It combines extreme sensitivity of the skin of the thighs, pain and tenderness of the thigh muscles, and weakness. Muscle bulk decreases, making it difficult for the person to arise from a chair or climb stairs. Loss of appetite and loss of body weight are common. This condition is treated carefully by treatment of the diabetes and use of pain relievers and nerve-quieting medication. Sometimes a preliminary period of nearly absolute rest may be needed, but ultimately an increase in physical activity or actually undergoing physical therapy helps restore muscles to their previous condition. Recovery is slow, however, and overnight changes should not be expected.

Occasionally a single nerve that operates a muscle or group of muscles is affected. This type of neuropathy can cause *double vision* if the muscles of the eye are affected. These symptoms may continue from three to six weeks. Complete recovery is the rule. The condition may appear more than once in the same person, but often different muscles are involved.

Another example of neuropathy is *foot-drop*. The muscles responsible for raising the foot become weakened and the foot slaps with each step. Should the muscles not regain strength, a brace may be worn. Fortunately, recovery usually does take place.

A less common type of neuropathy is radicular (radiating) pain, which causes an encircling or girdle-type pain in the chest or trunk nerves. It is a sharp, shooting, burning pain that is constant, excruciating, and sometimes defies definition. Sometimes patients mistake this for angina. It usually disappears gradually.

The stomach, small bowel, large bowel, and urinary bladder empty their contents by a series of rhythmic contractions of the muscles within their walls. When the nerves that operate these muscles become "neuropathic," a delay in the contractions takes place. The patient experiences fullness, bloating, vomiting of undigested food, infrequent but voluminous urination, and constipation. Sometimes medication that stimulates smooth muscle function helps.

Neuropathic damage can also affect the nerves that control the contraction of blood vessels. As a result, the blood pressure can fall when the person gets up from a lying position. This condition is called *orthostatic hypotension*. The severity of the symptoms can vary. Some medications can minimize the blood pressure drops if they are severe.

Impotence is the loss of the ability to have erections and is more common in men who have diabetes than in men who do not. Although it usually occurs after one has had diabetes for a number of years, it has been seen earlier in some individuals. It is thought that the primary cause of impotence is neuropathy, although hardening of the arteries in some men may have a role. Impotence that is due to diabetes begins gradually, but occurs with all attempts at sexual activity. Sexual desire (libido) is usually still present, although it may wane as lack of functional ability progresses. Psychological problems can play an enormous part in any man with impotence (Chapter 17). For men with diabetes, the fear of failure may make the impotence due to diabetes a self-fulfilling prophecy.

Men with diabetes and impotence should discuss the problem with their physician. Sometimes medications used for other medical conditions are a cause. The sex hormones can be checked for normalcy. A complete evaluation by a urologist is also advised, and a psychological screening may be recommended.

Nevertheless, diabetic autonomic neuropathies—neuropathy affecting the nerves that control erections—are often the cause of impotence in men with diabetes. Normally, psychic stimuli for sexual function travel out of the brain and down to the groin area through nerves. These nerves control small valves called polster valves which are located on the blood vessels leading to and from the penis. The sexual stimulus causes the polster valves on the inflow vessels to open, permitting blood to fill spongy areas within the body of the penis. The outflow polster valves close, trapping the blood within the penis and keeping it erect. When sexual stimulus subsides, this process reverses, the blood drains out, and the penis becomes flaccid.

When impotence occurs in men with diabetes, it is probably due to damage of the nerve fibers that control the polster valves. As a result the polster valves do not function properly, and potency is reduced. Thus impotence is considered a form of diabetic neuropathy. Another theory, and actually another possible mechanism for impotency which may occur in some men with or without diabetes, is that the blood vessels become narrowed or blocked, similar to vascular disease that occurs in other parts of the body. The end result—impotence—is the same.

The development of impotence in men with diabetes tends to come on gradually. It does not occur suddenly one evening. The rigidity of the penis, or the duration of erection, tend to get less and less over time. Nocturnal and morning erections are also affected. With this decline, there is no reduction in sexual desire. While there is certainly a physical reason for impotence, fear of failure can worsen function even further. Impotence does not imply infertility, however.

Various treatments for this problem have been developed. The most effective is the insertion of a penile prosthesis. This involves insertion of two rods or balloon-type cylinders into the body of the penis. There are two basic varieties of prostheses. One is a permanently elongated variety. This model can be bent down when not in use, but the length and semirigidity remain. The second variety is an inflatable type. A small pump, placed in the scrotal sac under one of the testicles, is used to pump the balloon-like cylinders full of a fluid that is stored in a reservoir in the lower pelvic area. When not in use, this model allows the penis to appear normal size. The inflatable model requires more gadgetry and is therefore a bit more involved to have inserted. It therefore has more potential for difficulty. For men with difficulty with manual dexterity, the permanently elongated variety is preferable. Using either model, men who are otherwise fertile may be able to ejaculate normally. In general, both types have been widely and successfully used. These prostheses can be inserted by urologists (physicians who practice the surgical specialty relating to the urinary tract).

Another problem that some men with diabetes may face is a phenomenon known as *retrograde ejaculation*. Normally, during sexual activity, the semen is ejaculated outward in order to impregnate the partner. Some men with diabetes have a type of nerve damage that prevents the semen from moving outward. Instead, it flows into the bladder where it is destroyed. If this occurs, fertility can be reduced or prevented altogether. This can be a serious problem to young men wishing to start a family. The nerve damage that causes this problem is different from the damage resulting in impotence. Fortunately, retrograde ejaculation is quite rare. The beginnings of retrograde ejaculation do not necessarily mean that fertility will be a problem, but it may be an incentive to begin a family sooner rather than later. There are many other potential causes of infertility, and if there has been difficulty conceiving, both partners should be checked by a fertility expert.

Charcot's joint is a rare and little understood form of diabetic neuropathy which involves changes in the small bones of the foot and in the joints between them. The condition is relatively painless, but the bone structure may be injured unless walking is monitored during the acute period.

All forms of neuropathy are troublesome, and some are temporarily disabling. Rarely are they permanent. Most symptoms disappear completely or improve. Nevertheless, occasionally neuropathy can be so disabling, or persist for so long, that the person experiencing it begins to doubt reassurances of eventual improvement. It is a most distressing condition to treat and can be very frustrating to your physician as well.

What Causes Neuropathy? The cause of neuropathy is not completely known, but there have been many theories over the years. It has been blamed on insufficient nutrition or destruction of the nerves, thrombosis (plugging) of the blood vessels leading to the nerves, insufficient vitamins, and many other reasons.

The current theory is that the nerves may be injured or destroyed due to the metabolic changes of diabetes. Nerves are like electric wires. Just as a wire is surrounded by a plastic sheath to protect it (and you), nerves are surrounded by a sheath of cells to protect them. In people with diabetes, the excess sugar gets into the sheath cells and undergoes a series of chemical changes (the "polyol" pathway) to produce sorbitol. These reactions are stimulated by an enzyme called aldose reductase. Sorbitol is thought to make the cells swell. This swelling leads to irritation of the nerve, and, if present long enough, to death of the nerve cell. Although irritated nerves may recover, function does not return to dead nerves.

Recently, experimental medications known as aldose reductase inhibitors have been used to treat neuropathy. These are chemicals that slow or stop the enzyme aldose reductase, blocking the reaction that leads to neuropathy. Further research trials will tell whether these substances are effective tools in the prevention and treatment of this complication.

Treatment. For neuropathy, there are many attempts at therapy. Most of these are "nonspecific"—that is, they treat symptoms such as pain or other discomforts and are not a treatment for the specific reason for the disease.

One of the most effective longterm measures is improved control of diabetes. However, this improvement may take weeks, months, or even years. Some measures may be helpful in the short term to relieve some of the discomfort. Heat or bed rest may help some, while activity may help others. Various types of medications have been used, largely analgesics (pain relievers) and other types of compounds that may work directly to reduce inflammation or irritants of the nerves. The use of narcotics should be discouraged in all but the most severe cases. In future years, if aldose reductase inhibitors or similar medicines are perfected, they may be a more "specific" treatment for the cause of the pain. As with many other medical problems, there is continuing research to solve these. Look what has happened in the treatment of eyes, feet, and the heart, to mention a few. Somewhere someone will find a solution to this problem.

Cardiovascular Complications

The cardiovascular (circulatory) system includes the heart and blood vessels. Diseases of this system have many effects on the body. Blockage of the coronary arteries which supply blood to the heart can cause angina—the pain due to insufficient blood (ischemic heart disease)—or a myocardial infarction (heart attack) when the blood supply is blocked altogether. Blockage in the circulation to the brain can cause what is referred to as a cerebrovascular accident (CVA, or "stroke"). This blockage can be caused by blood clots building up in the blood vessels (thrombosis), a blood clot breaking off of a blood vessel and traveling to the brain where it lodges in a smaller vessel and blocks it (embolus), or a blood vessel that leaks and bleeds into the surrounding tissue (hemorrhage). Blockages in the blood vessels that supply blood to the legs and feet can lead to leg or calf pain when a person walks some distance. This condition is called *claudication*. Poor circulation in the legs can also make it harder for wounds to heal and makes infection more likely. Indeed, cardiovascular disease affects all parts of the body.

The mechanism by which diabetes has an effect on the cardiovascular system (heart and blood vessels) is not entirely clear, but it does appear that people with diabetes have a greater likelihood of developing problems with circulation than people who do not have this disease. Arteriosclerotic heart disease, with or without diabetes, is the greatest single cause of death in the United States, and certainly many of the more than half a million people who die each year from this condition have diabetes. In some studies, a third to a half of those who have had a recent heart attack have had an abnormal glucose tolerance test, at least temporarily. It is difficult to determine which disorder came first.

Although all of the factors connecting heart disease with diabetes are not known, myocardial infarction (heart attack) is the chief cause of death in people with onset of diabetes after the age of 30. Unfortunately, heart disease symptoms in many people with diabetes are less definite than they are in those without diabetes, and many do not get the usual warnings such as pain (angina) until very late in the course of this disease. The Framingham (Massachusetts) Heart Study has helped identify various risk factors that contribute to heart disease. These include elevated blood pressure, smoking, overweight, elevated cholesterol, and diabetes. Among the factors protecting the cardiac system are normal weight, normal blood pressure, low cholesterol, and high HDL (high density lipoproteins, the "good" cholesterol) levels.

In addition to improved medical care for all cardiac patients, improved surgical treatment, such as the coronary artery bypass operation, has been one of the greatest success stories for ischemic heart disease (insufficient blood flow through the coronary arteries to the heart muscle). Recently, a technique called angioplasty has been developed. This allows the unblocking of some arteries using a catheter tube fed into the heart vessels without the more extensive bypass surgery. Medications are becoming available which prevent the need for surgery by dissolving blood clots in blood vessels. Even day-to-day medications for treatment of various kinds of heart disease are improved so that people with these ailments can lead more normal, productive lives. At one time a certain amount of high blood pressure was tolerated. A recent medical journal headline stated that even small amounts of hypertension are inexcusable. We can say this now because many new medicines are effective and available.

Blood Vessel Changes. Thickening of parts of the walls of the large blood vessels is the underlying event that produces most cardiovascular diseases. It is believed that diabetes makes this thickening worse. This is already a phenomenon of aging and is speeded up by diabetes. Insulin deficiency, reflected by elevated blood sugar levels, may bring about changes in the metabolism of vascular tissue. Increased blood levels of lipids (fats) are also harmful to blood vessels. Good control of diabetes can help reduce the amount of fat, especially the blood triglycerides. An eating plan with reduced intake of saturated fats is the primary treatment of elevated blood lipid levels. If diet alone is not sufficient, additional medications are available to help lower blood fat levels. The smaller blood vessels of the eyes and kidneys are also susceptible to the metabolic changes of diabetes. These were discussed earlier in this chapter.

Infections

It is true that people with diabetes may have more infections than those without diabetes. However, the old adage that "people with diabetes do not heal as well as others" is not necessarily true.

It all depends on circulation and diabetes care. For example, young people with excellent circulation and reasonably good control of their diabetes heal just as rapidly as anyone else. The healing problem occurs more often in older people with poor circulation in the feet and legs and in those whose diabetes is poorly controlled. It is now also known that bodily defenses against invading bacteria are unable to perform at their best ability when diabetes control is negligent. Phagocytes (the white cells that help to fight infection) appear to be much less effective in uncontrolled diabetes. However, their activity is restored to normal with good treatment that lowers blood glucose levels.

Fifty years ago, the bane of the person with diabetes, and a frequent cause of death, was carbuncles. These are rarely seen now. This is true of many infections that were common before the discovery of antibiotics and the availability of insulin. However, infections are still a hazard to the unwary person with diabetes. High levels of blood glucose can provide a better breeding area in the skin and mucous membranes for some bacteria and fungi. As a result, people with poorly controlled diabetes more readily acquire skin and nail infections, especially the annoying fungal infections of the feet and groin areas. With their increased risk of infections, which may also be more severe than in people without diabetes, people who have diabetes should consider receiving injections of vaccines against pneumococcal pneumonia infections and influenza. The pneumococcal vaccine, called *pneumovax*, is given once only. It is recommended for people with long-standing diabetes and for people who have diabetes and may also have lung, heart, or vascular diseases. Influenza immunization injections are recommended for these same individuals, plus those who are likely to receive a high exposure to this infection—for example, medical personnel, school personnel, or parents of young children. Older people should also consider both of these injections, as serious illnesses can be more debilitating in this group of individuals.

Feet

Problems with the feet are one of the most common longterm complications of diabetes, and possibly the most crippling. Because there are about 12 million people with diabetes in the United States, there are, as Dr. Marvin Levin of St. Louis, Missouri, has pointed out, "120 million very vulnerable toes on 24 million feet."

The foot is often the "Achilles' heel" for those with diabetes.

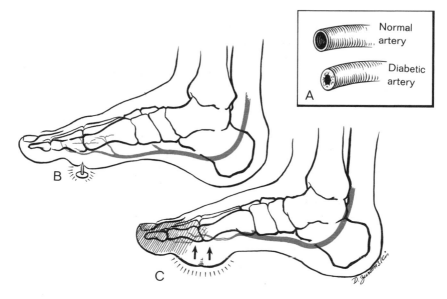

FIG. 16–8. Foot complications are often caused by diminished blood supply. (A) The thickened artery of the person with longterm diabetes permits less blood to circulate than a normal artery. (B) An injury that causes inflammation requires an even greater blood supply, which is often unavailable. (C) The infected foot swells, compressing the arteries and thereby further diminishing the blood supply.

Although many people have foot problems, the feet of those with diabetes are particularly vulnerable for several reasons (Fig. 16–8): (1) the circulation is very often decreased in older people, especially where the blood vessels become narrow at the lower end of the foot; (2) in people with diabetes, the degree of blood vessel narrowing may be even greater for their present age; (3) in diabetes, sensation is often decreased because of neuropathy. These factors, along with increased tendency for infection in poorly treated diabetes, provide a background for impending trouble.

Any precipitating infection or mechanical impediment, such as an ingrown toenail, an infected callus or corn, trauma, untreated athlete's foot or tight, poorly fitting shoes, may damage the tissues and serve as an opening for infection. As the infection spreads, inflammation and swelling occur, with greater demands for blood supply which is not available. A chain of events takes place in which each thing worsens the other. The infection spreads, aided by inadequate circulation. The person has diminished pain sensation and continues to walk on the injured part, so the foot crisis deepens.

The commonest lesions are corns, calluses (especially on the toes and soles of the feet), ingrown toenails, fungus infection (athlete's foot), and ulcers caused by pressure—indeed injuries or infections of any kind. Then, of course, deformities due to neuropathic changes may exist. Some of these are shown in Figure 16–9.

> **Principles of Good Foot Care:**
> 1. **Give your feet good preventive care.**
> 2. **Look at your feet regularly or have someone else do so.**
> 3. **Avoid injury to your feet.**
> 4. **Wear well-fitting shoes.**

Skin Care. Most of the common foot problems involve the skin. Feet should be washed, but *not soaked*, in warm (*not hot*—test the temperature with your hand or elbow first), soapy water daily. Soaking the feet softens the skin and makes it more susceptible to infection. People with dry skin on their feet should apply a

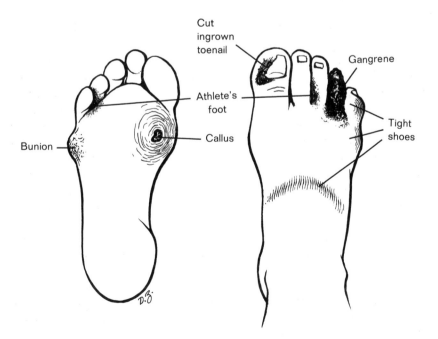

FIG. 16–9. Some common foot problems in people with diabetes caused by improper care.

moisturizing lotion containing lanolin nightly to the feet. However, the web spaces should not be saturated with lotions, which may cause the skin to weaken and break apart. Lotions such as Nivea, Dermassage, Alpha-Keri, Polysorbhydrate, and many others are appropriate. When the skin is too moist, apply talcum or baby powder daily to absorb the moisture. Never nick the skin with scissors or sharp instruments.

Nail Care. It is a good rule never to cut nails. File them down instead. Any instrument that will cut your nails could also cut your skin. If the nails are extra thick owing to fungal infections or previous injury, or if you have poor vision and cannot see them, have them trimmed by a podiatrist (foot doctor). Never file your

---

FOOT INJURY CAN RESULT FROM MANY CAUSES
1. **Heat (this includes sunburn, electric heating pads, hot or warm water bottles, walking barefoot on a hot pavement, or bath water that is too hot).**
2. **Cold and frostbite.**
3. **Pressure from shoes, wrinkled stockings, sandal straps, or nails in the shoes.**
4. **Chemicals and strong patent medicines (for example, alcohol or iodine).**
5. **Adhesive tape.**

---

nails shorter than the ends of your toes. Shape them according to the contours of your toes and the toes next to them. Avoid bathroom surgery!

Some PHARMACY ITEMS for good foot care are:

Emery boards for filing nails.

ST-37, a mild but effective antiseptic.

A moisturizing or a water-attracting agent for moistening dry feet (Nivea, Dermassage, Alpha-Keri, or Polysorbhydrate. Do not use perfumed lotions because they contain alcohol, which can further dry the skin.

A nonallergenic paper tape that will not pull off or irritate the skin if bandages are needed.

Bacitracin or other ointments for infected areas.

FOOT FIRST AID measures include the following:

1. Always rest an injured or infected foot. The foot does not

have to be elevated, but needs only to be extended straight on a hassock, bed, or lounge-type chair.

2. Use only mild cleansing agents and antiseptics. Never use iodine, Lysol, or colored agents. Dry after using soap. Use nonallergenic tape if a dressing must be applied (paper tape is good).

3. Limit all dressings to simple, sterile "cling" bandages. These should be loosely applied when the foot is at rest.

4. Antibiotic ointments may be used sparingly.

5. Do not be deceived by the absence of pain in an infected foot. Spreading infection can go unnoticed when normal sensation is impaired by neuropathy. Signs of infection are redness, swelling, drainage or pus, or slow healing.

6. Stay off the foot as much as possible until it has been seen by a doctor.

7. IF IN DOUBT CALL YOUR PHYSICIAN.

Shoes. Unfortunately, foot types are often not considered in the average measurements of shoe size. A 10C size does not consider problems of the instep, a narrow heel, or even fifth toe deformity. A podiatrist can often help you obtain shoes with the proper fit.

Shoes should be chosen which protect and cover your feet. Do

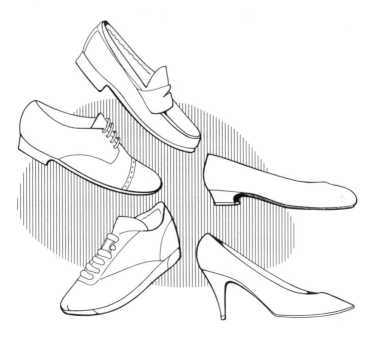

TEN COMMANDMENTS OF FOOT CARE

1. *Never apply heat of any kind to the feet.*
2. *Never soak the feet.* Soaking the feet often allows too much time for the skin and underlying structures to come in contact with excessive heat, and if the skin is macerated, the barrier against infection is broken.
3. *Never cut your own toenails; only file them.* The nails should be filed so that they are straight across and filed diagonally at the corners. People with U-shaped nails may develop ingrown toenail problems. Periodic podiatric care along with good shoes is the best investment against foot problems.
4. *Never wear ill-fitting shoes.* Vanity and style have often allowed the medical aspects of good fitting to go unemphasized.
5. *Never go barefoot.* Injuries often occur in the home when people do not wear footgear, be it shoes or slippers.
6. *Never assume that sensation or circulation is normal in the feet.* Often a vague numbness or tingling is the only sensation that patients with severe neuropathy describe. Healing of painless ulcers of the feet sometimes requires more than 3 weeks of complete bed rest. These ulcers are not innocent lesions.
7. *Never use strong or colored medicines on the feet.* Strong medicines burn. Medicines with color, such as Betadine or iodine, can make the skin look red and mask areas of inflammation.
8. *Never permit calluses or corns to develop.* In general, this requires a careful analysis of your particular foot problems, and properly fitting shoes.
9. *Never perform "bathroom surgery" on your own feet.* About as common as the problems from ill-fitted shoes or injuries from walking barefoot are the self-inflicted wounds that occur when people cut corns or use sharp scissors to cut the nails (especially if they have poor vision).
10. *Never keep the feet too moist or too dry.* Overly moist feet promote skin infections, while extremely dry skin allows fissures and cracks to develop resulting in infections. Keep a balance between powdering and lubricating the feet.

not routinely wear sandals, clogs, or flip-flops when shoes would be more appropriate. Make certain your shoes allow room for your toes to rest in their natural position. Avoid pointed shoes that squeeze the toes together. Break in new shoes gradually to prevent blisters. When you wear slippers around your home, make certain they have sturdy toes in order to prevent stubbing your toes. DO NOT GO BAREFOOT FOR ANY LENGTH OF TIME!

Cotton and wool socks and stockings are preferable but any machine washable hosiery is satisfactory. Wear a clean pair daily. Socks and stockings should be the correct size and free of seams and darns. Never wear socks or stockings with constricting tops. Constricting garters should also be avoided. An exception to this is if your physician recommends support hosiery, especially if you have problems with dropping blood pressure (orthostatic hypotension). If this is the case, be sure that the pressure is even and the stockings are fitted properly. Very high heels may appear flattering to the legs, but they give poor support and make for unstable walking. It is amazing that people go to great lengths for the rest of their wardrobe but put almost anything on their feet.

> **Are you considering investments? Stocks and real estate have their place, but a really good, well-fitting pair of shoes may pay better dividends.**

Athlete's Foot. Athlete's foot (dermatophytosis) is a common fungus infection of the feet and is not limited to athletes. It may remain scaly, dry, and unnoticed, or can break out as an inflamed area with broken skin, often between the toes. Feet that perspire heavily are more susceptible. The fungus can be acquired in locker rooms or from bathroom floors.

Athlete's foot is serious for the person with diabetes because of its potential for further infection. The treatment of athlete's foot includes the following measures:

1. Treat both the skin area involved and the insides of shoes. Wet footwear can be a source of reinfection.
2. Antifungal ointment (Desenex and Tinactin are commonly used medications) must be used on the affected skin for an extended period of time. Using antifungal powder in shoes as a general preventative at least twice a week after the acute infection has ended is a good idea.
3. Wear clogs or thongs in the bathroom or shower rather than

walking barefoot, especially in gymnasiums and health clubs.
4. Keep feet dry with regular powder, especially when feet are likely to perspire profusely.

Problem Prevention. The tragedy is that so many foot problems are preventable. In one year in the New England Deaconess Hospital, 417 of almost 5000 people with diabetes who were admitted had severe foot problems. These 417 people remained in the hospital for a total of 10,742 days, a much longer average than that of other patients.

In a recent study, the average cost of a hospital stay for people with diabetes and foot infections which resulted in an amputation was about $20,000! These tend to be shorter admissions than admissions for people whose leg or foot is saved, as it takes longer, with more expense for hospital days, to nurse these infected limbs back to health. For these people, the costs are often greater. These costs do not include physician or surgeon fees and do not take into consideration the pain, time lost from work, or the impact of illness on the patients' families. This study of hospitalized patients with foot disorders showed that one-third of these disorders *could* have been prevented, while another third *might* have been prevented. This finding suggests that half might have been helped. Observation and earlier good care might have saved much pain and money. Education is also vital.

Many patients, particularly older people, do not look at their feet routinely although they may have decreased sensation and decreased peripheral circulation. One preventive measure is to have a husband and wife look at each other's feet, 3 or 4 times each week—or more—especially between the toes, searching for areas of infection or other suspicious findings. Prevention is an absolute necessity. The feet must be examined by both those people with diabetes and their physicians. The "Ten Commandments of Foot Care" appear in the box on page 298.

Damaged feet that previously would have been lost are now being saved because of better care of diabetes, the use of antibiotics, and improved surgical techniques. Blood vessels that are clogged and cannot transport blood down to the legs and feet can be replaced surgically by utilizing grafts of blood vessels from other parts of the body or synthetic vessels. Better foot care is available through physicians, podiatrists, nurses, and even family members who are taught to monitor the feet. THE BEST TREATMENT IS PREVENTION. The quotation, "For want of a nail, the shoe was lost; for want of a shoe, the horse was lost; for want of a horse, the rider was lost" applies to foot care. The physician should be consulted at the first sign of inflammation, infection, trauma, or discoloration. FEET CAN BE SAVED.

Skin Problems

The skin covers the package known as the body, and if the body has problems, the skin is likely to share these. People with diabetes have the same skin problems as others, as well as some problems specific to diabetes. One of these is excessively dry skin caused by dehydration in poorly controlled diabetes. Sometimes tiny areas known as "shin spots" (dermopathy) appear on the front of the legs. These are quite harmless, although worrisome. The increased incidence of athlete's foot and the possibility of fungus infection have already been discussed.

Fatty plaques called xanthomas, orange-yellow in color, sometimes appear around the eyes or on the shins or elbows; they are usually related to high blood levels of fat (cholesterol or triglycerides). Some people with poorly controlled diabetes have elevated blood fats that return to normal levels with proper diabetes control. If they do not, medications can be given which further lower blood lipid levels. Once these come down, the xanthomas often disappear.

Probably the most specific problem for people with diabetes is a relatively harmless but cosmetically disfiguring condition with the jaw-breaking name of necrobiosis lipoidica diabeticorum (NLD). This probably results from an inflammation of the skin which ultimately leads to its thinning out so that it becomes discolored and dimpled. Actually, there is destruction of the layer of fat in the skin. It occurs more often in girls than in boys, generally during the teens, and although it may be found in other areas, it occurs most often on the front of the legs between the knees and ankles in what is unfortunately a highly visible area. It appears first as a pink or red discoloration and later becomes shiny and tight, much like the skin of an apple. This condition, while harmless, may be very disturbing, especially to young girls. Parents of young children become alarmed as they fear that this stigma will cover the child's entire body—not so. It is not usually dangerous, and the lesions often improve, although this improvement may take years. Healing generally starts in the center of the lesion and then gradually extends to the sides.

The main danger of this condition is that the area may break open to form an ulcer and become infected.

There is no satisfactory treatment for NLD. Ointments are generally useless, although some have improved with cortisone treatment. Skin grafts are sometimes necessary. Cosmetics are often used to hide these unsightly blemishes. Wearing slacks or pants helps hide them. However, the important thing is to recognize the presence of this condition.

Recently, it has been proposed that a cause of NLD may be clumping of platelets (a part of the blood-clotting mechanism), which can lead to blockage and inflammation of blood vessels and the beginning of NLD. Some physicians suggest using antiplatelet medications to slow the progression of this condition. At this time this is purely experimental, but there may be hope for the future.

Is It Caused by My Diabetes?

When people with diabetes develop a medical problem, it is common for them to ask, "Is this problem related to diabetes?" In fact, diabetes is blamed for many things not related to it at all. Too often patients are told, "It is probably due to your diabetes"! Of course, it may be, but sometimes this is an excuse or a "cop-out." Some people are actually reassured if something is expected to go along with diabetes, rather than being the sign of new, more disastrous problems that were not expected.

Complications of diabetes may be categorized into three groups: (1) problems that are particularly due to diabetes, (2) those that occur more commonly in people with diabetes but also occur in people without diabetes, and (3) problems not related to diabetes which occur in people with or without diabetes.

Some specific problems are diabetic retinopathy, diabetic neuropathy, and diabetic nephropathy (kidney disease). These can be direct complications of diabetes.

Examples of problems that occur more frequently in people with diabetes are heart disease, elevated blood pressure, and decreased circulation in the legs. Although more common with diabetes, the treatment is the same whether or not diabetes is present. The final category includes everything else—most peptic (gastrointestinal) ulcers, asthma, osteoarthritis, and many others. While no more common in people with diabetes, these may be *found* more readily in these people because they are seen more often by their physicians. This may be one reason people with diabetes are living longer. The incidental diseases are found and treated earlier. The physician who treats these other conditions need not be an expert in diabetes, but it is important that he or she knows that you have it, so that if anything that is recommended affects your condition, the proper precautions can be taken.

As a general rule, if you are unsure whom to consult about a particular problem or whether it is related to your diabetes, ask your physician.

Summary

The longterm complications of diabetes may be threatening. However, many of them are not as frightening as they once were. Eye problems continue, but with earlier detection of retinopathy, the new generation of lasers, and more sophisticated research, much has been learned and the eyesight of many people with diabetes is being preserved. There is also hope for people with kidney conditions. Neuropathy remains something of a mystery, but, although disabling and painful, it often improves with time. Remarkable advances have been made in vascular surgery to improve circulation to the feet. Thus, while there is much yet to learn about long-standing complications, the recent improvements in treatment are remarkable. Dr. Priscilla White of the Joslin Clinic spoke of this progress in a statement included in the last edition of this manual (1978). When asked whether she was discouraged about the problems faced by people with long-standing diabetes, Dr. White paused, and then answered that if one considers only an individual person, one might be discouraged, but if one considers people with diabetes as a group, they live longer and better than they did 25 years ago, and even 10 to 5 years ago. Proud as she was, then, of how far we had come in the treatment of diabetes and its complications, we are prouder still of the progress made since that time, and of the progress now being made to make the future even brighter.

17

Living with Diabetes

This is one of the most important chapters in the book. You now know what diabetes is, how it should be treated, problems that might develop, and how to overcome them. Now we must think about how you live with diabetes—how you can handle it day in and day out and live a good life.

The treatment of diabetes requires a whole new life-style for most people. It can also affect your family and friends. How long you live is important, but that is not enough. How well you live is also important.

Adjusting

What helps people adjust to diabetes? No one with diabetes can live quite as freely as someone without it. Ignoring diabetes and taking poor care of it does not free anyone from its control even for a short time. Poor control inevitably leads to not feeling well and perhaps having frequent insulin reactions or hyperglycemia. By neglecting the condition the person is even more controlled by it.

Complete freedom to eat and do as one pleases is restricted by the need to follow the action pattern of the daily insulin injection. It is a life full of needles, syringes, a new or revised diet, home testing materials, and continued concern over infections, skin care, and health in general. Living with these things can stir strong emotional feelings. Yet the response to diabetes varies greatly, ranging from anguish, depression, and a feeling that life can't be worthwhile, to a sense of accomplishment in adapting to the new and complex problem that has been thrust upon one. Some do this with a feeling of victory!

Age also affects the process. Small children get confused and do not understand what is happening. Yet they see things happening to them—injections, blood tests, reactions—and they want to understand. Information must be appropriate to the level of the child's development and understanding. For example, young children may be upset by occasional separation from parents caused by hospitalization. This fear must be recognized and understood before these children can properly deal with their diabetes.

Older people may view diabetes as a sign of early and premature aging. The elderly, as they often do with illness, see it as the "beginning of the end." They remember "Aunt Mary" and comment, "Oh, yes, she had diabetes just before she died." Family, friends, and health care providers must recognize these feelings. They are not correct, but may seem to be the right thing to the person with diabetes. Understanding and support are a must if the individual is to adjust successfully to diabetes.

Interest and involvement of others is important in helping many people adjust to their diabetes. Someone who lacks support can feel quite alone. Frequently, other life events can also have an effect on how one adapts to diabetes. Problems at work, the death of a loved one, financial burdens, and family stress can be distractions from the interest and attention to self-care.

Most important, the ability to cope has a profound effect on whether diabetes becomes an overwhelming burden in an already difficult life, or a challenging and time-consuming task that can be taken in stride. All too often, people already having adjustment problems are told by a well-intentioned health care professional or friend, "I understand your anguish now, but don't worry. With time, you will learn to accept diabetes." Such statements may be true for many in the situation, but not everyone accepts diabetes "with time." Many harbor lingering guilt, resentment, or anger and cannot really adjust. Diabetes may make other problems worse or more difficult to deal with. As time passes, this can lead to difficulties within a family as well. While acceptance is certainly a worthy goal, the inability to accept diabetes is not an *abnormal* response. There is nothing fundamentally wrong with you if you can never fully be comfortable with or accept this condition. You are better off recognizing the lingering emotions early and seeking help in dealing with them than letting them continue and destroy family relationships or friendships unnecessarily.

Denial. Why should people really want to accept something they don't like? It is not surprising that people frequently approach diabetes the way they deal with any undesirable situation—by denying it. DENIAL IS A STATE IN WHICH THE PERSON SUBCONSCIOUSLY BEHAVES AS IF THE UNPLEASANT SITUATION DOES NOT REALLY EXIST. THUS THE INDIVIDUAL ACTS AS IF HE OR SHE DOES NOT HAVE DIABETES.

Sometimes, denial can be healthy, enabling an individual to keep a positive view despite adversity. "We shall overcome!" This might be considered optimism—seeing only the positive side of things. Such a person will think of diabetes as having a positive effect on his or her approach to health. "I have diabetes, so I will take better overall care of myself. I will be O.K." To some degree, this attitude is essential. We all need to maintain some optimism in the face of difficulties; otherwise we would be overcome by every problem and accomplish nothing in life.

Unfortunately, denial can also be a great problem when it prevents people from taking an active role in caring for their diabetes. When this occurs, denial can lead to a subconscious attitude that the diabetes does not exist and to the neglect of good health advice. Fortunately, few people dare deny the existence of diabetes enough to actually skip insulin or take the wrong dose, although this has happened. However, many people effectively neglect their diabetes by ignoring warnings of poor treatment.

Social pressures make it easy to deny the problem: "How can I take better care of my diabetes—when I eat out with my friends, they will not let me follow my diet," or "My work schedule interferes with the timing of things." These people often subconsciously deny that the diabetes is a part of their lives for more than the few minutes in the morning that it takes them to inject their insulin. Yet when asked, they proudly state that they are doing all that they have to do. When these people go to see their physician, they tend to remember the compliments such as, "Oh, you are looking well," and report to their families that the doctor found "things were good." They forget that the physician also commented that "your diabetes is not in very good control."

Sometimes, friends and family notice the denial in a person's actions, although the person with diabetes may be too involved to be aware of the denial. Helping the person face denial is one important way that others can provide support.

Education is often a helpful tool in prying people away from their denial. Ideally, people with diabetes should learn enough to say, "Now I know I can lead a better life by taking responsibility for my care and improving it." Group experiences with others who have diabetes can help break patterns of denial. Whether at camps for children, counseling for adolescents, or discussion groups, talking with others and seeing how others face their diabetes can help an individual confront the diabetes and learn to live with it.

Fear. Information about diabetes often confuses people. Some of the statistics about diabetes or examples of individuals with diabetes who fared poorly may produce fear. Many families recall the experiences of a relative who had a difficult time with diabetes, even though the situation is completely different from the present one. Often these memories have a negative influence on the newly diagnosed person's view of his own condition. As a result, this person who was diagnosed with diabetes a year or two ago and is otherwise perfectly healthy sits cringing at each examination with the expectation that a leg will need to be amputated or that blindness will affect him shortly, all because he "knew someone to whom this happened."

Anxiety that is a result of this type of influence can be quite destructive to self-care and the quality of life. Because of this fear, these people panic and freeze in their tracks, unable to perform even the simplest tasks needed for diabetes care.

Some early success in treating diabetes can generate hope. Using correct insulin dosages that really make the person feel better, learning about diabetes so it is understood, knowing what to expect as well as seeing the success of others, and the sweet smell of personal success can go a long way toward reducing fears and restoring calm. If positive influences do not help, anxiety can become all-consuming and extend beyond the diabetes itself. This can affect relationships with family, spouse, and co-workers. Some people surrender to this fear and anxiety and live dull, defeated lives that so muddle their thinking that they are incapable of making important decisions.

Fear and anxiety about the effects of diabetes can affect others close to the person with diabetes as well. When the parents of young people with diabetes are filled with fears of the possible complications, they may become overbearing and overprotective. This in turn can lead to rebellion by the young person and worsening of care.

Fear and anxiety are poor motivators. To show someone who is not taking care of himself another person who is blind or has lost a limb will not motivate him. Too often, it terrifies him, so he does almost nothing. More often, people respond to fear by denying that this could happen to them. As a result, they do nothing. So fear is not a good way to get someone motivated.

Guilt. Guilt is the third common response to the diagnosis of diabetes. If parents realize that neither they nor anyone else can control the traits they pass on, or think they pass on, to their children, then there is no reason for them to have a sense of guilt about their child's diabetes. Too often, husbands and wives blame each other's "side of the family" for bringing diabetes to their offspring. Some people, as in a more primitive society, think they are suffering for previous misdeeds or sins. This feeling depresses people and makes them less able to handle the tasks of living with diabetes. *People should remove diabetes from the realm of morals.* As we mentioned earlier, it is important to avoid using the terms "good blood sugar" and "bad tests." Instead we should say "normal blood sugar levels" or "high blood sugar levels."

If the person with diabetes can discuss these feelings of denial, fear, and guilt, he may develop a better outlook and achieve acceptance. Overcoming the natural emotional feelings about having diabetes is a major concern of doctors, nurses, and family members trying to help their relatives who have diabetes.

"How Long Will I Live?"

This is a question that many people diagnosed with diabetes ask the physician. Others wonder but don't ask. Older statistics about the duration of life for people with diabetes do not help reduce feelings of anxiety. These data, however, are often misquoted or misinterpreted and certainly are not understood. Coldly quoting numbers can cause severe anxiety. The real question should be, "What will happen to me?"

The plain facts are that with the proper use of insulin, antibiotics, and other modern treatments and medications, people with diabetes are living longer than ever before—and each year the picture improves! Each new development may further extend life. While it is not quite correct to say that on the average, people with diabetes live as long as people without it, unquestionably the statistics have improved.

In the past, a factor that discouraged those with diabetes was the attitude by many that one can do little to influence the future. This is now incorrect. Those with diabetes can definitely influence their future in at least three ways:

1. Find the diabetes as early as possible and start treatment. If you think you or a family member may have it, find out and do something about it!

2. Do not neglect the treatment of diabetes. And accept only the best treatment.
3. Do not neglect other overall health factors such as high blood pressure, overweight, smoking, or high blood fat levels. These may shorten your life.

There is another interesting reason why people with diabetes can live longer. How often do many people without specific symptoms see their physicians? Those with diabetes who are checked regularly can find out about high blood pressure or some other abnormality early and have it treated and corrected. This is an advantage in the game of life.

You *can* make a difference. Better self-care *can* decrease the chances of diabetic ketoacidosis and severe hypoglycemic reactions as well as other problems. Proper control, with steadier glucose levels, can make you feel better. Yes, we talk in terms of chances, likelihood, and probabilities. Diabetes is not a predictable condition. But as with any game of chance, you want the odds to be in your favor. You can influence your own odds.

Using the Medical System

The medical system has changed and will continue to change. It is certainly getting more complex and confusing. The way in which "health care" is "delivered" barely resembles the way "medicine" was "practiced" when Elliott P. Joslin's practice was in its heyday. For example, today there are newer, computerized tests and devices to help you. For the person with diabetes, it can be a challenge to find the best possible health care setting.

Choosing a Physician. Who should be your doctor? The vast majority of people with diabetes have been and will continue to be treated by a personal physician, whether a family practitioner or an internist, even in the newer group settings. This is the way it should be. In fact, throughout the world, over 90% of those with diabetes will be treated by their general practitioner or internist.

The internist or family practitioner tends to take an overall approach to health care delivery, treating the whole person, which is good because diabetes is not limited to the pancreas. The physician who cares for your diabetes should be both experienced and interested in the care of this condition. The sign of a good physician is that he knows his limits and will refer to specialists if needed. This approach is very important. Certainly, not everyone diagnosed with diabetes needs a specialist; but one should be available if needed.

> **The doctor you need is one whom you like and who likes you, understands you, and cares for you and the details of your diabetes treatment.**

If you choose to seek care from someone who specializes in treating diabetes, fine, but it is important to have a physician who knows you well and is your "primary care physician." While some who specialize in diabetes may also fill this primary care role, others may not, preferring to act as a consultant to assist you and your home physician in managing your diabetes. A consultant living a distance from the patient cannot be the primary care provider. You need someone near for the sudden emergencies of life!

Some people with a number of medical problems requiring attention prefer to see multiple specialists for each area. This approach may result in excellent care for each specific area of expertise, but vital routine health care—checking cholesterol levels, giving "flu shots" and doing pap smears—may be forgotten. Be sure that you and your physicians fully understand what each person's role will be in providing your total health care. Remember, it is still important to have one physician who is in charge overall, the quarterback who calls the signals!

Choosing a diabetes "expert" can be difficult. In general, most endocrinologists are knowledgeable about diabetes, but things can get confusing because endocrinologists may specialize further in a particular gland or system. There are also many physicians who have specialized training in the care of diabetes without formal training in the rest of endocrinology. These physicians can provide very good care for people with diabetes as well. Therefore, titles and credentials tell only part of the story. A good recommendation from a trusted physician or knowledgeable friend can be a good guide. Ultimately, however, the decision is made by you, the informed consumer of health care. Therefore, having some idea of what good care of diabetes is all about will help you recognize a good physician when you find one.

You do not want to see a physician only when an emergency threatens. In addition, you do not want to have your diabetes regulated only in an emergency room or facility. These are oriented toward the care of urgent or immediate problems, but they are not the locations for longterm management. This should be provided by a physician who is able and wants to care for you on a longterm, regular basis.

How Often to See Your Physician. This depends on many factors. If you live a distance from a diabetes specialist whom you see as a consultant, then your visits to this physician will be less frequent than to your primary physician. During periods of poor control or when adjustment is needed, visits may be weekly or monthly. People with stable diabetes who have sufficient knowledge and are able to take responsibility for much of their own care may need to be seen only a few times a year. Certainly with self monitoring and proper guidelines on when to call for help, you can make more frequent visits if problems arise.

What You Can Do to Help Your Physician. What your physician can do for you depends a great deal on what you can do to help your physician. Some people consider a medical visit to be a game of secrecy and let the doctor try to find out what is wrong. Others talk about everything except what is wrong and needs attention. Still others make this a treasure hunt, dropping clues to see if the physician really is astute. One woman said about her physician, "He wasn't very smart. He asked me a lot of questions and never found out what I came for!" Come with a list of medicines, insulin dose, and reactions (if any). It is also helpful to bring your blood or urine test results for the past several weeks. Sometimes people bring in test results from a year or two ago. This is well intended, but not very useful except to show diligence in testing. If you have specific problems, speak up. Mention them first. If the doctor is explaining something important to you, don't interrupt with another question or change the subject. The discussion may never get back to that point, and you might lose some vital information. If you don't understand something, ask! You are entitled to know the reason for things and most present-day physicians are delighted to explain and, more important, make you part of the health care team, since you are living with the problem.

Health Insurance. Obtaining health insurance continues to be difficult for people with diabetes, who often find that health insurance available to them is either very expensive or full of restrictions or exclusions. Insurance carriers consider "chronic diseases" such as diabetes to be a "high risk" based on the number of claims that they have or expect to pay. The problem is that these statistics are based on their past, often unhappy, experience. Unfortunately, this approach affects all people with diabetes, even if their personal history is one of good control and health maintenance.

Many people with diabetes are able to obtain adequate coverage through the group plan at their place of employment. These group plans through large companies or associations usually offer the most comprehensive coverage with a minimum of exclusion clauses and at low premiums. If you are not affiliated with such a group, the insurance carrier may request medical records from a physician to determine whether your diabetes control has been maintained at a good level for a period of time so that the premiums might be lower. Even so, restrictive clauses may be included limiting benefits for treatment of diabetes and related problems either for a period of time or completely.

Insurance plans differ widely in what they allow, and you must familiarize yourself with the details of your own particular policy to determine what is included, what is limited, and the amount of the deductibles.

Some states offer pooled risk plans which provide insurance for high-risk individuals unable to obtain coverage elsewhere. Check with your state's insurance commission to see if they have instituted such a program.

Health maintenance organizations (HMOs) provide health care at a lower cost. Their emphasis on prevention may be an advantage. With an HMO, the health care providers are selected from a specific and limited group of enlisted health care professionals, and most often you are limited to that group. If services are sought from physicians who are not members of that HMO group, expenses incurred are usually the responsibility of the individual unless the HMO agrees to a referral. If you are considering getting your care from an HMO, be sure that you are satisfied with the diabetes care provided by that organization because you will have to get your care from them.

> One of the best things you can do to improve your odds of getting health insurance is to keep your diabetes under the best possible control and be able to prove it.

State and federal assistance programs (Medicaid, disability insurance, Medicare, etc.) are available to provide care for individuals with low incomes or physical handicaps and who are unable to get insurance and cannot afford health care costs on their own. The standards for eligibility vary with each state and municipality, and application is through local agencies who determine eligibility. When applying for such assistance, it is advisable to have medical records and financial statements prepared to document probable need.

Medicare is available to people when they reach the age of 65 and will pay up to 80% of allowed medical costs after deductibles have been paid. Many people seek an extension of their medicare coverage through commercial insurance companies so that the balance of their medical expenses such as prescriptions and deductibles can be paid for. These supplementary coverage plans vary. Shop carefully to see which ones offer the most benefits at the lowest premiums, based on your needs. In particular, check what frequency of medical examinations is covered, completeness of hospital coverage, and medication cost coverage.

With the growing complexity of medical coverage, it is more important than ever before that you and your family keep informed about health insurance issues. The health insurance industry is undergoing many changes to adapt to the changing health care delivery system and to respond to competition. It is likely that changes will continue. Frequently, your local American Diabetes Association and related groups are a good source for updated information. Your physician, or the person in your physician's office who handles insurance issues, may also be able to assist you.

Life Insurance

Life insurance is increasingly but slowly becoming available to people with diabetes. However, getting it at premiums which are not excessively high may not be easy. Many people with diabetes can find life insurance if they are otherwise in perfect health, but they are still charged high premiums. Nevertheless, most companies now offer such coverage. Factors they consider include age at onset of diabetes, duration of diabetes, its severity as measured by the treatment required, and, of course, known complications. Other unfavorable factors include overweight or a history of other medical problems. The decision as to insurability is often made by the insurance company's medical department based on information from the individual's personal physician. Unfortunately, old out-dated actuarial tables still may be used which may reduce the likelihood of insurability. The American Diabetes Association, through its affiliates, can be a source of information on life insurance for those with diabetes.

The Economics of Diabetes

Diabetes can be expensive. Medical care can be costly, especially if your health insurance does not cover all expenses. Insulin, injection supplies, oral hypoglycemic agents, and self testing materials are an unceasing expense. And the economic impact of diabetes can be felt in many other aspects of life as well.

One way to cut expenses is to get prescription medicines—which means most of what those with diabetes need—through prescription plans that are provided by various groups or organizations as part of a benefits or health care package. Some employers have access to these along with their insurance policies. Similarly, AARP (American Association for Retired Persons) has discount services. Some states offer special assistance for children or even older people with diabetes. This may be important for the person who needs special care and vocational counseling or training to become employable.

April 15 of each year can be less taxing also if you keep careful records of the cost of medications, prescription items, appliances, and other health necessities. Many of these items are tax deductible. As with all special medical aids, regulations vary and you should check the rules in your own area.

Diabetes and Employment. Job discrimination against people with diabetes still exists and unjustly reduces the income potential for many people. Some employers hesitate to hire people with diabetes because of ignorance, a bad previous experience, or fear that the person with diabetes will cost extra in employer-paid health insurance premiums. For years, people who work in the field of diabetes care have fought to eliminate discrimination against people who are otherwise healthy, solid citizens but who happen to have diabetes. Diabetes should not be an excuse not to hire someone. Similarly, diabetes is not a reason for disability from most jobs or occupations. Increasingly, strong antidiscrimination laws are being passed by the various states.

Data from employers such as Ford and DuPont have shown that people with diabetes have a remarkably good work record. Dr. Paul S. Entmacher of the Metropolitan Life Insurance Company says that the job applicant who has diabetes should not conceal his diabetes under any circumstances and suggests that it is helpful to bring to the employment office a physician's report of diabetes control or, for younger people, a good school attendance report. Glycohemoglobin records, with explanations to employment officers as to what they signify, can be excellent documentation of control.

The employment office of your work place should certainly be aware of your diabetes and the medications you use. Co-workers should also be aware of the possibility of hypoglycemic reactions and how to treat them. Accidents may occur if you have a hypoglycemic reaction and fellow employees, unable to recognize it, allow you to continue working. A "buddy" system is often useful to be sure that someone is keeping watch for symptoms of hypoglycemia and can provide prompt help if needed.

Thankfully, the tide against employment discrimination for people with diabetes is turning. The rules have been very irregular. Taking over 20 or 25 units of insulin daily would disqualify people from some jobs. This is nonsense because some people take 50 units daily and have no reactions while others who are careless can have reactions with 10 or 15 units. Recently, several airline cabin attendants who had been disqualified because of insulin-requiring diabetes were, after threatening court action, returned to their jobs when it was shown that they had taken excellent care and that insulin reactions were avoidable. The American Diabetes Association policy states, "Any person with diabetes, whether insulin-dependent or non-insulin-dependent, should be eligible for an employment for which he or she is individually qualified." This statement stems from the 1973 Federal Rehabilitation Act. More and more, court decisions are protecting those with diabetes. A recent one in Los Angeles upheld the right to a job by a local truck driver, stating that if a person having a "handicap" is qualified to do a job, it is up to the employer to prove that the employee cannot do the job.

Some jobs are still denied to people who use insulin. The U.S. armed forces have this policy as does the Federal Bureau of Investigation for its field agents. These make some sense because people in those categories may be on isolated duty in strange places where their medications may not be available. Also, the military likes to feel that all of its people are completely interchangeable at all times. The Department of Transportation does not allow insulin-dependent truck drivers to drive interstate for fear of reactions while driving for long hours. Many states permit driving with insulin *within* the state, but some do not. Airline pilots have not been permitted the use of any medication (insulin or pills) for diabetes. While insulin will probably still be prohibited, the medical authorities of the Federal Aviation Administration (FAA) are now reviewing the possibility of some pilots being permitted to fly using oral agents under careful supervision. The big danger, of course, is that of hypoglycemic reactions, some of which might occur without warning.

Educational Opportunities

As children with diabetes become adults, they will seek further education of various types. Colleges do not exclude young people with diabetes, nor do most postgraduate programs, although some may still have some prejudice as a result of past unrewarding experiences or misconceptions. In reality, properly treated diabetes should have *no* detrimental effects on your ability to learn and acquire educational credentials. There is no question that people with diabetes can and do successfully attend colleges, postgraduate school, technical training, and business schools. Many states financially support these young people in full or in part, usually through a department of rehabilitation.

Career Guidance. Career guidance is important for people with diabetes. Certain jobs are understandably less appropriate for people with insulin-requiring diabetes, as we discussed earlier. For example, some cities, towns, and states have regulations regarding public transportation jobs, prohibiting insulin users from driving passenger-carrying vehicles. By a strange quirk of fate, one streetcar driver, displaced because of this restriction, was reassigned to work as a chauffeur for the director of the transportation system. Apparently the director considered him a good risk for himself if not for paying passengers. Many prohibitive regulations are based less on likely difficulties than on the risk of legal problems.

Certain other occupations are not ideal for people requiring insulin treatment. These include jobs in which sudden loss of control due to hypoglycemia could be dangerous. Such jobs include work on scaffolding at great heights or work with high-tension wires.

On the positive side, young people with diabetes should be encouraged by the vast expansion in the variety of employment opportunities which have opened many new possible fields of endeavor. Occupations in electronics, computer programming, data processing, and other high-tech fields are becoming more numerous, and these provide excellent career opportunities for people

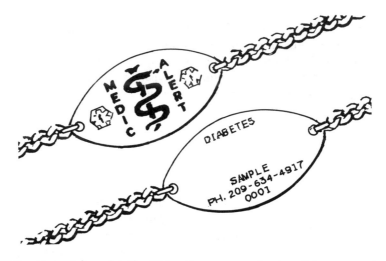

FIG. 17-1. A bracelet identifying the wearer as having diabetes.

with diabetes. In addition, with few exceptions, most civil service jobs are now available to people with diabetes. New regulations state that all people with diabetes "who have achieved reasonable control of the condition are eligible for Federal employment with proper placement to be based on the severity of the diabetes and the medication required for control." Further information can be obtained by writing to the Medical Director, United States Civil Service Commission, Washington, DC 20415. While the career situation is far from perfect, it is improving.

Identification Jewelry and Cards

All people with diabetes should understand the need for carrying identification concerning their diabetes. Some people carry cards, while others rightly prefer bracelets or neck chains with an inscribed message. Unconsciousness or injury can result from many causes unrelated to diabetes as well as from diabetes-related conditions such as hypoglycemia or ketoacidosis. The person with diabetes should be instantly identified so that a low blood glucose reaction or other problem can be treated immediately. Sometimes people with hypoglycemia due to diabetes are mistaken for being intoxicated and, despite protests, lose time being arrested instead of being given the needed carbohydrate. Identification cards can be obtained from the American Diabetes Association or your own diabetes clinic. The Medic Alert Foundation International of Turlock, California, makes up bracelets, necklaces, and anklets engraved with medical information (Fig. 17–1). This type of identification has an advantage over cards because wallets can be lost or stolen, and emergency medical personnel tend to look first for this

---

Some people are hesitant to carry identification because they think it makes others look down on them. Not so. Many people now carry such identification for allergies and sensitivity to certain medications. It is increasingly common.

---

type of medical alert information. Nevertheless, even a simple card is better than nothing and can be life-saving (Fig. 17–2). It carries a simple message, or, for travelers, can say in whatever language you wish that you have diabetes. There is no excuse for anyone with diabetes to be without identification.

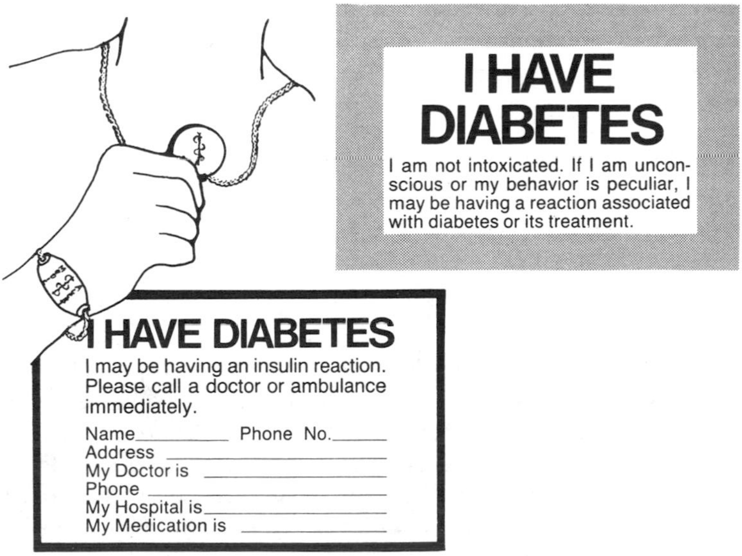

I HAVE DIABETES

I am not intoxicated. If I am unconscious or my behavior is peculiar, I may be having a reaction associated with diabetes or its treatment.

I HAVE DIABETES

I may be having an insulin reaction. Please call a doctor or ambulance immediately.

Name_____   Phone No._____
Address _____
My Doctor is _____
Phone _____
My Hospital is_____
My Medication is _____

FIG. 17–2. An identification card indicating that the person with the card has diabetes. The card should be carried in the wallet in case of emergency.

Driving Automobiles, Boats, and Other Vehicles

Today, driving an automobile is not a luxury but, in the United States, a prime means of transportation, vital to making a living. It calls for special precautions on the part of those with diabetes. The same cautions apply to power boats, motorcycles, and snowmobiles, among other potentially harmful vehicles. The operation of automobiles by people with diabetes has come increasingly under the surveillance of state licensing authorities. While the federal government is involved where commercial interstate travel is concerned, such as with trucks or trains, driving regulations vary with each state. Most states require identification of the diabetes on the license application. Some states pose bizarre, poorly worded questions such as, "Do you ever have fits or fainting spells?" No one with diabetes treated with oral hypoglycemic agents or insulin should ever drive without a readily available snack such as sugar or candy. Nor should anyone ever skip or delay a meal while driving. An accident, even though caused by low blood glucose, is still the responsibility of the driver. People with diabetes must be especially careful because, if enough of them have poor driving records, legislatures and registries of motor vehicles may restrict their driving privileges as a group. This is especially true because there is growing public concern about auto casualties and safety on the highways. Regulations concerning boats and other powered pleasure vehicles are ill-defined, but accidents involving such vehicles are no less dangerous.

Parties and Special Occasions

Parties and special occasions are major events in the lives of everyone. This is especially true for most children and adolescents. It is important to many people with diabetes, and especially these youngsters, that they not be stigmatized as being "different." The poorest possible approach is to have the host or hostess in any way make an issue of the diabetes. The daily diet can be adjusted to permit ice cream, cake, or other goodies on this special occasion. In fact, with our growing understanding of glycemic indexes (the effect on the blood glucose levels that certain foods or combinations of foods may have), ice cream may indeed be allowed as part of a full meal for some people with type I diabetes as long as they do not have a weight problem. Supplemental insulin could be used before or after the party, as needed. Unless one makes a career of partying, the resentment engendered, especially in a young person, is probably more harmful to the diabetic career than the temporary allowed-for alterations in "control" on unusual occasions. Common sense on the part of the parents of youngsters, and understanding by the child and adult party-goer alike, are better than an impossibly rigid set of conditions.

Alcohol and Diabetes

Back when Elliott P. Joslin started in practice, the general opinion of physicians was that anyone with diabetes should never, ever have even one drop of any alcoholic beverage. In an earlier edition of this manual, he stated, "I think it far easier for a diabetic to exercise self-restraint without the use of alcohol than with it. It is certainly not needed in the diabetic dietary." This statement, in its pure sense, is still true, but there may be some exceptions.

Even today, there is no doubt that excessive use of alcohol is a problem that affects all of society. This problem is never so acute as when it affects youth and when it affects all people, with or without diabetes, who operate motor vehicles. Yet many people can consume some alcoholic beverages responsibly, and drinking is a fact of our society that should be recognized. For people with diabetes, it is important to understand how alcohol can affect diabetes so that they can make an intelligent decision about how to use it.

How Alcohol Affects Diabetes. When alcohol is consumed, it is absorbed rapidly into the bloodstream from the stomach. What is not absorbed in the stomach passes into the small intestine, where it is absorbed more slowly. When alcohol is used with other foods, the presence of this food in the stomach prevents some of the alcohol from being absorbed in the stomach, favoring the slower small intestine and reducing the apparent intoxicating effect.

More than 90% of the alcohol that enters the body is completely metabolized, mostly in the liver. This is why the liver can be damaged in people who consume large amounts of alcohol. The healthy adult metabolizes alcohol at the rate of 7 to 10 grams of alcohol per hour (or about 1 oz. of liquor) per hour.

Alcohol is generally classified as a depressant to the central nervous system rather than a stimulant, despite its legendary reputation to the contrary. In the past, physicians sometimes prescribed whiskey because they thought it might protect cardiac patients by relieving tension and help angina by dilating small blood vessels. Recent studies have not resolved this issue. While some suggest that small amounts of alcohol might actually help the heart, no study suggests that excessive alcohol is beneficial.

The greatest short-term danger for people with diabetes is its effect on low blood glucose reactions. When someone with diabetes drinks, the liver's ability to create new glucose from the carbohydrate (glycogen) that it stores (this process is called gluconeogenesis) is almost completely blocked. In the presence of alcohol, competition for the liver enzymes stops this process. Because sugar is not freely available when needed, the low blood sugar that follows can be quite profound and prolonged, and the effects of insulin or oral agents can be intensified. Also, drinking can mask the usual signals of low blood glucose. There are also more practical considerations, such as the danger of insulin reactions while driving, to say nothing of the direct effect of alcohol on driving and other important activities.

Alcohol may pose a problem for people using some first-generation sulfonylurea oral hypoglycemic agents. The combination of alcohol with some of these—particularly chlorpropamide (Diabinese)—can cause an intense flushing of the face due to the engorgement of the surface blood vessels. Some people experience headaches or nausea. These phenomena are harmless, although they may be disquieting or embarrassing!

Calories from Alcohol. Although it produces calories, alcohol is not a food. It furnishes no carbohydrate, protein, or fat, and it is not helpful in nutrition. Nevertheless, 1 gram of alcohol provides 7 calories, so that it is a readily usable fuel. The amount of alcohol in a drink is determined by the "proof." One-half of the proof represents the percentage of alcohol in a drink. For example, 80-proof whiskey contains 40% alcohol. One ounce of straight whiskey contains about 85 calories. An alcohol drinker adds significant calories to the diet. Adding sweetened liquids such as ginger ale or cocktail mixes, and the usual hors d'oeuvres, means still more calories.

The alcohol content of U.S. beer averages about 4%; it is as high as 12% in beer from other parts of the world. Beer also contains a little more than 4% sugar and 0.6% protein. Overall, beer provides about 13 calories per ounce or about 156 calories per 12-ounce can or bottle. The so-called light beers usually have 90 to 110 calories per 12-ounce can or bottle.

Wines vary greatly from high-calorie, fortified wines to dry table

Table 17–1. AMOUNTS OF CARBOHYDRATE, ALCOHOL, AND CALORIES IN ALCOHOLIC DRINKS
Use of alcoholic beverages should be discussed with your physician

Alcoholic Drinks	Household Measure	Total Grams	Grams of Carbohydrate*	Grams of Alcohol†	Calories (Approx.)
Whiskey— Bourbon, Irish, rye, and Scotch	1 brandy glass (1 oz.)	30	none	10½–12	75–85
Brandy, gin, and rum	1 brandy glass (1 oz.)	30	none	10½–13	75–90
Liqueurs and cordials	1 cordial glass (⅔ oz.)	20	4–10	4—7	50—80
Malt liquors— ale, beer porter, and stout	1 glass (8 oz.)	240	7–14	7–14	80–150
Light beer	1 glass (8 oz.)	67	0	9–10	65
Wines— Sweet, domestic	1 wineglass (3½ oz.)	100	8–14	13–15	140–165
Sweet, imported	1 wineglass (3½ oz.)	100	3–20	10½–18	110–175
Dry, domestic	1 wineglass (3½ oz.)	100	½–4	10–11	75—90
Dry, imported	1 wineglass (3½ oz.)	100	½–3	8–14	60–110
Cider— Sweet	1 glass (8 oz.)	240	25	trace	100
Hard (fermented)	1 wineglass (3½ oz.)	100	1	5	40

*Every gram of carbohydrate supplies 4 calories.
†Every gram of alcohol supplies 7 calories.

wines, which are lower in sugar and alcoholic content. If wine is consumed with a meal, the probability of a hypoglycemic reaction is less. "Dry," generally white wines, such as Chablis, Chardonnay, Reisling, Sauternes, and Sauvignon blanc are safest for people with diabetes. Sherry, although "dry," still provides about 30 calories an ounce. Burgundies can be difficult to judge because the manufac-

---

TABLE 17-2. RECOMMENDATIONS FOR PEOPLE WITH
DIABETES WHO WISH TO DRINK ALCO-
HOLIC BEVERAGES

---

1. No person should drink alcoholic beverages who has any medical
   condition that would be harmed by the consumption of alcohol.
   You should always discuss your desire to drink alcoholic beverages
   with your physician.
2. No person should drink alcoholic beverages who is following an
   eating plan for weight reduction.
3. No person should (a) drink alcoholic beverages to excess, (b) drink
   if under age, (c) drink on an empty stomach, or (d) drink in
   association with driving an automobile or any other type of motor
   vehicle or operating any dangerous machinery.
4. Assuming none of the above applies, alcohol should be consumed
   sparingly and intelligently. Often wine or beer with a meal is
   acceptable. Avoid more than 2 "alcohol equivalents" at one time (1
   "equivalent" equals 1 1/2 oz. liquor, 4 oz. dry wine, or 12 oz. light
   beer). Avoid drinks that contain a large amount of sugar. A drink
   with 1 1/2 oz. whiskey should preferably be consumed with water,
   soda, or "on the rocks" as a before dinner drink.
5. Know how the alcohol affects your daily caloric intake. Although
   there is no fat in such drinks, they are considered a "fat
   exchange," because this is the simplest way of measuring the
   calories. One "equivalent" (from item 4 above) equals 2 fat
   exchanges. (Regular beer, rather than light beer, is 2 fats plus one
   bread exchange.)
6. Always wear or carry identification that says you have diabetes.

---

turers sometimes add a sugar solution to help the fermentation
process. Some dry sparkling wines may have a lower sugar content.

Liqueurs have high carbohydrate values and should be avoided.
A list of calories in alcoholic beverages without the addition of any
mixers is given in Table 17–1.

In summary, alcohol in every form, even without mixers, yields
an abundance of calories with little nutritional value, if any. The
harder spirits such as whiskeys have a high alcohol content and
provide more calories than, for example, unsweetened wines.
Alcohol is prohibited in most weight-reduction diets because, for
example, in a 1200-calorie daily meal plan, one drink may contain
10% of the daily intake. Because alcohol is very easily burned as fuel
but has no lasting food value, the drinker is caught on the horns of
a dilemma. If one does not eat while drinking, the alcohol is
absorbed at a faster rate, and if one does not become intoxicated,
one might still have a low blood glucose reaction. On the other
hand, if a person drinks and eats considerably, the calorie intake is
great and the food is more likely to be stored for the future in
unflattering places such as the classic "beer belly."

Recommendations for those who need occasional social drinks

Table 17-3. IF YOU MUST DRINK!

1. You must be in control of your diabetes.
2. You must not be an alcoholic.
3. You must not be pregnant.
4. Drink only "dry" drinks, avoiding all sweet wines and liqueurs.
5. It is better if you are not overweight.
6. Do not use sweetened mixes.
7. Drink sparingly and immediately before or with meals.
8. *Never* drink before driving under *any* circumstances.

From M.A. Schneider, M.D., *Practical Diabetology*, March/April 1986.

are listed in Table 17–2. Guidelines for drinking are listed in Table 17–3.

Smoking

There is very convincing evidence that cigarette smoking is hazardous to anyone's health, with or without diabetes. In addition to the usual reasons for not smoking, the risks of vascular diseases resulting from diabetes are significantly increased in people who also smoke. Most physicians will agree that smoking, especially by people with diabetes, is a tremendous health hazard.

While some physicians are not as forceful as they should be on the subject, a health authority recently said, "We must appreciate the obvious fact that the time and effort spent by physicians in convincing their patients not to smoke cigarettes will produce more meaningful and useful years of life than all the cardiac transplants have produced." The increased risks of cancer and emphysema for the smoker in the general population are well known. For people with diabetes, the fact that their risk of cardiovascular complications is greater should be an added deterrent to smoking. Tobacco smoking also increases constriction of the smaller blood vessels, further impeding circulation. Older people as well as people with diabetes of long duration already have decreased circulation in their extremities, so for them, smoking seems to add insult to injury.

Smoking is a habit that is most difficult to break, and people can best avoid this struggle by not starting. As to the number of cigarettes required to cause damage, it is impossible to say that 3 cigarettes won't and 20 will. There is no way to determine the precise danger point. For people with diabetes, the number of daily cigarettes should be *none*!

Stopping smoking is easier said than done, as many will attest. Prescribed medications such as Nicorette gum can be helpful for some people. Biofeedback or hypnotism is useful for others. Many people simply make up their mind to quit and do it, either gradually or "cold turkey" (all at once). If you wish to quit and are having difficulty doing so, your physician may have some helpful advice, especially if he or she doesn't smoke.

The Drug Culture

The term "recreational drugs" is an invitation to disaster and should never be used. The use of any of these substances is a social ill of major concern to physicians, government officials, law enforcement officers, and, indeed, all concerned citizens. Needless to say, the use of these substances is not recommended for any human being, and people with diabetes are certainly members of this group of humans!

Unfortunately, many people, including people with diabetes, are consuming various substances for alleged "recreational" purposes. When confronted, most drug users are not likely to cease readily. They made the decision to use drugs, and they must make the decision themselves to stop. Some, however, may need help making this decision to stop. Help is usually available, but people must *want* to stop for it to work. Proper education on the effect of drug use—especially the effect on diabetes—is helpful.

Unfortunately, the effect of drug use on glucose metabolism is something that has been poorly studied. Some drugs can directly increase blood glucose levels. Others may decrease them. Some substances can interact with the medications used to treat diabetes to change glucose levels as well. Urine testing may become inaccurate with some of these substances. However, the effect of recreational drugs that is of the most concern is the impairment of the mental processes and judgment required to keep the diabetes schedule, remember the medications, and follow an eating plan— the things so important in maintaining proper diabetes control.

Of the specific substances, *marijuana*, in high doses, probably causes hypoglycemia, but if marijuana use causes "the munchies" (the urge to eat frequently), it may lead to hyperglycemia. Altered mental capacity and judgment are also a problem. The longterm use of marijuana has been associated with the so-called drop-out syndrome of apathy and lack of interest—two traits that are a problem for people caring for their diabetes. Marijuana may hide symptoms of hypoglycemic reactions. The American Cancer Society says that smoking a cigarette of marijuana may be more dangerous than one made from tobacco as far as cancer is concerned. Marijuana contains more tar and other by-products. Marijuana cigarettes are also inhaled more deeply, are held in the lungs longer, and are often smoked to the very end, where the carcinogens are maximal. It may cause an increased breakdown of glycogen with a resultant increase in the insulin requirements.

Opiates, such as *heroin, cocaine,* and *morphine,* cause euphoria which impairs judgment. They also increase blood glucose levels. Cocaine may impair the appetite, however, and eating less would decrease blood glucose levels. Stimulants such as *amphetamines* (speed) and *caffeine* (in large amounts) can increase blood glucose levels. Amphetamines are used by some individuals as "diet pills" to help them lose weight—a tempting idea to many people who are overweight and have type II diabetes. Unfortunately, they are not effective in weight reduction and have a hyperglycemic effect as well as increasing nervousness. Some people who have used these for weight loss find that they regain the weight once they try to "get off" these medications. Other drugs that alter the perception and the ability for self-care include the sedatives-hypnotics and the psychedelic drugs.

Many legitimate drugs and medications can be misused. For example, "sleeping pills" and tranquilizers can lead to dependence and the need for stronger medications with occasional tragic results. Their use in combination with alcohol is especially dangerous.

> PEOPLE WITH DIABETES ALREADY HAVE ONE SETBACK IN THEIR COMPETITION WITH OTHERS. THEY DO NOT NEED ANYTHING FURTHER SUCH AS DRUG ABUSE THAT TAKES THEM OUT OF REALITY OR ADDS TO THEIR PROBLEMS.

Approaching any person who is abusing drugs, with or without diabetes, is difficult. One of the most difficult tasks is getting a person to realize that drug use is detrimental to his or her health. People often deny their drug abuse is a problem and make no attempt to stop. It is sometimes useful to find out why they have turned to drugs. Are they trying to escape something? (Is it their diabetes?) Do drugs help them deal with a painful situation? Is it a "status" symbol or a means of acceptance by their peer group? By determining why the individual is using drugs, one may begin to be able to deal with the problem and, perhaps, get the individual to realize the seriousness of the situation. Frequently, however, help from professionals skilled in dealing with people who have problems with drug dependency is required.

There is no easy answer to the problem of drug abuse. Suffice is to say that the person with diabetes must overcome the numerous problems that having this condition presents in order to lead a successful life. To achieve this success, this individual must be able to deal with reality at all times. Anything that is used to avoid dealing with reality puts a person with diabetes at even greater risk of failing to achieve life's goals.

Usable Medications

Those with diabetes can use almost any medication that people without diabetes can use. Exceptions are medications that use highly sweetened or concentrated syrups for a base. Even these may be used on occasion, on advice of your physician, but you must know how to compensate for the increased blood glucose levels. Cortisone and related substances such as prednisone and dexamethasone raise blood glucose levels and should be used only under the direction of a physician.

People with diabetes are concerned about medicines such as those used for relief of cold symptoms. These may have labels that state "Not to be used in case of hypertension, diabetes. . . ." These medicines often contain minute amounts of drugs that have an adrenaline-like action; they tend to raise blood glucose levels, although usually slightly, if at all. The warning is a simple legal one, much like a sign reading "road officially closed." Yet with care, the road can often be safely traveled. The purpose is to protect the highway authorities from real or imagined responsibility. If they really thought there would be a problem, the road would be barricaded. Similarly, the drug warning may be overlooked if the individual's physician indicates that the medication is safe when judiciously used. Most medications that may cause difficulties are "barricaded" by being obtainable only with a physician's prescription.

Other Problem Medications. *Birth control pills* may elevate blood glucose levels slightly, but this would be a concern only for the person with "borderline" diabetes. *Epinephrine* (adrenaline) raises the blood glucose level and in the past was used to treat low blood sugar reactions. *Diuretics* (used to remove excess fluid from the body) impair glucose tolerance in many people with diabetes. Other problems may arise from medications that tend to decrease blood glucose levels either by their own action or by potentiating medications used for this purpose.

Another thing to be wary about are "sound-alike" medications. The *Pharmacy Times* publishes lists yearly warning of as many as a thousand medications that sound alike (or even look alike). Examples are glucagon and glucotrol, Orinase and Ornade, Visidex and Vistaril, and Dymelor and Demerol. Not knowing the difference could be dangerous.

In conclusion, because one medication may interfere with or increase the action of another, it is important to consult your physician when taking several medications.

Surgery and Diabetes

Today, with better preparation and care of diabetes, necessary surgery can be performed on most people with diabetes. If the diabetes has been neglected, it may be necessary to postpone the surgical procedure long enough to bring the diabetes under better regulation to insure the best results.

Traditionally, people with diabetes were hospitalized two days prior to the scheduled time of surgery to make sure that the diabetes was controlled, as well as to check their general health. In this age of cost containment, this practice is no longer possible. People are often hospitalized one day before surgery, the morning of surgery or not at all, with more and more operations being performed on an outpatient basis. This practice may create problems for people with diabetes.

If you have any concern about your diabetes control, or have not seen your diabetes physician for some time, inform your surgeon so that an outpatient evaluation of the diabetes and your general health can be arranged. If you have surgery in a hospital other than the one your diabetes physician visits, an outpatient visit to meet the physician responsible for your diabetes care can be helpful.

For people undergoing "day surgery" (surgery without being hospitalized) it is important to know how to manage your diabetes in anticipation of that event. Plan with your diabetes physician what you will do on that day. You will need to know whether you must not eat before surgery and, if so, for how long, what time the operation will take place, how long it will take, and how long it will be before you can eat again after the surgery. Under no circumstances should you omit your insulin altogether unless your diabetes physician tells you to do so. Usually the insulin dose is reduced prior to surgery, with the remainder being given after the operation is complete.

For people undergoing day surgery, be sure you are able to eat once you go home. If there is any question about being able to eat after surgery, you should remain at the hospital until you do so. Once at home, you should treat the next few days as "sick days," testing frequently and giving additional insulin if necessary.

Dental Problems

It should not be too surprising that diabetes can affect the teeth too. The types of dental problems affecting people with diabetes do not occur only in these individuals. However, when dentists note that someone's teeth and gums are in poor condition, the thought that the person may have diabetes crosses their mind. Uncontrolled diabetes seems to accentuate disease of the gums (peridontal disease), the second most common cause for the loss of teeth. Certainly poor general mouth care may precede the diabetes and influence some of the problems. However, when diabetes is grossly uncontrolled, it appears that patients lose their teeth at a faster rate (perhaps even a decade earlier) than they should. There are many reasons for this. One is the formation of *dental plaque* (collections of bacteria that cling to the teeth surface). There is also a loss of collagen (supportive connective tissue). Studies have shown that even *prediabetes* (elevated blood glucose before diagnosis) can cause increased caries (cavities). Poorly controlled diabetes also causes poorer healing. These are the reasons your dentist is concerned with your diabetes!

Acupuncture

With increased contacts with the People's Republic of China, there has been widespread interest in acupuncture, and many people with diabetes have hoped that this technique might solve some of their problems. Unfortunately, there are few well-researched studies on the subject; it is not well-documented, even in China. Acupuncture is based on a theory of flowing nerve energy and the release of nerve impulses.

A Joslin physician who has been in China observed this technique. It is not generally used for treatment of diabetes. It is used mostly as a rather good local anesthesia and for treatment of various nerve-related ailments. It is interesting that in many of the large hospitals there, Western style medicine and acupuncture are used side by side.

The danger is that if reliance on this acupuncture causes a person with diabetes to neglect accepted treatment, it could indeed be harmful. However, it has been used as a treatment of stress, which, if successful, might be helpful to the person with diabetes.

Biofeedback, Meditation, and Relaxation Therapy

The exact effect of stress on diabetes is still unknown. While most people agree that acute stress—the death of a relative, losing a job, etc.—will directly increase blood glucose levels to some degree for a short period of time, it is unlikely that chronic stress has the same effect. However, many people note worsening blood glucose levels while they are experiencing the more chronic types of stress—a family problem, preparing for exams, or just a difficult time at work. Whether the stress directly causes the elevations in blood glucose levels, or whether the stress causes the person to be careless with diabetes care, is unclear. The actual effect may vary from person to person.

Many people agree that stress can be a health problem. If nothing else, it makes life less enjoyable, can raise the blood pressure, promote heart disease, and stimulate peptic ulcer formation in addition to the effects on diabetes. It is safe to say that there is nothing good about stress. Various techniques such as biofeedback, meditation, and relaxation therapies have been developed in hope of reducing stress. Some people advocate these methods to help reduce or stabilize blood glucose levels, especially in the person with non-insulin-dependent (type II) diabetes. If you are a person who suffers the ups and downs of stress, it may be beneficial to explore these techniques to see if they will help. Even if you do not notice much improvement in your diabetes control, you may feel more at peace with life and happier about yourself. Of course, these therapies are only an adjunct to your usual diabetes treatment, not a replacement for it.

Contact Lenses

People with diabetes often ask about the use of contact lenses. One reason for this concern is that in many people with diabetes, the outer layer of cells on the cornea (corneal epithelium) does not adhere to the underlying tissue as it should. In people with diabetes, contact lenses are more likely to scratch off these cells if the lenses do not fit properly. In addition, people with diabetes may take longer to heal from these injuries ("corneal abrasions"). Some with diabetes may have less acute nerve endings and lack the ability to sense discomfort on the cornea, which normally would warn of ill-fitting lenses.

Despite these concerns, if the outside of the eye is healthy and the lenses are well fitted by an expert, they can be used by people with diabetes. People who may be subject to unconsciousness for any reason may wish to use one of the longer wear lenses so that they will not suffer corneal damage should they lose consciousness, not have the lenses noticed, and wear them much longer than they should before they are removed.

> WHEN TRAVELING, YOU SHOULD HAVE IDENTIFICATION SAYING THAT YOU ARE WEARING CONTACT LENSES. IN SOME COUNTRIES, CONTACT LENSES ARE UN-HEARD OF, AND, IN CASE OF ACCIDENT, THE HEALTH CARE PEOPLE SHOULD KNOW!

Yet, the *very long* ("constant wear") lenses are not recommended. Anyone who may be subject to periods of difficult diabetes regulation should wait until the diabetes has stabilized before being fitted for contact lenses. People with diabetes may be subject to increased susceptibility to infection, and lenses should be rechecked and cleaned at regular intervals.

Contact lenses are now available after cataract surgery. These replace the old-fashioned very thick and heavy lenses, and are an alternative to intraocular lens implants, which must be sutured into place.

Ear Piercing

Ear (and in some cultures, nose) piercing usually involves punching a small hole through the ear lobe (or wherever) and having wires or studs inserted immediately to prevent closing. When healed, a permanent canal exists for use with better grades of earrings or other jewelry. If the procedure is skillfully done with proper precaution against infection, the person with diabetes should be able to undergo this procedure with no more difficulty than someone who does not have diabetes.

Camps for Youngsters with Diabetes

Special camps for youngsters with diabetes are now widely available. Certainly the young person with diabetes has unique problems, both physiologically and especially psychologically. These camps are for health, recreation, and fun, and can help these young people live with diabetes very effectively. Camps are discussed in more detail in Chapter 12.

Summertime

The "good old summertime" can also affect diabetes—and why not? To be sure of getting the maximum out of summer fun, certain precautions must be taken.

Sunburn can be a serious problem. Remember, a burn from the sun is like any other burn, except it is milder—but often covers more of your body. Go into the sun gradually for a slow tan. Don't try to do it all at once, or you can have real problems. Protective sunscreen lotions are available. Increasingly dermatologists warn about the danger of too much sun causing skin cancer in later years.

Poison ivy, poison oak, and other lovely looking plants lie in wait for people who want to be close to nature. Try to avoid them. If you do get involved, wash carefully with lots of soap and water as soon as you come in from the outdoors. If there is swelling, itching, and oozing from the skin, contact your physician for appropriate ointments. Infection from these plants is no better than other infections.

Insect stings can spoil a lot of picnics. Many cause a localized reaction. Rarely are they serious, although bee and wasp stings have been known to be fatal to those very allergic. Stay away from any of

332 LIVING WITH DIABETES

these along with honeybees and yellow jackets. Do not provoke them. You may be friendly, but they may have had a bad day. If you are stung and the swelling is more than minor or if you have a generalized reaction, seek your health care team members' assistance. Flies, mosquitoes, and flying ants are in season too, but are not too dangerous. Near the water, beware of things that float. The most likely offenders are the *Portuguese men-of-war*. They travel in fleets through the waters of the Pacific and Atlantic Oceans and are very common off the southeast coast of Florida in winter and spring. They can be a foot and a half across and float on the waves in the wind. It is the trailing mass of tentacles that can be dangerous. The tentacles can still have some burning venom even after the man-of-war has washed ashore and died. Stay away!

Sports

Sports are encouraged for people with diabetes. Exercise of any sort (Chapter 5) can improve diabetes control as well as overall health. Indeed, diabetes has not prevented some dedicated and motivated individuals from becoming professional athletes. Football players have played professionally despite diabetes. Bobby Clarke, one of the greatest hockey players, has type I diabetes. Hamilton Richardson and Bill Talbert of tennis fame and Ron Santo, the baseball player, and numerous others, all achieved excellence in their sports while having diabetes. The main danger is the possibility of low blood glucose reactions. Injuries pose no greater risks for people with diabetes than for those without diabetes. However, coaches, teammates, and others who play with the person with diabetes should be aware of the hypoglycemic potential. Extra carbohydrate must be used as needed, and insulin dose adjustments may also be required beforehand.

Marriage, Childbearing, and Sexual Function

As with many aspects of our lives, diabetes may affect the decision to marry, making it that much more complex. Diabetes forces both the person with diabetes and his or her partner to face certain issues early on in their lives, especially if childbearing is part of the long-range plan.

Marriage Counseling. The desire to marry and have children is a normal goal for most people in our society. One of the more urgent questions asked by people with diabetes facing marriage and childbearing is, "Will my children have diabetes?" The hereditary aspects of diabetes have been discussed earlier (Chapter 1). Beyond childbearing, however, there are other issues that must be considered.

Marriage to a person with any chronic condition poses problems that may require patience and understanding by the spouse. What may be an intolerable burden to some marriage partners may be no problem to others. Although facts and data usually do little to change minds where human emotions are involved, the person contemplating marriage to someone with diabetes should do so with complete knowledge. If you understand all of the potential problems that may affect the marriage, you will be better able to handle them.

The following should be considered:

1. Complications may occur after a number of years. Disability or premature death may occur—not necessarily, but possibly.
2. Pregnancy in a woman with diabetes may be more difficult and will require much more attention than pregnancy in others (Chapter 13). Outcomes of pregnancies in women with diabetes have been very good in recent years with proper monitoring—and are improving.
3. The partner without diabetes must realize that the nature of diabetes requires medical care and understanding throughout life and that there is at present no "cure" for this condition.
4. Special problems with employment and insurance may arise.
5. The prospective spouse of a person with diabetes should learn about diabetes so that he or she can understand the disease and the problems that arise. There should be an understanding about how well or poorly the prospective partner has been controlling the diabetes and the nature of any complications already present.

Does it seem that the negative aspects of marriage have been stressed? Of course, there are many favorable features of marriage as well, but these are better known! With knowledge and understanding, aided and abetted by generous doses of love, there is a foundation for a stable and happy marriage.

Male Sexual Function. One aspect of marriage that is not discussed often enough with people with diabetes is sex. People often seek advice from those who know even less than they do. People with diabetes have the same sex characteristics and desires as others, are usually able to perform sexual activities normally, and can lead satisfying sex lives. The difficulties, if any, concern the eventual inability of the male with diabetes to achieve or maintain erections sufficient for satisfying sexual function. This problem is called impotence and is discussed in detail in Chapter 16.

Men with diabetes are subject to the same tensions and resultant lack of performance as men without diabetes. In the general population, the leading cause of impotence is psychological difficulties—tension, fear of failure, guilt, etc.—and the same problems can occur in men with diabetes as well. One of the problems with impotence, whether physical or psychological, is that no one knows what is really normal. Some men with diabetes can perform into their seventies while some who do not have diabetes have sexual dysfunction 20 or 30 years earlier. In modern life, with heavy emphasis on sex in news media and all types of literature, sometimes expectations are out of proportion to reality. However, among men who do become impotent, those with a solid basis for their emotional life, with numerous other interests, and with a happy married life are not as disturbed about this as they earlier thought they would be. It is not *their* fault. It is a medical or physical fact of life, and there should be no guilt.

Birth Control. In general, women with diabetes may use the same birth control measures as those without diabetes. The oral contraceptive medications can have the same contraindications (circumstances in which their use is not advised) for both groups of women, and these should be discussed with one's gynecologist or family physician. Statistics on birth control pills are improving. A recent study of 4774 women (age 20 to 54) by the U.S. Centers for Disease Control showed that pills containing some estrogen and progestin actually protected against ovarian cancer. Of course, further study is needed.

For women with diabetes, there is the additional consideration of the possible worsening (usually temporary) of the diabetes during oral contraceptive use. Indeed, some women whose diabetes is controlled by oral hypoglycemic agents may need to start treatment with or increase the dose of their oral agents or insulin while on "the pill." Oral contraceptives work by hormonally simulating pregnancy. Usually, physicians prescribe oral contraceptive pills for limited periods.

The long-used forms of birth control such as condoms and diaphragms are still widely used. Intrauterine devices (IUDs) have also been used, but require so much caution and close observation by a physician that they are being used less and less, often being replaced by other methods. Clearly, there is no one form of contraception that is perfect for everyone. The physician and patient should consider whether a particular contraceptive method or pregnancy represents the greater risk for a given person. Vasectomy in the male (excision of part of the sperm-carrying duct) or ligation (tying off) of the fallopian tubes in the female provide permanent protection. These are becoming more popular solutions. These procedures do not impair sexual function. In fact, freedom of the fear of pregnancy sometimes improves sexual performance!

Sexual Activity and Hypoglycemia. Some people with diabetes fear that the excessive exertion of sexual activity may cause them to have a hypoglycemic reaction. That worry can interfere with sexual function or enjoyment. If, indeed, sexual activity is like excessive exercise, it can have the potential to cause hypoglycemia. As with exercise, however, this varies from person to person. If you have had difficulty with this problem during sexual activity, it can be corrected as for any other type of exercise—adjustment of insulin or a snack in anticipation. Sugar-containing beverages just before may be appropriate, and possibly an additional snack afterward. Self blood testing before and after can help determine just how much food may be necessary. Unlike other forms of exercise, however, most people do not like to stop in the middle of this activity to test their blood glucose level! So, be prepared!

Traveling with Diabetes

Each year the world becomes smaller, and thousands of people who never traveled before go to faraway places. There is no reason why those with diabetes should not be among them. Most of the comforts and conveniences of home can now be found even in remote places. If diabetes is well controlled at home, travel should not be burdensome. However, if the person with diabetes is having trouble with control under ideal circumstances, the uncertainties of travel can cause further difficulties. People with very unstable diabetes should improve their control as much as possible before departing.

Before Leaving. It is almost impossible to begin preparing too early for a big trip. After the itinerary has been chosen and passports, visas, and tickets obtained, the detailed planning starts. It is important to make certain that your health insurance policy applies to the areas that will be visited. This is an important question that is generally overlooked. Not only do you need health insurance, but you may need "on-the-spot" insurance. For example, Medicare does not pay benefits for hospitalization abroad, but other supplementary insurances do.

At the International Diabetes Federation meeting held in Nairobi, Kenya, in 1982, a group of sightseers went to view the animal preserves. A sightseeing vehicle jammed with visitors turned over, and three of the passengers were hospitalized with fractured pelvises. They recovered but had a hard time because none of them was covered by insurance for that hospitalization.

Some insurance policies cover emergency hospitalization immediately and also will pay for your trip home. Sometimes people who are injured or have been ill require first class (expensive) travel home. Check your insurance policies before you leave, especially if you are going on an extended trip. Remember, many hospitals now require proof of payment before you can be discharged.

No special inoculations are needed for travel to commonly visited centers in Europe. When planning travel in Asia, Africa, or Central or South America, consult your physician about needed inoculations. These should be brought up to date as needed in advance, and proper documentation provided. Yellow fever, poliomyelitis, and malaria are endemic in some parts of the world, as are infectious hepatitis, tetanus, and cholera. Smallpox is rarely a problem these days and, in fact, vaccination certificates are not asked for. Protection against cholera and infectious hepatitis is short in duration, but protection against the other diseases lasts for reasonably long periods. For malaria it is now possible to take a preventive medication at weekly intervals for several weeks before and after the trip, which reduces the chances of acquiring malaria.

Inoculation requirements can change. Information concerning these diseases can be obtained from your local health department, the U.S. Public Health Service, or the Centers for Disease Control in Atlanta, Georgia. The pamphlet "Immunization Information for International Travel" can be obtained from the Superintendent of Documents, U.S. Government Printing Office, Washington, DC 20402.

Try to get your immunization injections early, so that if you have any reactions to them, you have them before you leave home. Also, it is no fun getting injections all at once!

Choosing Clothes. Like everyone else, people with diabetes often take too many clothes when traveling. However, because they must watch their feet scrupulously, they should tuck in an extra pair of comfortable walking shoes. Do not try to break in new shoes on the trip. Take old ones that you know are comfortable. *Simple baggage tip*: Put a large initial with adhesive or colored tape on the side of each piece of baggage. When the jumbo jet with 300 passengers unloads with 900 pieces of brown, blue, or gray baggage, the bags all look alike. This tip may help you spot yours more quickly.

Health Record and Identification. It is useful to carry a note from your physician stating your current medical condition and listing medications *by their generic* rather than trade names (which vary all over the world). For example, list tolbutamide instead of Orinase (also known as Artosin, Rastinon, etc.). Glucotrol would be glipizide, and Diabeta and Micronase would be glyburide (also known as glybenclamide in some places). Generic names are understood nearly everywhere.

Diabetes identification is important at home and even more vital for travel abroad. Although people with diabetes generally have no particular problems at customs, an identification card or bracelet

---

ANOTHER INSURANCE PROBLEM

When people travel and have an accident abroad, who covers the hospitalization? Many insurance policies do not. For example, Medicare does not, but Medex does. Does your health policy give you coverage?

Most hospitals worldwide demand ability to pay the bill *in advance*. Some policies give the admitting hospital a guarantee of payment. One such is WorldCare, which has a worldwide telephone and telex number. Address: 2000 Pennsylvania Ave., NW, Washington, D.C. 20006. There are others. Check with your insurance agent.

---

can be useful in placating a dubious official who is casting a baleful eye on the supply of syringes and needles. If you take insulin, a physician's note might be obtained which includes a statement regarding the need for syringes and needles because occasionally (rarely) customs agents might ask questions about why you need 200 disposable needles!

Personal Medication. For most trips, it is best to bring necessary medications with you. Aspirin or acetaminophen (Tylenol) and perhaps foot powder can be helpful. Also bring something for diarrhea: Lomotil and Kaopectate can be useful. Make certain that you carry your medications (especially the diabetes-related ones) in your carry-on flight bag in case your suitcases go to Bulgaria when you are going to Singapore! Although most medications are available throughout the world, the labels can be confusing, and you may need to wait for it. Do not worry about refrigeration for insulin. It can tolerate the same temperatures as you for several weeks or months. Be sure to take enough medication for the entire trip, and even some extra in case you lose or damage it. There is no evidence that the metal detectors used at most airports will harm any of the medications.

Diabetes during Traveling. Many travelers prefer the convenient strip urine testing methods (Chemstrip uG, Diastix, Tes-Tape, etc.) to the Clinitest tablets for traveling. Urine acetone test materials and blood testing supplies should be brought along as well. If you have a meter with rechargeable batteries, investigate whether the current where you are going is compatible with your meter. You may need to bring a current converter along or have enough batteries for the battery type meter. Be sure to have some blood test strips that can be read directly without a meter in case of difficulty.

Up, Up, and Away! Most international travel is now done by jet airplane. Certainly, this is the fastest and best way for people with diabetes to travel because it is less disrupting to the schedule. Many people need a day after a major jet trip to get back into the normal rhythm, and those with diabetes have the added problem of the proper timing of their medications and meals. Many trips require that you eat on an airplane, and most people with diabetes can choose a satisfactory meal from airline foods. Many airlines now serve special meals such as kosher, vegetarian, or even diabetic meals, but these must be ordered in advance. However, many airlines are cutting corners on shorter trips by serving "snacks," which may be insufficient or poorly timed. It is advised to check into this before the flight. A few airlines will honor a written menu recommended by your physician. If the diabetes is very unstable, the steward or stewardess should be reminded of your condition early enough so that if you require something sweet in a hurry or if there is a delay in serving, you can have some priority. Nevertheless, carrying a "just in case" snack is always a good idea. Plain granola, peanut butter or cheese crackers, 1-ounce bags of nuts or seeds, and small cans of juice travel well for this purpose.

Time Zones. While the speed of a jet shortens trips, it also shortens the day going east or lengthens the day going west (Fig. 17–3). For example, flying east from New York to Paris shortens the day by 6 hours. Going west from New York to Hawaii, the day is much longer. When returning to the United States from Europe, it is possible to get daytime flights, but flying to Europe from the East Coast almost always involves a night flight. People with diabetes worry about insulin adjustments. Most often the west-east flight disturbs them. Most flights to Europe start at an hour of the night when the person has already had his or her evening meal. About an hour after takeoff, a meal is usually served. After a short sleep, the traveler is landing in Europe at perhaps 8:00 a.m., which is actually 2:00 a.m. at home.

People with stable diabetes taking relatively small single doses (about 20 units) of insulin rarely have difficulty with overlapping of the insulin during this shortened day. People with unstable diabetes or who take larger or multiple doses of insulin may have difficulty and will need to talk with their physician to decide on an adjustment plan. This whole issue of insulin dose adjustments, however, has been greatly simplified with the advent of the self–blood testing methods, which have taken the guess work out of it.

Unless you travel constantly, the major concern of the occasional traveler with diabetes is to avoid hypoglycemia on the day of travel. It is unlikely that severe hyperglycemia will occur as long as a reasonable dose of insulin is taken, and slightly elevated blood glucose levels on the day of travel are not a major concern. Therefore, a general rule would be to lower the insulin dose on the day of departure when traveling east, thus anticipating a shortened day. For example, if you are traveling from New York to London, you lose about 6 hours, which is one-quarter of a day. Therefore, reduce your dose by about one-quarter. The most important thing to do is to check your blood glucose level periodically. If you are dropping too low, have a snack. (Food should be carried on board for this purpose in case you cannot get a snack from the cabin attendant in time.) If your glucose level is rising, either take a little more insulin at the next injection time, or, if it is quite high, take an additional injection of regular (clear) insulin.

If you are traveling west, which will add time to your day, take your usual insulin dose, but also monitor your blood glucose levels. Have extra snacks to cover the additional time period. Extra insulin can also be used to cover high glucose levels, if necessary. North-south travel is rarely a problem, as no major time shifts occur. It is frequently a good idea to review your travel plans with your

---

TEMPERATURE ANYONE?
Much of the world uses centigrade, while we in the United States use Fahrenheit.
While the true conversion formula from one to the other requires arithmetic with fractions, there is a quick and easy way to come close!
Double the centigrade temperature and add 30. For example, if it is 10 degrees centigrade, double it (2 x 10 = 20), then add 30 (20 + 30 = 50), to get 50 degrees Fahrenheit.
From Fahrenheit to centigrade, simply subtract 30 and divide by 2. While this conversion is not quite accurate in the extremes, it works well in the mid-ranges.

---

physician so that he or she can advise you specifically on how to handle your diabetes treatment during time zone changes.

Problems en Route. The chances of low blood glucose reactions occurring while flying, although the primary concern, are actually minimal because there is little activity and, frequently, large (almost too much) amounts of food are served. Airsickness is rare, but medication, if needed, will be useful only if taken before it is required. If you are susceptible to airsickness, you should obtain dimenhydrinate (Dramamine) or a prescription for another medication such as meclizine (Bonine), cyclizine (Marezine), or a scopolamine patch. It is advisable on longer flights to take occasional walks up and down the aisle to avoid possible blood clotting in the legs caused by inflammation of the veins; this is called "passenger phlebitis." It can result from continuous sitting with the seat pressing on the backs of the knees. Most jet planes are now pressurized to comfortable pressures, and there is rarely any problem with breathing. Air conditioning can be dehydrating, and drinking fluids during the flight can make one feel more comfortable.

Travel by Ship. While the number of transoceanic crossings by ship is decreasing, the relaxed life of a cruise can be tempting to anyone. Most large cruise ships have competent medical staffs, and some have hospitals. Although there are no problems with time zones, never was a ship built that didn't pitch and roll during stormy weather, at least a bit, especially on the North Atlantic. Seasickness,

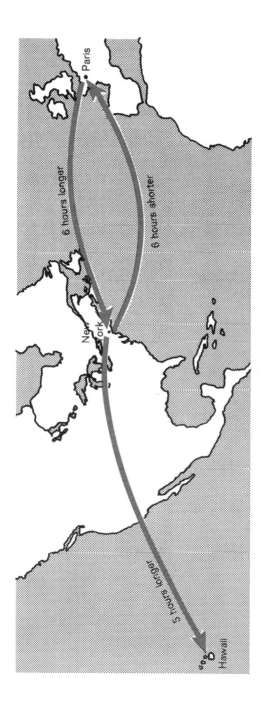

FIG. 17–3. When traveling, the day becomes shorter going east and longer going west. Going *east*, New York to Paris, the day is 6 hours shorter; Hawaii to New York, 5 hours shorter. Going *west*, Paris to New York, the day is 6 hours longer; New York to Hawaii; 5 hours longer. Japan is another 3,580 miles further west. Flying north or south doesn't usually make much difference.

for people without diabetes, can be a temporary inconvenience, but for those with diabetes, extended gastrointestinal upset can be a real problem. The remedies previously mentioned to prevent motion sickness can help, but they are not foolproof. It is always a good idea to alert the medical staff on the boat of your condition just in case you run into "rough sailing." When traveling by ship, note that time zones change only one hour each 24.

On Arriving. Avoid overeating, overdrinking, and overexerting, especially on the first day. Your "travel cycle" may not have caught up with you. The food and drinking water are usually quite safe in the major hotels in the developed countries. However, while the water may not contain dangerous organisms, it may differ from the water to which you are accustomed. Generally, in most hotels and certainly away from them, it is safest to use bottled water. Cooked foods are usually safe in accepted hotels and restaurants. Be cautious with raw food unless you have peeled it yourself. Generally, the hotel that caters to foreign visitors is the safest place to eat.

"Tourista"—The Curse of the Traveling Class! Not much is known about the very annoying condition known by the name "tourista" and other exotic names. This illness, usually not serious, is characterized by abdominal cramps, diarrhea, nausea, and, at times, chills and low-grade fever. It usually lasts only a few days. For United States visitors, it occurs most commonly in the Mediterranean areas, Asia, and some parts of Central and South America. The cause is not always known, although recent studies show that bacteria are responsible most of the time, whether or not it is actually detected. There are no satisfactory preventive measures except good sense and caution. After diarrhea develops, a bland diet consisting of tea, rice, and clear soup is usually adequate, although people with diabetes who take insulin must remember to use sweetened food or liquids to make certain that the carbohydrate intake is adequate. Any number of medications, such as Kaopectate or Lomotil, can be prescribed in advance by your physician and taken along for use in case of need. Pepto-Bismol has recently been shown to be effective as well. Antibiotics are rarely needed unless the condition persists more than a couple of days, in which case it is best to see a physician. Recent publications have recommended the use of doxycycline hyclate (Vibramycin) or trimethoprim and sulfamethoxazole (Septra) in appropriate doses, *not as a treatment of active diarrhea* but as a preventive medication against some of the diarrhea-causing organisms. Your physician can provide prescriptions for these.

Looking for Medical Help. Your own doctor may know of physicians abroad. In addition, many countries have diabetes associations affiliated with the International Diabetes Federation. You can contact the IDF or the American Diabetes Association (their addresses are given at the end of this chapter) in advance for a list of diabetes-trained physicians in countries you will visit. For foreign travel, the IDF knows of diabetes associations in about 85 countries. Most major hotels also have access to physicians who speak English, as does the United States embassy or consulate in each country. An organization called Intermedic (777 Third Ave., New York, NY 10017) lists English-speaking physicians who treat patients for a set fee. There are very few places in the world without adequate medical service, and into those very few areas only the person who is well trained and self-reliant on the care of his or her diabetes should venture.

Other Hints. As noted earlier, the insulins and other medicines most commonly used here not only are obtainable elsewhere around the world, but often are made by the same companies that make them for you. Oral agents available abroad are listed in Appendix 3. If you need to buy insulin abroad, you can show your insulin bottle to the pharmacist, who generally can find the equivalent. As a general rule, clear insulin is usually regular insulin, and cloudy insulins are usually intermediate-acting. As noted earlier, hypoglycemia is the greatest danger while driving for the person with diabetes who takes insulin or oral agents. Snacks and meals must be taken on time or a bit sooner, and something sweet should be available in the car. Bus or train travel requires advance planning because of the infrequency of the stops and the usually crowded conditions of terminals when you do stop. Carry snacks, and be sure to eat when you get the opportunity. Carry insulin with you.

It is wise to carry either an extra pair of eyeglasses with you or the prescription for your own in case a pair is broken. Tourists can be very helpless if they cannot see well. If you have spare dentures, bring them. Another important thing to remember in traveling is care of the feet—proper bathing, frequent changing of socks, and treatment of athlete's foot and minor infections. This care, along with plenty of rest, can do a lot to prevent foot complications and make your trip much more enjoyable.

In summary, at home or abroad, your diabetes training is your best friend, and with that, you can happily succumb to the wanderlust that infects all of us from time to time. Have a safe and happy trip!

For More Information

Most of us need all the help we can get in life. The following three organizations can give you information on living with your diabetes:

Joslin Diabetes Center. One Joslin Place, Boston, MA 02215, (617) 732-2400. The center has literature, pamphlets, and other sources of help and guidance. (Write for an updated publications list.)

American Diabetes Association, 1660 Duke St., Alexandria, VA 22314, (703) 549-1500. This is an organization that you should belong to because there are affiliates in every state. It is also a source of informative literature.

International Diabetes Federation, International Association Center, 40 Washington St., 1050 Brussels, Belgium, phone: 32-2/ 647 44 14. This is a group whose membership comprises all the world's national diabetes associations. The American Diabetes Association is one of about 85 such national associations that are affiliated with the IDF. Membership brings you the IDF *Bulletin* and partnership in the world of diabetes.

18

A Look Ahead

To look back today on the progress made in the treatment of diabetes during this century is to see miraculous changes in the outlook for people with diabetes mellitus. Before the discovery of insulin, the outlook for people with insulin-dependent diabetes, as has been mentioned several times in this book, was grim. The only treatment was slow starvation in hopes of merely postponing what appeared to be an inevitable death. Common colds were life-threatening, and influenza was almost certain death. Ketoacidosis and diabetic coma were commonplace. Dr. Elliott P. Joslin's early records document the cause of death as "coma," "coma," "coma."

The improved outlook enjoyed by people with diabetes today has come about through efforts by clinicians and researchers everywhere. The goals have been to find new ways to treat and educate people with diabetes. Survival today, although not guaranteed, is almost taken for granted. Today people strive for "normalcy," that is, making the life of the person with diabetes as close to normal as possible. Recent advances have allowed the lives of those with diabetes to be more flexible than ever, although they still must take insulin or tablets, monitor their blood glucose levels, and follow a prescribed eating plan. More people can now live lives that are close to "normal." Ultimately, the hopes for the future are that we can achieve true "normalcy" for all people with this condition.

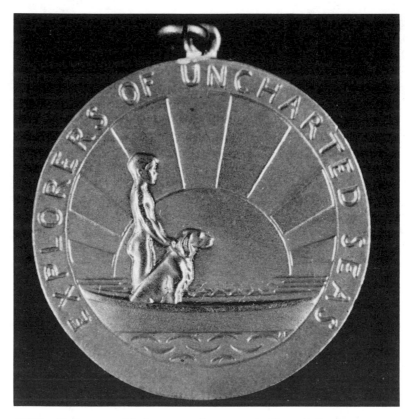

FIG. 18–1. A medal honoring those involved in diabetes research. (Original by Amelia Peabody.)

Where We Are Today

In this manual we have attempted to outline today's "state of the art" of diabetes treatment. This level of care came about because of a quiet revolution in diabetes treatment in the early 1980s. This period has seen the introduction of home blood glucose monitoring and glycohemoglobin measurements, and the availability of improved (purer and human-like) insulins and new oral hypoglycemic agents. We now have the ability to approach "normal" patterns of blood glucose levels more closely than ever before. As a result, people with diabetes can enjoy more flexibility in their activity and eating programs, and a more normal life-style as well.

The treatment of the complications has improved, as well. Laser treatment has dramatically reduced the frequency of significant vision loss. Renal dialysis and transplantation prolong the lives of many people with failing kidneys. Newer treatments of heart disease, both with surgery and with newer medications and treatments, prolong the lives of millions. Better treatment of circulatory disease saves countless limbs. Improved medications for the treatment of diabetic neuropathies are also improving the quality of life for many individuals. Awareness of risk factors for vascular (circulatory) diseases is prompting more vigorous efforts to treat high blood lipid levels and high blood pressure, as well as stimulating people to stop smoking. Education has become a part of treatment instead of just an accessory. That which was available to only a fortunate few is now available around the world. Indeed, we have come a long way. Yet we still have a long way to go.

Research Today, Hopes for Tomorrow

As important as the past accomplishments may be, even more exciting is the hope for the not-too-distant future. To paraphrase Neil Armstrong, many small steps are being taken so that diabetes care can take many giant leaps for humankind.

Researchers now have many pieces of the puzzle and are trying to fit them together. Because types I and II diabetes may indeed be caused by different factors, efforts to prevent and cure them often take different paths.

Prevention of Insulin-Dependent Diabetes. Before you can treat or prevent something, you must first find out what it is that causes that thing to happen. Today, much attention is being focused on preventing type I (insulin-dependent) diabetes and thus on why it occurs and how to identify those destined to get it. Much of this research, as discussed in detail in Chapter 1, has focused on the identification of certain genes that are more likely to be present in individuals who have type I diabetes. These genes may predispose a person to develop type I diabetes. However, because many people with these genes do not have diabetes, their presence does not always predict future developments. In addition, all of the genes that may play a role in the development of diabetes have not yet been identified.

There are other factors, however, which help predict who may get diabetes in the future. Many individuals destined to develop type I diabetes may have antibodies in their blood which are directed against the islet cells of the pancreas that make insulin. Antibodies, of course, are made by the body to help fight off foreign substances, such as viruses, but in some instances antibodies may turn against part of the body itself. There is evidence that certain antibodies may take part in the destruction of the islet cells, thereby causing diabetes.

When we have the ability to predict the candidates for diabetes, we will be able to start proper treatment sooner, when suggestive symptoms are noted, reducing the chances of ketoacidosis. However, the important breakthrough will come when methods are developed to stop the process that is destroying the islet cells, thus preventing diabetes from ever developing.

Some exciting research has used corticosteroids and cyclosporine in an attempt to prevent beta cell destruction that has been detected by the presence of islet cell antibodies. It was hoped that the use of these anti-immune drugs could preserve beta cell function and, as a result, insulin injections would not be needed. Early results suggested that these compounds have some effect, but there was some concern whether it was feasible to give these medications for prolonged periods of time because some of their side effects can be quite serious. Meanwhile, other similar and possibly less toxic substances are, as always, being developed. Overall, the entire premise of "shutting down" the developing diabetes shows some promise.

Prevention and Treatment of Non-Insulin-Dependent Diabetes.
Because you cannot choose your ancestors, the most effective method of preventing type II (non-insulin-dependent) diabetes is prevention of obesity. While seemingly simpler than preventing type I diabetes, it actually may be more difficult. People have been trying for years to devise ways to prevent obesity, and no really effective methods have yet been devised. Genetic factors, social pressures, psychological issues, and cultural trends in modern living all come into the picture. There is no quick fix here, as anyone who has tried to lose weight knows!

Research is continuing into better understanding the actual cause of type II diabetes. We have learned in recent years that this type of diabetes may be influenced by three factors. The first factor, insulin resistance, is invariably present in type II diabetes and seems to be getting the most attention in recent years. We are learning more and more about how the insulin transmits its message to the cells of the body so that they can allow the glucose to enter. We know that there are receptors on the surface of the cells to which the insulin attaches. Insulin then triggers a series of reactions which eventually permits the glucose to get into the cell. It is probably somewhere in this chain of reactions, starting with the insulin trying to attach to the receptor and ending with glucose entering the cell, that the key to the insulin resistance of type II diabetes will be found.

The second factor contributing to type II diabetes is probably a defect in the ability of the pancreas to secrete insulin properly. As a result, the quantities of insulin present are insufficient to overcome the insulin resistance. Thus we refer to this situation as "relative insulin insufficiency," which implys that whatever the amount of insulin present (even above normal amounts), it is still not enough to overcome insulin resistance and bring the blood glucose levels to normal. The third factor is a reduction in the number of beta cells (the cells that produce insulin).

We have known for years that type II diabetes is an inherited disease. It is common to see numerous people in a family, especially if they are overweight, with type II diabetes. Just how this condition is inherited, and how these three potential causes of type II diabetes may be passed on to the next generation, is a fertile area of research.

As we learn more about the causes of type II diabetes, we can treat it more effectively. The oral hypoglycemic agents used to treat type II diabetes are considered to work by, among other things, reducing insulin resistance, although the exact mechanism for this is not fully understood. Some of these compounds may also encourage the pancreas to secrete insulin. In the future, we can anticipate newer, more effective medical therapy of this disease, as we learn more about insulin resistance and insulin secretion.

Insulin Treatment of Diabetes. A growing understanding of the normal patterns of insulin secretion and action have allowed the design of insulin treatment programs that more effectively mimic the normal situation (Chapters 9 and 10). However, we still are unable to achieve total normalcy, and the prospect of doing this is an eternal challenge to diabetes researchers.

Transplanting the Pancreas. Since the first pancreas transplant was performed in 1966, there have been high hopes that this operation would lead to the "cure" for their disease. Unfortunately, the success of this operation is limited, despite improvements over the last 10 years. One major problem is the need to suppress the body's efforts to "reject" the foreign pancreas (that is, suppress the immune system). The side effects of this immunosuppressive therapy can be as bad as the diabetes itself. To subject a healthy person to a risky transplant operation for a chance for a "cure" that is far from certain, and which carries potentially serious side effects, would be offering a "cure" that was worse than the disease itself. Therefore, transplants are being performed for the most part on people who have already received a kidney transplant, a truly life-saving procedure. These people are already receiving immunosuppressive therapy to protect their transplanted kidney. Transplants of this type are being done, but are still experimental, with only about 20% of the transplanted pancreases functioning successfully for a limited period of time.

It is hoped that eventual improvements in transplant techniques will reduce the risks of this treatment so that it can be useful in treating more people with type I diabetes before they develop life-threatening complications, rather than after they have the problems.

Islet Cell Transplantation. It is the islet cells that actually make the insulin. Transplantation of these cells alone would seem to be simpler than transplantation of the pancreas. However, obtaining enough cells and implanting them so that they will survive is indeed a great challenge. The major problems that must be faced include isolation of "pure" human islet cells in sufficient quantity for transplantation, preventing rejection of these "foreign" cells by the patient's immune system, and avoiding a return of the diabetes due to factors which probably destroyed the original beta cells and caused the diabetes in the first place. Recent research efforts have led to improvements in isolation of these cells, but, despite some remarkable progress in this one area, there are problems that continue to hamper the best efforts of those doing the research.

One possible solution to the rejection problem is to implant the cells in a filter capsule to prevent rejection. The holes in the filter would be small enough to let the insulin out and the nutrients in, but too small for the antibodies and the destructive white blood cells to pass through and thus destroy the cells.

The Artificial Pancreas. The insulin pumps that are in use today, as discussed in Chapter 10 are "open loop" pumps that cannot determine blood glucose levels and cannot determine the proper insulin dose. The pump user must perform these functions, thus "closing the information loop" by telling the pump how much insulin to deliver and how often. A true artificial pancreas would be able to sense the glucose level, and then after deciding how much insulin is needed, deliver it.

The good news is that such a machine exists. The bad news is that it is a computerized machine used only in research which is about the size of a large television set, much too big to be practical for those with diabetes. One such machine is known as a Biostator (Fig. 18–2). It can be attached to a person for a short period of time. Blood flows out of the body and into the Biostator, which measures

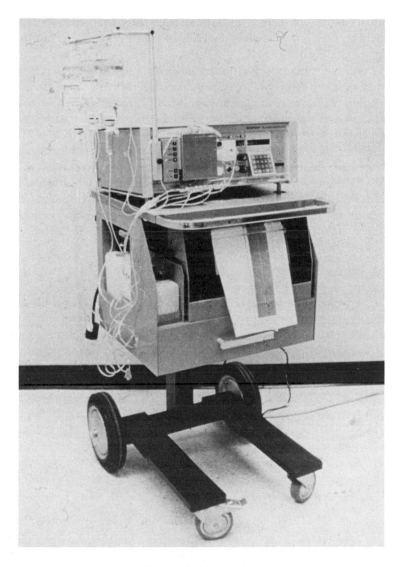

FIG. 18–2. A Biostator. This machine can automatically adjust the blood glucose level of a person with diabetes to a predetermined level using computerized technology to control a constant flow of a glucose solution and insulin. It is useful for research studies.

the glucose level and determines the precise amount of insulin to be added, and then the blood is returned to the body. The complexity of this procedure, to say nothing of the size of the machine, prevents any longterm practical use. It is currently used for a short period of time to study the effects on metabolism of normalizing the blood glucose levels of people with diabetes. Occasionally, it is used to help decide on the daily insulin requirements for a person with type I diabetes who has extremely unstable blood glucose levels, but this is not common practice.

Recent advances in electronics, however, have brought us closer to having a self-contained, implantable, closed-loop pump. In fact, such devices have been designed and built (Fig. 18–3). The key to this device is the glucose sensor (Fig. 18–4), which measures the blood glucose level and then feeds this information into the computer. Unfortunately, herein lies the stumbling block. The problem has been that the sensors, which must come in contact with body fluids, become ineffective because clotting blood attaches to the surface of the sensor. Work is being done to overcome this problem so that implantable devices (closed-loop pumps) can become a reality. Indeed, there are many being tried, and hope

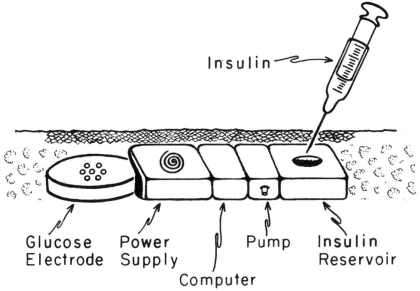

FIG. 18–3. A proposed model for an artificial miniature "beta cell," which would be implanted beneath the skin of the abdominal wall. The reservoir would be refilled with insulin by injection. (From Soeldner, J.S., et al.: Progress towards an implantable glucose sensor and an artificial beta cell. *In* Urquhart, J. and Yates, F.E.: Temporal Aspects of Therapeutics. New York, Plenum Publishing Corp., 1973.)

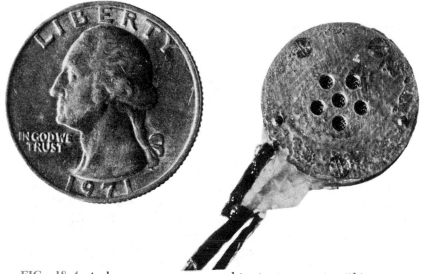

FIG. 18-4. A glucose sensor, compared in size to a quarter. This sensor could be implanted in subcutaneous tissue. (From Soeldner, J.S., et. al.: Progress towards an implantable glucose sensor and an artificial beta call. *In* Urguhart, J. and Yates, F.E.: Temporal Aspects of Therapeutics. New York, Plenum Publishing Corp., 1973.)

continues that these implantable pumps may be available in experimental trials soon.

Newer Insulins. Less dramatic than transplantation or artificial pancreases, perhaps, are efforts to devise newer insulins that are even more effective than those now available. The recent development of technology that allows the manufacture of synthetic "human" insulin represents a spectacular scientific achievement. This synthetic human insulin, already available, is a purer, less antigenic (less likely to stimulate allergic responses), and more predictable insulin than animal-based insulin. And it has an even more important benefit from a worldwide viewpoint. Many of the approximately 100 million people with diabetes in the known world do not have, cannot get, or cannot afford insulin. Before the development of synthetic insulins, everything depended on pancreases from pigs, cattle, sheep, etc. So insulin supplies in a given area depended in large part on what meats were eaten for food. Eventually, the new purer synthetic insulins might provide insulin for the world, and with large-scale mass production techniques, it is hoped that it will be at a price the underdeveloped world can afford.

Proinsulin is the natural precursor of insulin. The body manufactures proinsulin first, from which an extra piece, called C (for connecting) peptide is broken off, and the insulin is "ready for action." Synthetic proinsulin has been manufactured by methods similar to those used to manufacture human insulin. Initial attempts to use proinsulin itself, which acts similarly to NPH, as a diabetes treatment were put on hold pending further investigation. However, biosynthetic human insulin is currently made first as proinsulin, and then the C peptide is chemically removed, leaving the insulin molecule itself.

Efforts to develop nasal insulin have also been under way. Contrary to the impression given in some newspapers and magazines, this insulin would not replace injections, but would be given in addition to a reduced number of injections to improve overall control. Efforts to make an insulin that could be taken orally and not be destroyed in the gastrointestinal tract are also being made, but the availability of such a product is still a distant hope.

Treatment and Prevention of Complications. Since the discovery of insulin brought life to those with type I diabetes, the issue of diabetes complications has attracted much attention. Once it was realized that certain conditions were indeed associated with diabetes, the challenge focused on two major issues: (1) what it was about diabetes that caused these complications to occur and (2) how they could be prevented and/or treated. These two issues are still, today, fertile areas of research.

Diabetes Control and Complications Trial (DCCT). This study, supported by the National Institutes of Health, is trying to answer two questions regarding the control of diabetes and the development of complications: (1) using the technology that we have available today, is it possible and safe to achieve close to normal blood glucose patterns in most people with type I diabetes, and (2) Is achieving such near-normal glucose patterns likely to reduce the chances of developing certain diabetes complications?

Few physicians who specialize in diabetes treatment would disagree that good diabetes control is needed to reduce the likelihood of developing acute and longterm complications of diabetes. It is difficult, however, to determine what is meant by poor control. Everyone knows what normal blood sugar levels are, but where is the dividing line between "healthful" and "nonhealthful?" Standards of control have been published for normal or near normal blood glucose values, although achieving these standards is often impossible, especially in a person with true type I diabetes who has no insulin secretion. The term "tight control" has been used in some studies, implying that the blood glucose levels were "tightly held close to normal." What often happened, however, was that more insulin was given at the price of frequent, severe hypoglycemic reactions. In reality, the minute-by-minute movement of blood glucose levels did not at all resemble normal. Now, with the glycohemoglobin measurement and self monitoring of blood glucose (SMBG), it is possible to measure such control more accurately. Self monitoring can also be used to chart more precisely the daily glucose patterns, and with newer insulins and insulin delivery schemes (pumps, etc.), treatment can be tailored more accurately to the person's needs.

The DCCT is the largest and most extensive attempt to answer these important questions about controlling diabetes. It is a nationwide study that is comparing good, standard diabetes control with intensive control in a large group of young people (adolescents and young adults) with type I diabetes. The people taking part in the study are using intensive therapy as outlined in Chapter 10 hoping to keep their glucose patterns normal. This study is expected to run until about 1993.

Aldose Reductase Inhibitors. There is much research under way to determine the exact mechanism by which excessive blood glucose is involved in the development of the complications of diabetes. As discussed in Chapter 16, one possible mechanism for glucose's involvement is by its changing into sorbitol, a sugar alcohol. This action is stimulated by an enzyme called aldose reductase. This changing of glucose to sorbitol may be involved in the development of some forms of diabetic neuropathy, retinopathy, and kidney disease. As pointed out, a substance called an aldose reductase inhibitor blocks aldose reductase's actions. Several compounds of this type are under trial as a treatment in people with painful diabetic neuropathy. It is also being tried in a longterm study to see if it can reduce the chances of developing retinopathy. The actions and possible uses of other aldose reductase inhibitors are also being studied in the hopes that these will eventually be useful in blocking or treating some of the more devastating complications of diabetes.

Eye Research. Through the Early Treatment of Diabetic Retinopathy Study (discussed in Chapter 16), researchers are studying the effectiveness of argon laser photocoagulation therapy in treating certain types of eye disease in diabetes. They are also observing the effect of aspirin on eye diseases. Aspirin is said to reduce the aggregation of platelets (a form of blood clotting) in the blood vessels of the eye. Other research has advanced techniques of eye surgery and perfected procedures such as vitrectomy.

Kidney Research. There is a great deal of research under way on how diabetes causes damage to the kidneys, how to prevent this damage, and how to treat it once it occurs. The harmful effects that result from elevated blood glucose levels may be due to the binding of glucose to proteins.

Glycohemoglobin is an example of glucose binding to a protein—hemoglobin—in this fashion. The glomerular basement membrane (the inner lining of the kidney filtering tubes) may be another area where glucose binds to protein. This process may start the mechanism that leads to kidney damage. It is well known that high blood pressure (hypertension) also damages the kidneys, and when combined with diabetes, can lead to serious difficulties. Researchers are working to find ways to predict which people with diabetes are more likely to develop hypertension and thus be more susceptible to kidney disease as well. This knowledge would allow physicians to monitor these people more closely and treat developing problems earlier and more aggressively. For example, although it is known that albumin in the urine is an early sign of a failing kidney, newer techniques such as the measurement of microalbuminuria can detect the changes much earlier.

Researchers are also working to find ways to slow down the progression of kidney disease in people who have already developed it. Diets high in protein can also promote kidney damage, and experiments with low protein diets show some promise. Similarly, new medications are being tried. These dilate the blood vessels in the kidney, reducing the blood pressure in this organ and possibly preventing further damage. For those people whose kidneys have, indeed, failed, improvements are being seen in both dialysis and kidney transplantation, which, for a time at least, provide a cure. Research is also focusing on the causes for heart problems, which now rank first as the cause of death in those with diabetes.

Other Research. So much work is being done on diabetes and its causes that it is safe to say that in the last 10 years researchers have learned more than was found in the 20 or more years before that. Research into the relationship of insulin with other hormones is continuing in hopes of discovering interrelationships that may affect the way we metabolize sugar. Dramatic progress in molecular and cell biology are bringing us closer to the day when we can truly replace the lost insulin-producing beta cells. Recent research aims at making non-beta cell tissues produce insulin by means of genetic instruction. Science is moving very fast indeed, and diabetes research is a fertile field of effort!

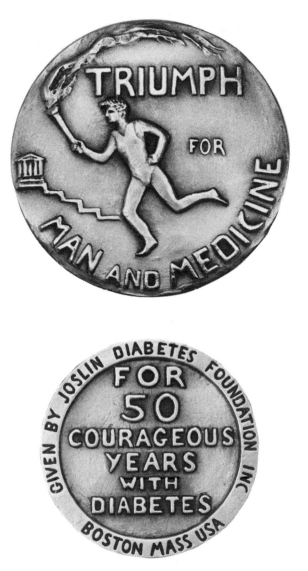

FIG. 18–5. The Fifty Year Duration of Diabetes medal. This medal is given to reward the courage and endurance of people who have lived 50 years or longer since the onset of their diabetes.

"Lest We Forget"

It has been a long trip from the starvation treatments of the early 1900s to the open-loop pumps, laser treatments of the eyes, harvesting crops of beta cells, and the other wonders we have become quite used to. However, there is a more practical measure of success and what it means to those with diabetes.

About 25 years ago in the New England Deaconess Hospital, several floors in the old Deaconess Building were reserved for patients with severe foot problems, many of whom later had amputations. Of course, there still is occasional need for surgery of this type, but much, much less often than previously. Today more preventive and reparative surgery can be done with vessel transplants and other means of *saving* feet. Patients with retinal hemorrhage 25 years ago were given little hope except the advice, "take the best possible care of your diabetes." Now, the miracle of the lasers is here. The problems of pregnancy in diabetic mothers was enormous, but better diabetes and obstetrical care has reduced the morbidity and mortality among the infants of women with diabetes to almost (but not quite) the same as those without diabetes. The rate of admission for treatment of "diabetic coma" has almost disappeared.

One of the most dramatic changes is that at that time, when a person had lived with diabetes for 20 years, he was greeted as if he were a distinguished visitor from abroad. In fact, medals were given for 25 years without complications. Dr. Elliott P. Joslin would introduce the person to the clinic physicians in order for them to hear how the patient did it. Now, almost any day in the clinic, it is common to see patients with 25, 35, 40, or 50+ years of diabetes (Fig. 18–5). Most of them are in remarkably good physical and mental condition. And consider that if such a person who has had diabetes for 50 years took insulin once daily for the first 25 years and twice daily for the second 25 years, this adds up to almost 30,000 injections! The interesting part of the story is that no one pays any exceptional attention to them beyond routine needed medical care. That is the price of success. The miracle has become commonplace. Isn't that the goal of medicine?

19

What To Do Until You Can Reach Your Physician

Accidents happen to everyone. With or without diabetes, there are worrisome emergencies or problems that come up. However, fears are compounded and emergencies seem much worse to people with diabetes or those close to them. Questions might nag in their minds. Few of these issues are serious, but those inexperienced with diabetes such as relatives or friends sometimes panic needlessly. When in doubt, call your physician. However, if you cannot reach medical assistance, there are things you can do which may solve the problem.

1. *How should I treat diabetes during acute illness?*

People with diabetes, like everyone else, sometimes have illnesses that are not necessarily related to their diabetes. These are quite common and are not terribly serious—usually a cold or "flu" or a stomach upset—but they make diabetes more difficult to treat. Those people who treat their diabetes with diet alone, or with oral hypoglycemic tablets, or even those using simple insulin programs may not experience much change in their diabetes control during such an illness. However, people with less stable diabetes (type I) may have difficulty with the control of their diabetes. Indeed, *anyone* with diabetes can have problems with diabetes control which could become dangerous if not well treated. At such a time, many people need *more* insulin, not less, even though the appetite may be poor. Insulin is often less effective during an illness, in much the same way that inflation weakens money's value. The blood or urine tests must be checked more frequently, and often extra doses of insulin are needed. At these times, urine specimens must be tested for acetone as well as for glucose. If acetone is present in any amount during an acute illness, contact a physician. Tables 15–3 through 15-5 outline sick day guidelines.

2. *How should you treat a person with diabetes who becomes unconscious?*

This depends somewhat on whether the unconsciousness was sudden (if related to diabetes it is most likely the result of low blood glucose reaction) or gradual over a period of time (possible acidosis on some other medical problem) as there are various reasons for someone to lose consciousness. Older people may be subject to "strokes" or other cerebrovascular disorders (because of changes in the circulation to the brain). However, if the onset is sudden in people treated with insulin or oral hypoglycemic tablets, the cause is likely to be hypoglycemia. (Table 15–6 outlines characteristics of hypoglycemic reactions.) While waiting for medical help or an ambulance, it is safe to inject glucagon because other problems not involving low blood glucose levels will not be affected by this. A discussion of the use of glucagon can be found on page 255. Do *not* try to force liquids or nourishment into a person incapable of swallowing. These may go into the respiratory tract and cause worse difficulties.

Nevertheless, for anyone who becomes unconscious, either slowly or rapidly, and especially if they have not responded to glucagon, immediate, emergency medical help should be sought.

3. *What can you do for convulsions?*

Most seizures are self-limited, meaning they will often stop on their own. If these are due to low blood glucose levels, the individual usually responds rapidly to intravenous glucose or some-times to glucagon injected beneath the skin, as insulin is given. When the victim can drink, sweet liquids such as orange juice or sugar-containing drinks should be given.

In the event of a true epileptic seizure, objects near the victim should be moved to prevent injury. Often these episodes pass quite rapidly. Once the seizure is over, the person should be turned on one side until consciousness is regained. This prevents aspiration of any vomited substances into the lungs. Even if a seizure passes and the person returns to normal, it is important to discuss the event with the person's physician to confirm the cause and to prevent future seizures.

4. *I have been sick with the "virus" and can't keep anything down. Since I am not eating, should I eliminate my insulin?*

NO! ABSOLUTELY NOT! Insulin should be taken and the blood or urine checked very carefully for glucose and acetone levels.

Generally, these acute episodes of nausea and vomiting do not last very long; if not much is taken by mouth, the nausea often improves rapidly. When the acute nausea disappears, it is safe to start taking small sips of bouillon, soup, or even regular ginger ale. Do not take more than a tablespoonful at a time until you are certain that the liquid can be kept down. Dry mouth and throat can be helped by sucking cracked ice, which melts and is swallowed gradually. If the blood or urinary levels of sugar are significantly increased, and especially if acetone is present in the urine, contact your physician. You should also contact your physician if you cannot hold down food or liquid for more than a few hours. A common error is to try to drink too much at once. A glass of orange juice can be very nauseating at a time like this. Ginger ale at room temperature taken a mouthful at a time, is better tolerated.

5. *Suppose I find acetone in my urine?*

Urinary acetone is sometimes found in small amounts. For example, it can appear in children without diabetes on hot days when they are playing hard because they do not have enough available carbohydrate and they break down fats. It also occurs during illness or fever and may represent a potentially serious problem if it is accompanied by a significantly elevated blood or urine glucose level. In such a case, it may be a prelude to acidosis and should be treated with extra insulin.

If your physician or nurse has not given careful instructions about how to treat the finding of acetone in the urine, its presence along with elevated blood glucose, should be treated using sick day guidelines to get you started until you reach your health care team. You should be sure to discuss insulin adjustment plans with your medical team as soon as they can be reached, however.

It is important to remember that the presence of acetone does not always signal problems. Acetone is sometimes found in the urine when someone is on a weight loss diet, resulting from the metabolism of fat. At this time, the blood glucose level is usually normal. Acetone may also be seen after a hypoglycemic reaction and resultant rebound. The reasons for the reaction need to be examined, rather than just giving more insulin to chase the rebound.

6. *Suppose I find a lot of sugar in my urine?*

Finding lots of sugar in the urine is not unusual with diabetes. It usually means poor regulation of the diabetes at this time—perhaps from too much food, not enough exercise, or possibly from an infection. At any rate, at least at this time, there is not enough insulin or insulin action. If there is no significant acetone present in the urine (i.e., trace or none), a bit of extra regular insulin might be useful (see the insulin adjustment guidelines in Chapter 9). If this happens often, you should check with your physician to make needed changes in your treatment. People not using insulin who find a lot of sugar in the urine should be extra careful in following their diet and should contact their physician if the tests do not improve.

7. *Suppose I get a sudden blurring of my vision?*

In the absence of any trauma or damage to the eye, the commonest reason for temporary blurred vision (presbyopia) is a rapid change in the blood glucose level—often a level that is low. Table 15–6 will help you differentiate between high and low blood glucose levels, but home blood glucose testing can answer the question rapidly. If the level is low, drink something sweet as soon as possible (*not* a diet drink). People being treated vigorously with insulin and who were previously uncontrolled may have periods of blurred vision. These are usually temporary and intermittent. They can be annoying and sometimes may last for several weeks. (See Chapter 15 (for a discussion of presbyopia.)

A marked loss of vision in a person known to have eye hemorrhages is another problem. In this case, the best immediate treament is to remain as quiet as possible and consult your eye physician (ophthalmologist) as soon as possible.

8. *I awakened this morning with a wedge-shaped red spot in the white of my eye. What is this?*

This usually is not related to diabetes and can happen to anyone. It is most often a subconjunctival hemorrhage due to irritation from rubbing the eye or some other such cause. If not aggravated further, this tends to fade in several days.

9. *How should cuts and bruises be treated in a person with diabetes?*

The same as they would be treated in a person without diabetes! In the case of bleeding, use pressure to stop the bleeding. Wash the area carefully with soap and water and apply a mild antiseptic such as ST-37. If the bleeding is severe or difficult to stop, medical attention is necessary. Infection in people who have well-controlled diabetes and good circulation is not a greater risk than in anyone else.

10. *I have a painless black toenail.*

If the dark area is limited to the toenail itself and there are no signs of redness or infection around the nail, it is usually due to hemorrhage beneath the nail caused by bruising the toe. Such an area usually fades and disappears, although it may take a few days to a few months for this to happen. If the foot is painful, inflamed, or discolored near or around the nail, consult a physician.

11. *What should a person with diabetes do after exposure to poison ivy, poison oak, or poison sumac?*

Which one you have been exposed to depends somewhat on the area in which you live. Poison ivy is commonest on the East Coast, and poison oak is commonest on the West Coast. In any case, the treatment is the same, and is the same as for anyone else. Wash the affected areas with large amounts of soap and water as soon as possible. In case of severe rash or eruption, see a physician.

12. *How should a sudden insulin reaction be treated?*

Ordinarily, low blood glucose reactions are not a severe problem and are often more frightening and annoying than dangerous. However, too much insulin, too much activity, or not enough food intake can cause the blood glucose level to drop too low or too rapidly. At that point, symptoms may become severe enough that confusion, disorientation, or even unconsciousness develop. (This problem is discussed in detail in Chapter 15.) Certain steps should be taken at once. Insulin reactions are nearly always preventable and when recognized should be treated immediately. If a person is able to swallow, give the nearest available sweet drink. Liquid is easier to swallow and is preferable to food. It is also absorbed more quickly. Do not waste time looking for a particular drink such as orange juice, Coca-Cola, or ginger ale; use any sweetened liquid. Do not use diet (calorie-free) drinks. Table 15–1 lists the things that are useful to treat low blood glucose reactions. If the person cannot swallow or does not respond, inject glucagon from a 1-cc vial and repeat with a second 1-cc vial shortly afterwards. If the person still does not respond, take him or her to the *nearest* hospital emergency room for intravenous glucose. Insulin reactions that are short in duration or minor are not harmful, but they should not be permitted to become prolonged without treatment.

13. *While traveling, I arrived in a distant city and discovered that I had left my insulin syringes and needles at home. What should I do?*

This is not an uncommon problem. In earlier times a similar problem occurred when glass syringes were used and were dropped and broken. First, always carry a diabetes identification card with you. Seek out the nearest hospital emergency room and tell your story. While some pharmacies might accommodate you, they are less likely to because they are vulnerable to people seeking syringes for other purposes. Many emergency rooms will provide you with an insulin dose. A better solution is to have your physician's or clinic's phone number with you and offer to pay for the phone call. This may help solve the problem! Many places have diabetes societies that might be helpful. Best of all . . . don't forget this vital equipment!

14. *I took too much insulin by mistake. What should I do?*

If you took just a little extra insulin in error, no severe problem should develop as long as you eat well and watch for symptoms suggestive of hypoglycemia. Sometimes people misread the insulin syringe and take twice as much insulin or a lot more than they should, or accidently take the larger morning dose at night. Don't panic! Simply take more carbohydrate or larger meals that day, supplementing these with orange juice or regular ginger ale and crackers between meals. In emergencies like this, ice cream, which has carbohydrate, protein, and some fat, may be a good choice. Self blood glucose testing can help you keep track of the blood glucose levels and can warn you if they are sinking too low. Even those who do not use self blood glucose testing regularly should know how to do so for emergencies of this kind. It is better to eat and drink a little too much rather than too little at times like this. If too much nourishment has been taken, the increased blood and urine glucose is temporary. Supplemental insulin can always be used later if needed. Small amounts of oral carbohydrate taken frequently are better than a single large meal. Frequently, setting the alarm clock and getting up during the night is useful.

15. *I took too many oral hypoglycemic pills by mistake. What should I do?*

Proceed the same as for insulin reaction, except that the action of the oral hypoglycemic agents is usually slower and does not lower blood glucose so deeply. However, some tablets may last longer, so increased nourishment may have to be taken for a longer period.

16. *What should I do if the needle comes off of the syringe, or for some other reason I lose some of my insulin and don't know how much insulin I have taken?*

Try to estimate how much insulin remains in the syringe and how much might have been taken. If you are reasonably certain about how much might have been lost, this can be replaced. If there is no way to determine how much has been lost, it is safest to check the blood glucose level (or urine sugar) before lunch, before supper, and at bedtime and add further insulin, usually regular, as needed.

17. *I don't remember whether I took my insulin.*

If doubt really exists about whether insulin was taken, carefully test the blood glucose levels or urine sugar at intervals of several hours throughout the day. You may need to take small amounts of regular, fast-acting insulin if the glucose level begins to rise. If the glucose level does rise and you need additional insulin, consult your physician for assistance.

18. *Many of the children in the school my child attends have colds and the flu. What can I do to prevent my child from getting it?*

At this point, there is very little you can do because your child has most likely been exposed to it already. It is very hard to prevent such exposure. The fact is that with sufficient rest, nourishment, and careful control of the diabetes using sick day rules, most of these infections are not serious. Most children get through these episodes without difficulty.

19. *How can I prevent insulin reactions during heavy exercise? I play tennis and frequently jog long distances?*

The first thing to do is to try to perform these exercises regularly or at about the same time each day. Then it is a matter of adjusting diet so that you take extra nourishment before the fact or can arrange your insulin appropriately. Several well-known professional tennis players with diabetes sip orange juice, ginger ale, or Gatorade while changing courts in the course of a match.

20. *If I cut my finger or step on a nail, will I heal?*

Just about everyone heals. Youngsters do quite effectively because they have adequate blood supply. Older people with diabetes who have decreased circulation in the feet might need more careful management. At any rate, treatment is the same as in question 9. But unless the diabetes is completely out of control, most people with diabetes heal quite well. In case of a puncture wound (e.g., stepping on a nail), the problem is a bit more serious because you have no idea what bacteria were residing on that nail. In that case, check with your physician because a booster injection for tetanus prevention may be needed.

In Summary. No matter what happens, do not panic! Look at the appropriate part of this manual. Do one step at a time and, if in doubt, call your physician, teaching nurse, clinic, or emergency room without delay.

Appendices

Appendix 1. Food Choice Lists 368

           Milk List   368
           Vegetable List   369
           Fruit List   371
           Bread (Starch) List 373
           Meat List   380
           Fat List   383
           Miscellaneous List 385

Appendix 2. Cholesterol and Saturated Fat Content of
           Some Foods 389

Appendix 3. Oral Hypoglycemic Agents Available
           Around the World by Generic and Trade
           Names 390

Appendix 4. Automatic Insulin Injectors 393

Appendix 5. Insulin Pumps 394

Appendix 6. White Classification of Diabetes in
           Pregnant Women 395

Appendix 7. Resources for the Elderly 396

APPENDIX 1. FOOD CHOICE LISTS

These food choice lists are to be used in conjunction with a diabetes meal plan that should be developed by a dietitian.

Milk List
(Includes non-fat [skim], low-fat and whole milk)

Milk is the main source of calcium for our bodies. Calcium is needed to build strong bones and teeth. Milk is also a good source of phosphorus, protein, some of the B-complex vitamins including folacin and vitamin B12, and vitamins A and D. Contrary to popular belief, milk is needed by our bodies throughout our lives.

Each of the milk items listed below, in the portion size indicated, is considered one (1) milk choice. Whenever possible it is best to use non-fat (skim) milk since it does not contain the saturated fat and cholesterol present in both 2% low-fat and whole milk. 1% low-fat milk is the next best choice.

Item	Portion
Non Fat Selections	
One Choice Provides:	
12 grams carbohydrate;	Non-fat (skim milk)	1 cup
8 grams protein;	Low-fat milk (½%)	1 cup
0 grams fat;	Powdered, non-fat (before adding liquid)	⅓ cup
80 calories.	Reconstituted powdered milk	1 cup
	Canned, evaporated skim milk	½ cup
	Buttermilk made from skim milk	1 cup
	*Sugar-free hot cocoa mix plus 6 ounces of water	1 cup

*Most cocoa mixes do not provide the same amount of calcium as one cup of milk. Mixes which do provide the same amount should indicate on the label that the product contains 30% U.S.R.D.A. for calcium. An example of a product which meets these calcium requirements is Alba™ sugar-free, hot cocoa mix.

Item	Portion
Low Fat Selections	
One Choice Provides:	
12 grams carbohydrate;	Low-fat milk (1%)	1 cup
	Yogurt, plain, unflavored, made from skim milk	1 cup

8 grams protein;
3 grams fat;
107 calories.

Medium and High Fat Selections

The following milk items should be used sparingly due to the high saturated fat and cholesterol content.

Low-fat milk (2%)	1 cup

One Choice Provides:
12 grams carbohydrate;
8 grams protein;
5 grams fat;
125 calories.

Whole milk	1 cup
Canned, evaporated whole milk	½ cup
Buttermilk made from whole milk	1 cup
Yogurt, plain, unflavored, made from whole milk	1 cup

One Choice Provides:
12 grams carbohydrate;
8 grams protein;
8 grams fat;
150 calories.

Vegetable List

(Includes fresh, frozen and canned vegetables)

Dark green and deep yellow vegetables are among the main sources of Vitamin A. Many vegetables such as asparagus, broccoli, brussels sprouts, cabbage, spinach and tomatoes are good sources of Vitamin C. Vegetables also provide potassium, folacin and fiber. Vegetables retain most of their vitamins and fiber when eaten raw, steamed or "lightly cooked" with a minimum of water.

Each of the vegetable items listed below, in the portion size indicated, is considered one vegetable choice. Unless otherwise indicated, the portion sizes are for both fresh and cooked vegetables.

One Choice Provides:
5 grams carbohydrate;
2 grams protein;
28 calories

Item	Portion	Item	Portion
Artichoke	½	Beet greens	1 cup
Asparagus	1 cup	Broccoli	½ cup
Bamboo shoots	½ cup	Brussels sprouts	½ cup
Bean sprouts	½ cup	Cabbage	1 cup
Beets	½ cup	Carrots	½ cup

Vegetable List (cont.)

Item	Portion	Item	Portion
Cauliflower	1 cup	*Tomato sauce, canned	⅓ cup
Celery	1 cup	Turnips	½ cup
Collard greens	1 cup	Vegetables, mixed	¼ cup
Eggplant	½ cup	*V-8 juice	½ cup
Fennel leaf	1 cup	Wax beans	1 cup
Green beans	1 cup	Water chestnuts	5 whole
Green pepper	1 cup		
Kale	½ cup		
Kohlrabi	½ cup		
Leeks	½ cup		
Mushrooms, fresh	1 cup		
Mustard greens, cooked	1 cup		
Okra	½ cup		
Onions	½ cup		
Pea pods, Chinese (snow peas)	½ cup		
Radishes	1 cup		
Red pepper	1 cup		
Rutabagas	½ cup		
Sauerkraut	½ cup		
Spinach, cooked	½ cup		
Squash			
summer	1 cup		
zucchini	1 cup		
Swiss chard	1 cup		
Tomato (ripe)	1 medium		
*Tomato juice	½ cup		
Tomato paste	1½ tablespoons		

Because of their low carbohydrate and calorie content, the following RAW vegetables may be used liberally.

Alfalfa sprouts		Parsley	
Chicory		*Pickles,	
Chinese cabbage		unsweetened	
Cucumber		Pimento	
Endive		Spinach	
Escarole		Watercress	
Lettuce			

*These vegetables are high in sodium (salt). Low sodium vegetable juices and sauces should be purchased if you are following a sodium restricted diet. Fresh and frozen vegetables are lower in sodium than canned vegetables, unless the canned product specifically states "low sodium."

Fruit List

(Includes fresh fruit, pure fruit juices, and canned, dried, cooked or frozen fruit without additional sugar)

Fresh fruit is a good source of Vitamins A and C as well as fiber. Fresh fruit contains more fiber than fruit juice. Fiber alters the absorption of food by your body and may cause less elevation of your blood glucose. Each of the fruit selections listed below, in the portion size indicated, is considered one fruit choice. USE ONLY CANNED FRUIT WHICH IS PACKED IN WATER OR IN ITS OWN JUICE. Use frozen fruit packed without additional sugar.

One Choice Provides:
15 grams carbohydrate;
60 calories

Item	Portion
Apple, 2 inch diameter	1 small
Apple, dried	¼ cup
Apricots:	
fresh	4 medium
*canned	4 halves
dried	7 medium halves
Banana, 9 inch length, peeled	½
Banana flakes or chips	3 tablespoons
Blackberries	¾ cup
Blueberries	¾ cup
Boysenberries	1 cup
Cantaloupe, 5 inch diameter	
sectioned	⅓ melon
cubed	1 cup
Casaba, 7 inch diameter	
sectioned	⅙ melon
cubed	1⅓ cup
Cherries, sweet	
fresh	12
*canned	½ cup
Cherries, sour, fresh	⅔ cup
Dates	3
Figs	2 small
*Fruit cocktal, canned	½ cup

Fruit List (cont.)

Item	Portion
Granadilla (passion fruit)	4
Grapefruit, 4 inch diameter	½
Grapes	15 small
Guava	1½ small
Honeydew melon, 6½ inch diameter	
sectioned	⅛ melon
cubed	1 cup
Kiwi (3 ounces)	1 large
Kumquat	5 medium
Lemon	1 large
Loquats, fresh	12
Lychees, fresh or dried	10
Mango	½ small
sliced	½ cup
Nectarine, 2½ inch diameter	1
Orange, 3 inch diameter	1
Papaya, 3½ inch diameter	
sectioned	½
cubed	1 cup
Peach, 2½ inch diameter	
fresh	1
*canned	½ cup
Pear	
fresh	½ large or 1 small
*canned	½ cup
Persimmon	
native	2
Japanese, 2½ inch diameter	½
Pineapple	
fresh, diced	¾ cup
*canned	⅓ cup
Plantain, cooked	⅓ cup

Plum, 2 inch diameter 2
Pomegranate, 3½ inch diameter .... ½
Prunes, dried, medium 3
Raisins .... 2 tablespoons
Raspberries .... 1 cup
Rhubarb, fresh, diced .... 3 cups
Strawberries .... 1⅓ cup
Tangerine, 2½ inch diameter 2
Watermelon, diced .... 1¼ cup

*Canned fruit should be drained of liquid when measuring portion size.

Fruit Juice

Fruit juice may elevate blood glucose rapidly, especially when consumed on an empty stomach or with a small amount of food such as a snack. Limit your intake of juice to no more than one meal each day or to times when you are engaging in vigorous activity or treating a low blood sugar.

Apple juice, unsweetened .... 4 ounces
Cranapple, low-calorie .... 12 ounces
Cranberry, low-calorie .... 10 ounces
Grape juice, unsweetened .... 3 ounces
Grapefruit juice, unsweetened .... 5 ounces
Lemon juice, unsweetened .... 6 ounces
Orange juice, unsweetened .... 4 ounces
Pineapple juice, unsweetened .... 4 ounces
Prune juice, unsweetened .... 3 ounces

Bread (Starch) List

(Includes bread, crackers, cereal, pasta, starchy vegetables and other selected items.)

Whole grain and enriched bread and cereals as well as dried beans and peas are good sources of iron, thiamine and fiber. Whole grain products have more fiber than products made from refined flours. Each of the following food items, in the portion size indicated, is considered one bread choice.

Bread (Starch) List (cont.)

One Choice Provides:
15 grams carbohydrate;
3 grams protein;
Trace of fat;
80 calories.

	Item	Portion
Breads (In general, one bread choice equals 1 ounce of bread)	White, whole wheat, rye, et cetera	1 slice
	Raisin	1 slice
	Italian and French	1 slice
	Reduced calorie (1 slice equals 40 calories)	2 slices
	Syrian	
	pocket, 6 inch diameter	½ pocket
	diet size	1 pocket
	Bagel	½ medium
	English muffin	½ medium
	Rolls	
	bulkie	½ small
	dinner, plain	1 small
	frankfurter	½ medium
	hamburger	½ medium
	tortilla, 6 inch diameter	1
Cereals To determine the appropriateness of other cereals, read the side panel on the container. If the number listed next to grams of sucrose is 5 or less, it is an acceptable choice. Contact your dietitian if you have	Cooked	½ cup
	Grits, cooked	½ cup
	Bran	
	*All Bran with Extra Fiber™	1 cup
	*All Bran™	⅓ cup
	*100% Bran™	⅔ cup
	*40% Bran Flakes™	½ cup
	*Bran Chex™	½ cup
	*Fiber One™	⅔ cup

additional questions regarding portion sizes of cereals not listed.

Buck Wheats™	½ cup
Cabbage Patch™	¾ cup
Cheerios™	1 cup
Corn, Rice Chex™	⅔ cup
Cornflakes™	¾ cup
Crispix™	½ cup
Fortified Oat Flakes™	½ cup
Granola	¼ cup
Grapenuts™	3 tablespoons
*Grapenut Flakes™	⅔ cup
Halfsies™	½ cup
Kix™	1 cup
Nutrigrain,™ corn	½ cup
Nutrigrain,™ barley	½ cup
Nutrigrain,™ rye	½ cup
Nutrigrain,™ wheat	½ cup
Product 19™	½ cup
Puffed Rice, Wheat	1½ cup
Rice Krispies™	¾ cup
*Shredded Wheat™ biscuit	1
spoon size	½ cup
*Shredded Wheat n' Bran™	½ cup
Special K™	¾ cup
Sunflakes™	⅔ cup
Team™	⅔ cup
Toasties Cornflakes™	¾ cup
Total™	¾ cup
*Wheat Chex™	½ cup
*Wheaties™	⅔ cup
Other cold cereals	⅔ cup

Cereals high in fiber

Bread (Starch) List (cont.)

	Item	Portion
Starchy Vegetables	Corn	½ cup
	Corn on the Cob, 5 x 1¾ inch length	1
	Lima Beans	½ cup
	Parsnips	½ cup
	Peas, green, canned or frozen	⅔ cup
	Plantain, cooked	⅓ cup
	Potato, white	
	mashed	½ cup
	baked	½ medium or 1 small (3 ounces)
	Sweet potato	
	mashed	⅓ cup
	baked	½ medium (2 ounces)
	Pumpkin	¾ cup
	Winter squash, acorn or butternut	¾ cup
Pasta (cooked)	Macaroni	½ cup
	Noodles	½ cup
	Spaghetti	½ cup
Dried Beans, Peas, and Lentils	Beans, peas, lentils (dried and cooked)	⅓ cup
	Baked beans, canned, no pork (vegetarian style)	⅓ cup
Prepared Foods	Biscuit, 2 inch diameter (1 ounce)	1 = 1 bread + 1 fat
	Cornbread, 2 x 2 x 1 inches	1 = 1 bread + 1 fat
	Croissant, 4 x 4 x 1¾ inches	1 = 2 bread + 2 fats
	Muffin, bran or corn, 2 inch diameter, 1½ ounces	1 = 1½ bread + 1 fat

Pancake, 4 inch diameter	2 = 1 bread + 1 fat
Taco shells	2 = 1 bread + 1 fat
Tortilla	
corn, 6 inch diameter	2 = 1 bread + 1 fat
flour, 7 inch diameter	1 = 1 bread + 1 fat
Waffle, 4 inch diameter	1 = 1 bread + 1 fat

Other

Barley, cooked	¼ cup
Bread crumbs	3 tablespoons
Bulgar, cooked	⅓ cup
Cornmeal	2½ tablespoons
Cornstarch	2 tablespoons
Flour	3 tablespoons
Kasha, cooked	⅓ cup
Potato or macaroni salad	½ cup = 1 bread + 2 fats
Rice, cooked	⅓ cup
Wheat germ	¼ cup = 1 bread + 1 lean meat

Occasional Choices

Due to the high saturated fat content of the following foods, they should be used only occasionally, i.e., not more than two times per week. Be sure to count the fat exchanges in your meal plan.

Ice cream	½ cup = 1 bread + 2 fats
Popcorn, microwave	4 cups = 1 bread + 2 fats
Popcorn, popped in oil	3 cups = 1 bread + 2 fats
Potatoes, french fries, 2 to 3½ inch length	10 = 1 bread + 2 fats
Potato or corn chips	15 = 1 bread + 2 fats
Stuffing mix, cooked	⅓ cup = 1 bread + 2 fats

Bread (Starch) List (cont.)

Item	Portion
Crackers Equal to One	
Bread Choice	
Animal Crackers	8
Crokine™ puffed crispbread	4 slices
Finn Crisp™	4
Gingersnaps	3
Graham crackers, 2½ inch squares	3
Matzoh	1 board (¾ ounce)
Manischewitz™ wholewheat matzoh crackers	7
Melba toast rectangles	5
Melba toast rounds	10
Norwegian flatbread such as Kavli™	
thin	3
thick	2
Popcorn, popped, no fat added	3 cups
Pretzel sticks	¾ ounce
Pretzel, Dutch type 2¾ x 2⅝ inches	1
Rice cakes	2
Rye Krisp,™ three triple crackers	3
Saltines	6
Sesame Ak-Mak	¾ ounce
Social Teas™	4
Soda crackers	7
Stella D'Oro Almond Toast™	1½
Stella D'Oro Egg Biscuit™	2
Stoned Wheat Thins™	2½
Uneedas™	4
Wasa Lite or Golden Rye Crisp Bread™	2
Zweiback™	3

Item	Portion
Crackers Equal to One Bread Plus One Fat Choice	Due to the fat content of the crackers listed below, they should be considered one bread choice plus one fat choice.*
Arrowroot™	4
Bordeaux Cookies,™ Pepperidge Farm	3
Butter crackers	
rounds	7
rectangular	6
Cheez-its™	27
Cheese Nips™	20
Club or Townhouse Crackers™	6
Combos™	1 ounce
Escort Crackers™	5
Goldfish,™ Pepperidge Farm	36
Granola bar, plain, raisin or peanut butter	1
Lorna Doones™	3
Meal Mates™	5
Oyster crackers	24
Peanut Butter Sandwich Crackers	3
Ritz™	7
Sea Rounds™	2
Sociables™	9
Stella D'Oro Sesame Breadsticks™	2
Stella D'Oro Breakfast Treats™	1
Stella D'Oro Golden Bar™	1
Stella D'Oro Lady Stella Assortment™	3
Sunshine Hi Ho's™	6
Tidbits™	21
Triscuits™	5
Vanilla Wafers™	6
Wasa Fiber Plus Crisp Bread™	4
Wasa Sesame™ or Breakfast Crisp Bread™	2
Waverly Wafers™	6
Wheat Thins™	12

*If your meal plan does not provide a snack fat choice, borrow one from another snack or meal.

Meat List

(Includes meat, fish, poultry, eggs, cheese and meat substitutes.)

All of the items listed in the meat list are good sources of protein. Many are also good sources of iron, zinc, vitamin B-12 and other B vitamins.

Cholesterol is a wax-like substance found in animal fats, dairy fats and egg yolks. Saturated fat comes from animal products and saturated vegetable oils. (See fat list for additional information about the differences between various kinds of fat.) Leaner selections of meat are recommended in order to minimize the intake of cholesterol and saturated fats. Trim off all visible fat before cooking. Bake or broil selections instead of frying. Weigh your portion after cooking. A three ounce serving of cooked meat is about equal to four ounces of raw meat.

Item	Portion
Low Fat Selections:	
One Choice Provides:	
7 grams protein;	
3 grams fat;	
55 calories.	
Cheese:	
Cottage, pot, 1% fat	¼ cup
*Lite-Line Cheese,™ * Nuform Cheese,™ Weight Watcher's cheese™	1 ounce
***Cooked dried beans	1 cup = 1 meat + 2 bread
Egg substitutes with less than 55 calories per ¼ cup	½ cup
Egg whites	3
Fish and seafood:	
Fresh or frozen	1 ounce
Canned	
Water packed salmon, tuna, crab, lobster	¼ cup
Imitation crab	1 ounce
Herring, uncreamed or *smoked	1 ounce
Water packed clams, oysters, scallops, shrimp	1 ounce
Sardines, drained	3
*Luncheon meat, 95% fat free	1 ounce

Item	Portion
Poultry: chicken, turkey or cornish hen, without skin	1 ounce
*Canadian bacon	1 ounce
Tofu	3 ounces

Medium Fat Selections
One Choice Provides:
7 grams protein;
5 grams fat;
75 calories.

Item	Portion
Veal, except for breast	1 ounce
Pork, except for deviled ham, ground pork and spare ribs	1 ounce
Beef, chipped, chuck, flank steak, hamburger with 15% fat, rib eye, rump sirloin, tenderloin top and bottom round	1 ounce
Lamb, except for breast	1 ounce
Cheese:	
Skim or part-skim milk cheese such as *Laughing Cow™ reduced calorie skim milk cheese, part-skim mozzarella, part skim ricotta, farmer, Neufchatel, diet cheeses with 50-80 calories per ounce	1 ounce
*Parmesan, *Romano	3 tablespoons
**Egg	1
Egg substitutes with 56-80 calories per ¼ cup	¼ cup
*Luncheon meat, 86% fat free	1 ounce
Peanut butter	1 tablespoon = 1 meat + 1 fat

High Fat Selections

Due to the high saturated fat and cholesterol content, the meat choices listed below should be used sparingly.

One Choice Provides:
7 grams protein;
8 grams fat;
100 calories.

Item	Portion
Beef: brisket, club and rib steaks, corned beef, regular hamburger with 20% fat, rib roast, short ribs	1 ounce

Meat List (cont.)

Item	Portion
Lamb: breast	1 ounce
Pork: deviled ham, ground pork,	1 ounce
spare ribs, sausage (patty or link)	
Veal: breast	1 ounce
Poultry: capon, duck, goose	1 ounce
Regular Cheese: *blue, brie, cheddar, colby,	1 ounce
*feta, Monterey Jack, muenster,	
provolone, Swiss, *pasteurized process	
*Luncheon meats: bologna, bratwurst,	1 ounce
braunschweiger, knockwurst, liverwurst,	
pastrami, Polish sausage, salami	
Organ meats: liver, heart, kidney	1 ounce
Fried fish	1 ounce

*These products are high in sodium.

**The American Heart Association recommends limiting your egg consumption to two per week.

***For additional information, ask your dietitian.

Item	Portion
High Fat Plus	
One Fat Selection	
Frankfurter (beef, pork or combination)	1 frankfurter (10 per pound)

Nuts and Seeds

The following nuts and seeds may be used as meat substitutes in the portion sizes listed. Remember to count the extra fat choices.

Almonds, dry roasted	1 ounce = ½ meat, 2 fat
Mixed nuts, dry roasted	1 ounce = ½ meat, 2 fat
with peanuts	
Peanut kernels	1 ounce = 1 meat, 2 fat
Pine nuts, Pignoli, dried	1 ounce = 1 meat, 2 fat
Walnuts, black, dried	1 ounce = 1 meat, 2 fat
Pumpkin and squash seed kernels, roasted	1 ounce = 1 meat, 1 fat

Meat List (cont.)		
Item		**Portion**
Sesame seed kernels, dried		1 ounce = 1 meat, 2 fat
Sunflower seed kernels, dry roasted		1 ounce = ½ meat, 2 fat

Fat List

(Includes butter, margarine, cream, mayonnaise, nuts, salad dressings, vegetable oils and other selected items)

One Choice Provides:
5 grams of fat;
45 calories

Fats are of both animal and vegetable origin and include both oils and solid fats. Oils are fats that remain in liquid form at room temperature and are usually of vegetable origin. Fats are divided into three groups: polyunsaturated, monounsaturated and saturated. These terms refer to the kinds of fatty acids found in various fats. Polyunsaturated fats tend to lower the level of cholesterol in the blood. Corn, cottonseed, safflower, soy and sunflower oils are polyunsaturated fats. Olive and peanut oil are monounsaturated fats. Recent research suggests these oils may lower cholesterol levels. Saturated fats increase the level of cholesterol in the blood. Palm and coconut oils are saturated fats. They, along with the other items listed below under the heading "More Saturated," should be used sparingly.

Item	**Portion**
More Polyunsaturated	
Avocado, 4 inch diameter	⅛
D-Zerta™ whipped topping	5 tablespoons
Margarine, soft, tub or *stick	1 teaspoon
**Mayonnaise	1 teaspoon
Nuts	
Almonds	6 whole
Brazil	2 medium
Cashews	1 tablespoon
Filberts (hazelnuts)	5
Macadamia	3 whole
Peanuts	
Spanish	20 whole
Virginia	10 whole
Pecans	2 large whole
Pignoli (pine nuts)	1 tablespoon
Pistachio	1 tablespoon

Fat List (cont.)

Item	Portion
Walnuts	2 whole
Other	1 tablespoon
Oils	
Corn, cottonseed, safflower, soy, sunflower	1 teaspoon
Olive, peanut (monounsaturated)	1 teaspoon
Olives	
green	5 small
black	2 large
Salad dressings	
**French, Italian	1 tablespoon
Mayonnaise type	2 teaspoons
Seeds (without shells)	
sesame, sunflower	1 tablespoon
pumpkin	2 teaspoons

More Saturated

Item	Portion
Butter	1 teaspoon
Bacon, crisp	1 strip
Chitterlings	½ ounce
Coconut, shredded	2 tablespoons
Coffee whitener, liquid	2 tablespoons
Coffee whitener, powder	4 tablespoons
Cool Whip™	3 tablespoons
Cream	
Half and Half	2 tablespoons
Heavy	1 tablespoon
Light	1½ tablespoons
Sour	2 tablespoons
Whipped, fluid	1 tablespoon
Cream, whipped, pressurized topping	⅓ cup

Cream cheese	1 tablespoon
Whipped	2 tablespoons
Lard	1 teaspoon
Margarine, stick	1 teaspoon
Oils, palm, coconut	1 teaspoon
Salt pork	¼ ounce

When using low calorie versions of fat choices, use amounts equal to 45 calories for 1 serving.

*Liquid corn, cottonseed, safflower, soy or sunflower oil should be listed as the first ingredient.
**Can be used with a fat modified diet if made with corn, cottonseed, safflower, soy or sunflower oil.

Miscellaneous List

Because of their ingredients, some foods are considered a combination of choices from several food groups. Pizza, for example, contains ingredients from four of the six food lists. These "mixed" foods can be incorporated into a meal plan by substituting them for choices from more than one food group. A sample list of combination or "mixed" foods appears below.

Item	Portion	Equals
*Canned Soup		
Rice or noodle with broth prepared with water	8 ounces	½ bread, ½ fat (Crackers can be added to make up the remainder of the bread choice. See page 379 for ½ portion.)
Chunky style, ready to serve	8 ounces	1 bread, 1 meat, 1 vegetable
Cream soup		
Made with water	8 ounces	½ bread, 1½ fat

386 Appendices

Miscelleneous List (cont.)	Item	Portion	Equals
	Made with 1% lowfat milk	8 ounces	½ bread, ½ milk, 1½ fat
	Clam Chowder, New England style, prepared with 1% lowfat milk	8 ounces	½ bread, 1 milk, 1 fat
	Lentil with ham, ready to serve	8 ounces	1 bread, 1 meat, 1 vegetable
	Minestrone, ready to serve	8 ounces	1 bread, 1 vegetable
	Split pea with ham, ready to serve	8 ounces	2 bread, 1½ meat
	Tomato, made with water	8 ounces	1 bread
Other Foods	*Plain cheese pizza	⅛ of 14 inch diameter	1 bread, 1 meat, 1 vegetable, 1 fat
	Lasagna, homemade	2½ x 2½ x 1¾ inches	1 bread, 3 meat, 2 vegetable, 1 fat
	*Ravioli, canned	1 cup	1 bread, 1 meat, 1 vegetable
	Beef stew, homemade	1 cup	3 meat, 1 bread, 1 vegetable
	Taco	1	2 meat, 1 bread, 1 fat
	Chili with meat and beans, homemade	1 cup	3 meat, 2 bread
	Frozen iced milk	½ cup	1 bread, 1 fat
	Pudding, sugar-free, made with skim or 1% low-fat milk	½ cup	½ milk, ½ bread
	*Spaghetti with meat, canned	1 cup	1½ bread, 1 vegetable, 1 meat, 1 fat

These products are high in sodium unless specially prepared without salt.

Free Food Group   The following foods contain very few calories and may be used freely in your meal plan. Items marked with an asterisk* should not be used, however, if you are on a salt (sodium) restricted diet.

Item	Portion
General	

*Boullion cubes	*Pickles (unsweetened)
*Broth (clear)	Postum™ (limited to 3 cups daily unless
Calorie free soft drinks	calculated as part of the total daily calories)
*Catsup (1 tablespoon daily—unless calculated	Rennet tablets
as part of the total daily calories	Saccharin
Coffee	Seasonings and condiments (See list below)
*Consomme	*Soy sauce
Cranberries (unsweetened)	Spices
Decaffeinated coffee	*Steak Sauce
Extracts (See list below)	Tabasco sauce
Herbs (See list below)	Taco sauce
Horseradish	Tea
Lemon and lime juice	Unprocessed bran (1 tablespoon)
Lemon rind/lime rind	Vinegar (cider, white, apple, wine)
*Mustard (prepared)	Yeast (dry or cake)
Orange rind	

Item	Portion
Spices, Herbs and Extracts	

Allspice	*Celery salt (seeds, leaves)
Almond extract	Chives
Anise extract	Chocolate extract
Anise seed	Cilantro (Mexican coriander)
Baking powder	Cinnamon
*Baking soda	Cloves
Basil	Cream of tartar
Bay leaf	Cumin
Black cherry extract	Curry
*Bouillon cube	Dill
Butter flavoring	Fennell
*Butter salt	Garlic
Caraway seeds	Ginger
Cardamom	Lemon extract

Item	Portion
Miscellaneous List (cont.)	
Spices, Herbs and Extracts (cont.)	
Mace	Peppermint extract
Maple extract	Pimiento
Mint	Poppy seed
Mustard (dry)	Poultry seed
Nutmeg	Poultry seasonings
Onion (1 tablespoon)	Saccharin
Orange extract	Saffron
Oregano	Sage
Paprika	*Salt
Parsley	Savory
Pepper	

Low or Reduced Calorie Foods

The labels of some foods contain the phrases "low calorie" or "reduced in calories." They will also state the number of calories per serving. *Try to limit the use of these foods to no more than 25 calories in addition to the foods on your meal plan.* Always read the labels carefully, however, before using these products. Consult your physician or dietician if you plan to use them regularly.

Some lower calorie foods you may use in limited quantities are:

diet jellies and jams;
diet syrups;
Equal™;
sugar free hard candy;
sugar free gelatin mixes;
sugar free gum.

Appendix 2. Cholesterol and Saturated Fat Content of Some Foods

Food	Cholesterol	Saturated Fat
Egg yolk	275 mg/oz	1.7 gm/oz
Egg white	0 mg/oz	0 gm/oz
Meat (trimmed of visible fat)		
Beef	25 mg/oz	1.6 gm/oz
Brain	606 mg/oz	*
Chicken, no skin	24 mg/oz	0.5 gm/oz
Kidney	114 mg/oz	*
Lamb	27 mg/oz	1.15 gm/oz
Liver	124 mg/oz	0.83 gm/oz
Pork	25 mg/oz	1.6 gm/oz
Sweetbreads	132 mg/oz	*
Veal	27 mg/oz	0.2 gm/oz
Dairy Products		
Butter	10 mg/tsp	2.4 gm/tsp
Cheddar cheese	30 mg/oz	6.0 gm/oz
Cottage cheese (creamed)	8 mg/¼ cup	6.4 gm/¼ cup
Cream cheese	31 mg/oz	6.2 gm/oz
Ice cream	35 mg/½ cup	5.9 gm/½ cup
Skim milk	6 mg/cup	0.4 gm/cup
Whole milk	34 mg/cup	5.0 gm/cup

*Data not available or unknown.

Appendix 3. Oral Hypoglycemic Agents Available Around the World by Generic and Trade Names

1. ACETOHEXAMIDE

Antrepar	Dymelor	Metaglucina
Dimelin	Gamadiabet	Ordimel
Dimelor	Hipoglicil	

2. AZEPENAMIDE

Betagon	Hexamyl
Betanase	Perinase

3. BENZYLSULFONAMIDE

Gludinase	Gondofo
Glycodiazin	Oisen
Glymidine	Redol

4. BUFORMIN
(Butylbiguanide)

Bumel	Gliporal Lentocaps	Sindatil
Diabetos B.	Munel TM	Tidemol Ret
Diabetun S.	P. 51084	Silubin, Retard
Diabrin	Probucal	

5. CARBUTAMIDE

Alentin	Diabetamide	Norboral Simplex
Antidiabeticum	Diabetoplex	Norboral Vit.
Butylsulfina	Glucidoral	Orank
Carbutamidum	Invenol	Retarden
Carbutil	Midisol	Sulfadiabet
Dia Tablinen	Nadisan	Yosulan

6. CHLORPROPAMIDE

Agnophenol	Diabetasi	Melormin
Apo-Chlorpropam	Diabetex	Nogluc
Bioglumin	Diabetics	Nogral
Catanil	Diabetil	Norboral
Chlopamide	Diabetoral	Novopropamide
Chloromide	Diabikyn	Orabet
Chloronase	Diabinese	Oradian
Chlorpropamida MK	Diabetex	P-604
Chlorpropamide	Dianese	Pamidin
Clordiabet	Galiron	Promide
Clordiasan	Glucopless	Propamid
Copamide	Glucosulfina	Shuabate
Diabinese	Glynese	Stabinol
Diabamide	Melitase	Sucrase
Diabet Pages	Mellinese	Toyomelin
Diabetas	Mellitos-C	

7. GLIBORNURIDE

Glinor	Gluborid	Glutril
Glitrim	Glutrid	Glutrim

8. GLICLAZIDE
Diamicron

9. GLIPENTIDE

10. GLIPIZIDE

Glibenese	Mindiab	Minodiab
Glucotrol	Minidiab	Minodial

11. GLIQUIDONE
Glurenor — Glurenorm

12. GLISOXEPIDE
Bay 4321 — Glucoben — Pro-Diaban

13. GLYBURIDE (glibenclamide)

Adiab	Euglucon-5	Glucoven
Armoniol	Euglyben	Glybenclamidum
Benclamide	Euglykon	Hemi-Daonil
Betanase	Gilamal	Lisaglucon
Clamid	Gliben	Maninil
Daonil	Glibenclamida MK	Micronase
Daopar	Glibenclamidum	Miglucan
Diabeta	Glidiabet	Pira
Diaboral	Glinor	Semi Daonil
Dimel	Glucolon	Semi Euglucon
Euglucan		

14. GLYBUTAMIDE
Glucidoral

15. GLYCODIAZINE
Gluconormal — Lycanol
Gondafon-28 — Redul-28

16. GLYCLOPYRAMIDE
Deamelin-S

17. GLYCYCLAMIDE
Agliral — Diaboral

18. GLYIBUZOL
Gluciase

19. GLYMIDINE
Redul

20. METAHEXAMIDE
Isodiane

21. METFORMIN
(dimethylbiguanide)

Diabetosan	Glucophage	Metformin
Diabex	Glucophage-Ret.	Metforminum
Diabfor	Glucophage Forte	Metiguanide
Diformin-Ret.	Gluformin	Orabet
Glafornil	Glyciphage	Risidon
Gleofago	Glycoran	Rythmes
Glucinan	Isotin	Stagid
Glucofago	Melbin	Tolubol
Glucofagos	Mellitin	Toulibor

22. PHENFORMIN (phenethyl biguanide)

Asipol	Diabiguan	Informin
Azucaps	Diabis Ret.	Insogen
Biguanida Ret.	Diaperos	Insoral
Cronoformin	Dibein	Lentobetic
DB Retard	Dibein Retard	Meltrol
DBI Ret. T.D.	Dibotin	Normoglucina
Debei	Dipar Retard	Oradiabeta
Debeina	Fegunide	Osmoform
Debeone	Glucopostin	Phenformin
Debynil	Glucopostin Ret.	Silubin
Diabetal	Glupostin	Silubin Ret.

23. TOLBUTAMIDE

Apo-Tolbutamide	Mobinol	Tolbutamid
Arcosal	Neo Norboral	Tolbutamid 500
Artosin	Neo Norboral Vit.	Tolbutamid Tabline
Artosina	Neobellin	Tolbutamid Ratio
Butamide	Novobutamide	Tolbutamida
Catanil	Oralin	Tolbutamide
Debetos 500	Oramide	Tolbutin
Diaben	Ordiabet	Tolbutone
Diabuton	Orinase	Tolgybuzamide
Diasulfon	Osdiabet	Tolnin
Diabetos	Pramidex	Tolurasi
Dolipol	Rastinon	Toluvaj
Edudine	Riboral	Tolvit
Guabeta N	Sinabetes	Varoxina
Mellitol	Tolbet	Yosulan T
Mellitos D	Tolbumid	

24. TOLAZAMIDE

Diabewas	Tolanase	Tolinase
Diabutos	Tolinas	Tolisan
Norglycin		

25. CARBUTAMIDE AND PHENFORMIN
Glucifrene

26. CARBUTAMIDE AND CHOLINBITARTRATE
Antidiabeticum

27. CHLORPROPAMIDE AND METFORMIN

Diabiformin	Mellitron	Obinese
Diabiphage		

28. CHLORPROPAMIDE AND PHENFORMIN

Bidiabe	Diabis Compositum	Insone
Biodiabes	Diabitol	Reobron
Chlorformin	Endiabin	Trane
Combinacin	Insogen Plus	Zacharol
Diabetoplex		

29. GLYBURIDE AND PHENFORMIN

Bi-Euglucon	Gliben F	Norglicem
Daopar	Gliformin	Suguan
Gli-Norboral Cpto		

30. GLYCYCLAMIDE AND METFORMIN

Agliral Compuesto	Diabomet	Diabone

31. GLYSOXEPIDE AND BUFORMIN
Sindiatil

32. TOLBUTAMIDE AND METFORMIN
Glucosulfa

33. TOLBUTAMIDE AND PHENFORMIN

Melus	Tolbusan	Ultra-Norboral, 500
Oraleo		

34. PHENFORMIN AND CHLOROBENZSULFOUR
Bidiabe

35. PHENFORMIN AND OXYPRODIOPHEN

DB Comb.	Prodiaben

NOTE: All are sulfonyluria derivatives unless otherwise designated.

Appendix 4. Automatic Insulin Injectors

Product	Description/Use	Source
Injection Devices		
Injectomatic	Use with Monoject syringe. Insert syringe, press against skin to inject needle. Patient pushes plunger.	Sherwood Medical, 1831 Olive St., St. Louis, MO 63103
Instaject	Similar to Injectomatic. Takes any syringe.	Jordan Enterprises, 1026 Brent Ave., South Pasedena, CA 91030
Diamatic	A full syringe is placed in this metal device, which injects the needle and pushes the plunger.	Ulster Scientific, P.O. Box 902, Highland, NY 12528
Autoject	Similar to Diamatic, but plastic.	Ulster Scientific (address above)
Jet Injectors		
Medi-Jector	2 sizes, up to 50 or 100 units (LV or II models).	Derata Corp., 7380 32nd Ave. North, Minneapolis, MN 55427
Preci-Jet	1 size, up to 50 units. Clicks for each unit to help the visually impaired.	Ulster Scientific (address above)
Vitajet	1 size, up to 50 units.	Vitajet Precision Instruments, Inc., 917 Gleneyre St., Laguna Beach, CA 92551
Button Infuser	Allows several days of injections into same site with only one puncture.	Markwell Medical Institute, Inc., P.O. Box 5173, Racine, WI 53405

Appendix 5. Insulin Pumps

NOTE: It is likely that this list will change as newer models are introduced and older models are replaced. You should discuss pump choice with your health care team.

Pump	Manufacturer
Betatron I	Cardiac Pacemakers, Inc. (CPI), 4100 North Hamline Ave., St. Paul, MN 55164 (800) 328-9588.
Betatron II	CPI (address as above)
Betatron IV	CPI (address as above)
Eugly	Travenol/Autosyringe, 1425 Lake Cook Rd., Deerfield, IL 60015. (800) 323-5490.
Minimed 504	Mini Med Technologies 12744 San Fernando Road, Sylmar, CA 91342 (818) 362-6822; 1-800-423-5611.
B-D 1000	Becton Dickinson & Co., 2 Bridgewater Lane, Lincoln Park, NJ 07035. (800) BECTON 6.

Appendix 6.   White Classification of Diabetes in Pregnant Women

Type	Description
Gestational Diabetes	Develops during pregnancy. Depending on the degree of blood glucose elevation, it may be managed by a carefully designed meal plan or by a meal plan and insulin injections.
Types I and II	
Class A	Any onset age and duration of diabetes. Managed by carefully designed eating plan.
Class B	Onset of diabetes age 20 years or older and duration less than 10 years. Managed by a carefully designed meal plan and insulin injections.
Class C	Onset of diabetes 10 to 19 years of age or duration of diabetes 10 to 19 years. Managed by carefully designed meal plan and insulin injections.
Class D	Onset of diabetes under 10 years of age, or duration of diabetes over 20 years, or minimal eye complications or hypertension (high blood pressure). Managed by a carefully designed meal plan and insulin injections.
Class R	Advanced eye complications. Managed by a carefully designed meal plan, insulin injections, and laser treatments for eye complications.
Class F	Kidney complications. Managed by a carefully designed meal plan, insulin injections, and close attention to condition of the kidneys.
Class RF	Both eye and kidney complications. Managed by a carefully designed meal plan, insulin injections, laser treatments for eye complications, and close attention to condition of the kidneys.
Class H	Heart complications. Managed by a carefully designed meal plan, insulin injections, and heart medications.
Class T	Prior kidney transplant. Managed by a carefully designed meal plan, insulin injections, and continuation of steroid and/or immunosuppressive medication (medication to suppress rejection).

Appendix 7. Resources for the Elderly

American Association for Retired Persons. 1909 K St., NW, Washington, DC 20049. (202) 872-4700.

American Council for the Blind. 1211 Connecticut Ave., NW, Washington, DC 20036. (800) 424-8666.

American Diabetes Association. 1660 Duke St., Alexandria, VA 22314. (703) 549-1500.

American Diatetic Association. 430 N. Michigan Ave., Chicago, IL 60611. (312) 280-5000.

American Heart Association. 7320 Greenville Ave., Dallas, TX 75231. (214) 750-5300.

Arthritis Association. 1314 Spring St., Atlanta, GA 30309. (404) 872-7100.

Children of Aging Parents. 2761 Trenton Rd., Levittown, PA 19056. (215) 547-1070.

Family Service Association of America. 44 E. 23rd St., New York, NY 10010. (212) 674-6100.

National Association of Area Agencies on Aging. 600 Maryland Ave., SW, Suite 208, Washington, DC 20024. (202) 484-7520.

National Council of Senior Citizens. 925 15th St., NW, Washington, DC 20005. (202) 347-8800.

Check in addition:
  Phone book yellow pages under social service organizations
  Phone book blue pages for government agencies
  Local diabetes societies
  Local hospitals
  Veterans' agencies
  Church or synagogue
  Local library

Index

Page numbers in italics indicate figures; page numbers followed by *t* indicate tables.

AARP; *see* American Association for
   Retired Persons
Abortion, spontaneous, 232
Abscess(es)
   infection site, 267-268
   intensive insulin therapy and, 185
Abuse of drug, 324-327
Accu-Chek II, 141*t*
Acetohexamide, 98, 390
Acetone
   odor of, 259-260
   urinary
      immediate treatment of, 361
      testing for, 148-149, 150*t*
Acidosis, 257-262
   pregnancy and, 232
Activity; *see* Exercise
Acupuncture, 328-329
Additive in food, 70
Adhesive, 184-185
Adipose tissue, 10, *11*
Adolescent, 210-211
Adrenal gland, 23
Adrenaline, 8, 326-327
   hypoglycemia and, 248
Aging, 22, 240-245
Air travel, 338-339
Alcohol, 319-323
Aldose reductase inhibitor, 355
Algorithm(s)
   illness and, 186-187
   intensive insulin therapy, 176, *177*,
      178-179
Allergy, insulin, 266-267
Alpha cell, 5
Alpha-fetoprotein blood test, 231
American Association for Retired Persons,
   313
Amino acid, 114-115
Amniocentesis, 225, 236

Amniotic fluid, 233
Amyotrophy, 286
Antibiotic, 282
Antibody, 115
Antigen, 21
Anxiety, 306
Artificial miniature beta cell, 352
Artificial pancreas, 350, 352
Ascorbic acid, 73*t*
Aspartame, 67-69, 67*t*
Atherosclerosis, 60
Athlete's foot, 298-299
Atony of bladder, 282-283
Atrophy, 267
Autoclix, 144*t*
Autoimmune reaction, 16
Autoject, 393
Autolance, 144*t*
Auto-Lancet, 145*t*
Autolet, 145*t*
Autolet-DTV, 145*t*
Automatic insulin injector, 393
Azepenamide, 390

Babysitter, 213-214
Background retinopathy, 223
Balanitis, 268
Battery, 184
B-D 1000, 394
Bee sting, 331-332
Benedict's solution, 147*t*
Benzylsulfonamide, 390
Beta cell(s)
   artificial miniature, 352
   function of, 3
   insulin production and, 6
Betascan, 141*t*
Betatron, 394
Biguanide, 103, 192
Bilirubin, 236

Biofeedback, 329
Biostator, 351
Biotin, 72t
Birth control, 334-335
    oral contraceptive and, 326
Black toenail, 362
Bladder, urinary, 282-283
Block testing, 152
Blood glucose; see Glucose; Monitoring of
        blood glucose
Blood pressure
    hypertension and
        kidney research and, 356
        mineral excess and, 76
    hypotension and, 286
Blurring of vision, 27-28, 265-266
    immediate treatment of, 362
Bottle feeding, 237
Bracelet, identification, 316-317
Brain, 248
Bread list, 373-379
Breast-feeding, 237
Brittle diabetes, 197
Bruise, 362
Buformin, 390
Burn, laser, 277
Button infuser, 393

Calcium, 76
Calories
    alcohol and, 320-323, 321t
    requirements for, 51-53
Camp, 214-215, 331
Candidasis, 27
Candy, 69
CAPD; see Continuous ambulatory
        peritoneal dialysis
Carbohydrate(s)
    diet and, 49-50, 57-58
    fuel and, 8-10, 9
    types of, 55-56
Carbuncle, 292
Carbutamide, 390, 392
Card, identification, 316-317
Cardiovascular complication, 290-291
Career guidance, 315-316
Cataract, 271, 273-274
Catheter, 184-185
Cerebrovascular accident, 290
Cesarean delivery, 236
Charcot's joint, 288
Chemstrip bG, 140t
Chemstrip UG, 148t
Child(ren), 195-217
    babysitter and, 213-214
    camps and, 214-215
    causes of diabetes and, 197
    goals for, 216-217

growth and development of, 211-212
hypoglycemic reaction and, 249-250
insulin-dependent diabetes and, 196-198
menstruation and, 213
metabolic abnormality and, 236
monitoring of, 205-207
psychological factors and, 209-211
stages of diabetes and, 198-199
survival skills for parent and, 207-208
treatment of, 200-205
types of diabetes and, 197-198
Childbearing; see Pregnancy
Chlorobenzsulfour, 392
Chlorpropamide, 98, 390, 392
Cholecalciferol, 73t
Cholesterol, 59, 61
    foods and, 389
Cholinbitartrate, 392
Chromosome, 19-20
Cigarette smoking, 323-324
Circulatory system, 290-291
Claudication, 290
Closed-loop pump, 352-353, 352
    intensive insulin therapy and, 172, 173
Clothing, 336-337
Cocaine, 325
Coldness, 285-289
Coma
    hyperglycemia and, 257-262
    immediate treatment for, 360
Committee on Food and Nutrition of
        American Diabetes Association, 50
Complication(s)
    acute, 246-268
        atrophy and, 267
        blood glucose and, 262-265, 265
        blurred vision and, 265-266
        chronic versus, 246-247
        hyperglycemia and, 257-262
        hypertrophy and, 267
        hypoglycemia and 247-257
        infection and, 267-268
        insulin resistance and, 268
    longterm, 269-302
        cardiovascular, 290-291
        eyes and, 270-280, 271, 277
        foot and, 292-300
        infection and, 291-292
        kidney and urinary tract and,
                280-284, 281
        neuropathy and, 284-290
        skin and, 300-301
    obstetrical, 232-233
    older patient and, 245
    research and, 354-356
Conjunctivitis, 271-272
Contact lens, 330
Continuous ambulatory peritoneal dialysis,

283
Continuous subcutaneous insulin infusion,
    182-186
Contraception, 334-335
    oral contraceptive and, 326
Convulsion, 360
Cortisol, 23
Counseling
    career, 315-316
    group therapy and, 77-78
    marriage, 333
C-peptide, 6
Cramp, leg, 27
Crystal, insulin and, 119-120
CSH; see Continuous subcutaneous insulin
    infusion
Culture, urine and, 227
CVA; see Cerebrovascular accident
Cyclamate, 67, 68-69
Cystitis, 281

Dawn phenomenon
    hormone and, 23
    intensive insulin therapy and, 170, 172
DCCT; see Diabetes Control and
    Complications Trial
Delivery of infant, 235-236; see also
    Pregnancy
Denial, 305-306
Dental problem, 328
Dermatophytosis, 298-299
Development, child and, 211-212
Dextrose, 65
Diabeta; see Glyburide
Diabetes Control and Complications Trial,
    354-355
Diabetic ketoacidosis
    hyperglycemia and, 257-262
    pregnancy and, 232
Diabetic Retinopathy Study, 278
Diagen, 141t
Dialysis, renal, 283
Diamatic, 393
Diarrhea, 342
Diascan, 141t
Diastix, 148t
Diatron Easy Test, 141t
Diet; see Nutrition
Dietitian, 62-63
Digestion, 7-8
Direct 30/30, 142t
Disability insurance, 311-312
Discrimination, job, 313-315
Disposable syringe, 121
Diuretic, 327
DKA; see Diabetic ketoacidosis
DNA
    insulin production and, 6

recombinant, 116
Dosing schedule, 169-170, 169
Double vision, 286
Down's syndrome, 225
Doxycycline hyclate, 342
Driving, 318
DRS; see Diabetic Retinopathy Study
Drug; see Medication(s)

Ear piercing, 331
Early Treatment of Diabetic Retinopathy
    Study, 278-279, 355
Easy Stik Lancet, 145t
Eating plan(s), 50-61
    pregnancy and, 234-235
Eclampsia, 233
Economics of education, 45
Edema
    insulin, 266
    macular, 278-279
Education, 34, 38-46
    child and, 201-202
    intensive insulin therapy and, 175
    opportunity for, 315-316
Eicosapentaenoic acid, 60
Ejaculation, retrograde, 288
Elderly patient, 396
Emergency insulin, 119
Emotional response of child, 209-211
Employment, 313-315
Endocrine gland, 3
Endurance training, 84-85; see also
    Exercise
Energy, 7-8
Epinephrine, 8, 326-327
"Equal" sweetener, 68
Erection, 287, 333-334
ETDRS; see Early Treatment Diabetic
    Retinopathy Study
Eugly, 394
Exactech, 142t
Exercise, 81-93, 86t, 87t
    adjusting treatment to, 89-93
    aging and, 243
    child and, 204-205
    endurance training and, 84-85
    insulin reaction and, 365
    nutrition and, 90-92
    program for, 84-88
    pumps and, 187
    sports and, 332
    type II diabetes and, 190-191
Exocrine function, 5
Eye(s), 270-280, 271, 277
    blurred vision and, 27-28, 265-266
    conjunctivitis and, 271-272
    contact lens and, 330

double vision and, 286
hemorrhage and, 271-272, 275
immediate treatment of, 362
pregnancy and, 223-224
research and, 355
retinopathy and; see Retinopathy

Fast sugar, 55
Fasting, 79-80
Fasting blood glucose
  diagnosis of diabetes and, 29
  intensive therapy and, 180
Fat(s)
  diet and, 58-61
  energy and, 10, 11
  food list and, 383-385
  fuel and, 12-13
  obesity and, 53-55
  pregnancy and, 220-221
  saturated, 389
Fatigue, 27
Fear, 306
Fetal development, 231-232; see also
  Pregnancy
Fiber, 56-57
Finger-pricking device, 143, 144-145t
Fluid, 92
Folic acid, 72t
Food; see Nutrition
Food choice list, 368-388
Foot, 292-300
  Charcot's joint and, 288
  immediate treatment of, 362
Foot-drop, 286
Framingham Heart Study, 290-291
Fructose, 65, 66
Fruit list, 371-373
Fuel, body; see Nutrition
Fungal infection, 298-299

Genital infection, 268
Gestational diabetes, 19, 221-222; see also
  Pregnancy
Gland, endocrine, 3
Glaucoma, 271, 272-273
Glibornuride, 390
Gliclazide, 390
Glipizide, 99, 101-102, 390
Gliquidone, 391
Glisoxepide, 391
Globin, 113
Glomeruli, 283
Glucagon, 8
  hormone and, 23
  hypoglycemia and, 255-256
  pancreas and, 5
Glucochek SC, 142t
Glucolet, 145t

Glucometer II, 142t
Glucosan 2000, 142t
Glucosan 3000, 143t
Glucose, 2-3, 13, 65-67
  breast-feeding and, 237
  carbohydrates and, 8-10
  diagnosis and, 28-30
  hyperglycemia and, 257-262
    exercise and, 90
    intensive therapy and, 179-181
  hypoglycemia and; see Hypoglycemia
  infant and, 236
  meter for, 139-140, 140t, 141-143t
  monitoring of; see Monitoring of blood
    glucose
  pregnancy and, 220-221, 235; see also
    Pregnancy
  sensor for, 353
  sulfonylurea and, 102-103
  urinary, 29-30
    immediate treatment of, 361-362
    testing for, 134, 146-149, 147t, 148t,
    149t
Glucose tolerance
  aging and, 241-242
  test for, 18-19
    diagnosis and, 29
    pregnancy and, 221-222, 222t
Glucostix, 140t
Glucosystem Lancet, 145t
Glucotrol; see Glipizide
Glybenclamide, 99
Glyburide, 99, 101-102, 391, 392
Glybutamide, 391
Glycemic index, 55-56
Glyclopyramide, 391
Glycodiazine, 391
Glycogen, 8-9, 10
  diet and, 57-58
Glycohemoglobin
  child and, 206-207
  kidney research and, 356
  measurement of, 135-137
Glycosuria, 198
Glycosylated hemoglobin; see
  Glycohemoglobin
Glycyclamide, 391, 392
Glyibuzol, 391
Glymidine, 391
Group insurance, 311
Group therapy for weight loss, 77-78
Growth of child, 211-212
GTT; see Glucose tolerance, test for
Guidance, career, 315-316
Guilt, 307
Gynecological problem, 27

HDL; see High-density lipoprotein

Healing, 292, 365
  necrobiosis lipoidica diabeticorum and,
    300-301
Health insurance, 310-312
Health maintenance organization, 311
Health record, 337
Heart disease, 290-291
Hemoglobin, glycosylated; see
  Glycohemoglobin
Hemorrhage
  retinitis and, 271-272
  retinopathy and, 275
  subconjunctival, 272
  immediate treatment of, 362
Heredity, 19-21
Heroin, 325
High-density lipoprotein, 60
HLA system; see Human lymphocyte
  antigen system
HMO; see Health maintenance
  organization
Home urine testing, 134; see also Urine
Honeybee, 332
Hormone, 23
Human insulin, 353;
  see also Insulin
Human lymphocyte antigen system, 21
Hyperglycemia, 257-262
  exercise and, 90
  intensive therapy and, 179-181
Hyperosmotic coma, 258-259
Hypertension
  kidney research and, 356
  mineral excess and, 76
Hypertrophy, 267
Hypoglycemia, 247-257
  exercise and, 365
  immediate treatment of, 363, 364
  infant and, 236
  intensive therapy and, 180-182
  ketones and, 149
  reactive, 257
  sexual activity and, 335
  symptoms of, 247-248
  treatment of, 160, 363
Hypoglycemic agent(s), oral, 94-106, 320,
    390-392
  classes of, 98, 99, 100-102
  exercise and, 89
  function of, 97-100
  older patient and, 243-244
  side effects of, 102-103
  sulfonylurea and, 94-106, 320
  type II diabetes and, 17-18, 191-194
  University Group Diabetes Program
    Report and, 104-105
  wrong dosage of, 364
Hypotension, 286

IDDM; see Insulin-dependent diabetes
  mellitus
Identification
  jewelry and, 316-317
  travel and, 337
IGT; see Impaired glucose tolerance
Illness, 24, 359-361
  insulin pump and, 186
  insulin requirement and, 262-264
  prevention of, 365
Immune reaction, 16
Impaired glucose tolerance, 18-19
Impotence, 27, 286-287
Infant, 212; see also Child(ren)
Infection(s), 24, 291-292
  abscess and, 267-268
  foot and, 293-294
  fungal, 298-299
  genital, 268
  kidney and, 283
  urinary tract, 282
  pregnancy and, 227
Inflatable penile prosthesis, 288
Infusion pump, 164-165
  closed loop, 352-353, 352
  intensive therapy and, 172-174, 172,
    173, 174, 182-186
  open-loop, 172, 173
Injection of insulin, 122-127, 128, 129,
    130, 130-131
  automatic injector and, 393
  child and, 203, 210
  injection site and, 130-131
  multiple daily, 175-182
  older patient and, 244
Injectomatic, 393
Insect sting, 331-332
Insoluble fiber, 56
Instaject, 393
Insulin, 107-131, 108, 109, 112, 113t,
    117-118t
  allergy to, 266-267
  antibodies and, 115
  characteristics of, 110-115
  child and, 202-203
  cloudy, 120
  coma and, 260-262
  conventional treatment and, 154-163,
    159t, 161t, 162t, 163t
  crystal and, 119-120
  definition of, 109-110
  edema and, 266
  emergency, 119
  exercise and, 90, 92-93
  food and, 204
  hyperosmotic coma and, 258-259
  illness and, 360-361
  infant and, 236

infusion pump and; see Infusion pump
injection of; see Injection of insulin
intensive therapy and, 164-188; see
    also Insulin-dependent
    diabetes, intensive therapy and
intermediate
    intensive therapy and, 170
    pregnancy and, 228-230t
    type II diabetes and, 166
lente, 113
newer, 116, 353-354
normal metabolism of, 7-8
older patient and, 243-244
pregnancy and, 220-221, 226,
    228-230t, 234-236
production of, 6
regular, 111
    cloudy, 120
    intensive therapy and, 170, 171
    pregnancy and, 229t, 230t
relative insufficiency of, 349
resistance to, 100
    hyperosmotic coma and, 258-259
    research and, 348-349
    type II diabetes and, 189-190
school and, 210, 213
storage of, 119-120
synthetic, 353
syringe and, 120-121, 121t
travel and, 120
treatment and, 35-37
types of, 116-119
ultralente, 113
    algorithm for, 177
    intensive therapy and, 170, 171
urine testing and, 151
Insulin reaction; see Hypoglycemia
Insulin-dependent diabetes mellitus, 15-17
    child and, 196-198
    exercise and, 89-90
    intensive treatment of, 164-188
        dawn phenomenon and, 170, 172
        definition of, 164-165
        dosing schedules and, 169-170, 169
        infusion pump and, 172-174, 172,
            173, 174, 182-188
        living with, 177-182
        need for, 168-169
        preparing for, 175-177
        reason for, 165-168
    prevention of, 347-348
Insurance
    health, 310-312
    life, 312-313
    travel and, 335-336
Intermediate insulin
    intensive therapy and, 170
    pregnancy and, 228-230t

    type II diabetes and, 166
Intrauterine device, 334-335
Iron, 76
Islet cell transplantation, 350
Islets of Langerhans, 3, 5
IUD; see Intrauterine device

Jet injector, 130, 393
Jet lag, 339-340
Job discrimination, 313-315
Joint, Charcot's, 288
Juice, 248-249
Juvenile diabetes, 197

Ketoacidosis
    hyperglycemia and, 257-262
    pregnancy and, 232
Ketone, 60
    exercise and, 90
    pregnancy and, 231
Kidney, 280-284, 281
    glycosuria and, 198
    pregnancy and, 224
    research and, 356
Kidney dam, 14, 14
Krebs cycle, 7-8

Labels on food, 64-65
Laceration, 362, 365
Lancet, 143, 144-145t
Laser, 277-279
LDL; see Low-density lipoprotein
Leg(s)
    cramp and, 27
    necrobiosis lipoidica diabeticorum and,
        300-301
Lens, contact, 330
Lente insulin, 113
Life insurance, 312-313
Life span, 307-308
Lipid, 58-61
Lipoprotein, 58-61
Low blood sugar; see also Hypoglycemia
Low-density lipoprotein, 58-61

Macrosomia, 236
Macular edema, 278-279
Male sexual function, 333-334
    impotence and, 286-287
Mannitol, 65
Marijuana, 324-325
Marriage counseling, 333
Maturity of fetus, 236
Maturity-onset diabetes of youth, 18, 198
    diet and, 203
Meals; see Nutrition
Meat list, 380-382
Medicaid/Medicare, 311-312

Medication, 324-327; *see also* Oral
    hypoglycemic agent(s)
  blood sugar and, 23-24
  cardiovascular complications and,
      291
  oral, 35
  travel and, 337-338
  type II diabetes and, 191-194
Medi-Jector, 393
Meditation, 329
Menstruation, 213
Mental stress, 25
Messenger RNA, 6
Metabolism, 7-8
  abnormality and, 236
  pregnancy and, 234-235
Metahexamide, 391
Meter, glucose, 139-140, 140t, 141-143t
Metformin, 391, 392
Microaneurysm, 275
Micro-Fine Lancet, 145t
Micronase; *see* Glyburide
Milk list, 368-369
Minerals, 75-76
Miniature beta cell, 352
Minimed, 501, 394
MODY; *see* Maturity-onset diabetes of
    youth
Moisturizing lotion, 295
Moniliasis, 27
Monitoring of blood glucose, 132-153
  child and, 205-207
  diabetes control and, 157
  fetal development and, 231-232
  glycohemoglobin measurement and,
      135-137
  history of, 133-134
  office, 138
  older patient and, 244
  pregnancy and, 227, 231
  reason for, 132-133
  self-, 139-146, 140-145t, 150-153
    Diabetes Control and Complications
        Trial and, 354-355
    intensive insulin therapy and, 175-176
  urine test and, 146-149; *see also*
      Urine
Monojector, 145t
Monolet Lancet, 145t
Monounsaturated fat, 59-60
Morphine, 325
Mortality, 307-308
Multiple daily injection, 175-182; *see also*
    Injection of insulin
Muscle wasting, 286

Nails, 295
Nasal insulin, 354

National Institutes of Health, 354-355
Necrobiosis lipoidica diabeticorum,
    300-301
Needle of catheter, 185
Neovascularization, 223
Nephropathy, 281, 283
Nervous system, 27
Neuritis, 266
Neuropathy, 266, 284-290
  pregnancy and, 224
Niacin, 72t
NIDDM; *see* Non-insulin-dependent
    diabetes mellitus
Nonfunctioning bladder, 282-283
Non-insulin-dependent diabetes mellitus,
    15, 17-18, 189-194
  child and, 198
  exercise and, 89
  prevention of, 348-349
Non-nutritive sweetener,
    67-69, 67t
Nonstress test, 231-232
Nonstrip urine glucose test, 147t
Numbness, 285-289
Nursing, 237
Nutrisweet, 67-68
Nutrition, 22-23, 47-80
  aging and, 241, 243
  body fuel and, 47-48
  child and, 203-205
  coma and, 259
  diet control and, 48-50
  dietetic foods and, 69
  dietician's role in, 62-63
  eating plan and, 50-51, 61, 63-64
    pregnancy and, 234-235
  exercise and, 90-92
  fasting and, 79-80
  food additives and, 70
  food choice lists and, 368-388
  food labels and, 64-65
  food quantities and, 51-53
  food types and, 55-61
  intensive therapy and, 182
  kidney and, 283, 356
  minerals and, 75-76
  organic foods and, 79
  pregnancy and, 234-235, 235t
  saturated fat and, 59, 389
  sick days and, 264t
  sweeteners and, 65-69
  treatment and, 34-35
  type II diabetes and, 190
  urine testing and, 151
  vegetarianism and, 78-79
  vitamins and, 70-75, 72-73t
  weight-loss and, 76-78
Nutritive sweetener, 65-67

Obesity, 22, 53-55
Obstetrical complication, 232-233; *see also* Pregnancy
Odor of acetone, 259-260
Office blood glucose measurement, 138
One Touch, 143*t*
Open-loop pump, *172*, 173
Opiate, 325
Oral contraceptive, 326, 334
Oral hypoglycemic agent(s), 35, 94-106, 390-392
    exercise and, 89
    function of, 97-100
    older patient and, 243-244
    side effects of, 102-103
    sulfonylurea and, 94-106, 320
    type II diabetes and, 17-18, 191-194
    University Group Diabetes Program Report and, 104-105
    wrong dosage of, 364
Orange juice, 248-249
Organic diet, 79
Orthostatic hypotension, 286
Oxyprodiophen, 392
Oxytocin challenge test, 232

Pain, 286
Pancreas
    artificial, 350, 352
    function of, 3-6, *4*, *5*
    transplantation of, 349-350
Pancrease, 114
Pan-retinal photocoagulation, 278
Panthothenic acid, 72*t*
Penis
    infection and, 268
    prosthesis and, 288
Penlet, 145*t*
Peripheral neuropathy, 285-286
Phenethyl biguanide, 391
Phenformin, 103, 391
    sulfonylurea agents and, 192
Phenylketonuria, 67-68
Photocoagulation laser, 277-279
Pituitary hormone, 23
PKU; *see* Phenylketonuria
Plaque, dental, 328
Pneumovax, 292
Poison ivy, 331
Polster valve, 287
Polyhydramnios, 233
Polyunsaturated fat, 59-60
Portuguese men-of-war, 332
PotAGT; *see* Potential abnormality of glucose tolerance
Potassium, 76
Potential abnormality of glucose tolerance, 18

Preci-Jet, 393
Preeclampsia, 233
Pregnancy, 19, 218-239, 219*t*, *220*
    breastfeeding and, 237
    complications of, 232-233
    delivery and, 235-236
    diet and, 234-235, 235*t*
    glucose tolerance and, 221-222, 222*t*
    intensive insulin therapy and, 227, 231
    ketones and, 231
    monitoring fetal development and, 231-232
    oral medications and, 192
    stress test and, 232
    urinary tract infection and, 227, 232-233
    weight and, 234
    White classification and, 223, 395
Presbyopia, 265-266
Prevention
    of diabetes, 347-349
    of illness, 365
Proinsulin, 6, 353-354
Proliferative retinopathy; *see* Retinopathy
Prosthesis, penile, 288
Protamine zinc insulin, 111, 113, *113*
Protein
    diet and, 58
    fuel and, 11
Psychological factors, 209-211
Pump, insulin infusion, 164-165
    closed-loop, 352-353, *352*
    intensive therapy and, 172-174, *173*, *174*, 182-186
    open-loop, *172*, 173
Pyelonephritis, *281*
Pyridoxal, 72*t*
Pyridoxamine, 72*t*
Pyridoxine, 72*t*

Quick carbohydrate, 55

Radiating pain, 286
Radicular pain, 286
RDA; *see* Recommended Daily Allowance
Reactive hypoglycemia, 257
Rebounding
    hypoglycemia and, 250
    insulin treatment and, 160
    ketones and, 149
Recombinant DNA, 116
Recommended Daily Allowance, 71-74, 72-73*t*
Record keeping, 150-151
Recreational drug, 324-327
Registered dietitian, 62-63
Regular insulin, 111
    cloudy, 120

intensive therapy and, 170, *171*
  pregnancy and, 229*t*, 230*t*
Relaxation therapy, 329
Renal function, 280-284, *281*
  glycosuria and, 198
  pregnancy and, 224
  research and, 356
  transplantation and, 282-284
Research, 347-358
  Diabetes Control and Complications
    Trial and, 354-355
  eye and, 355
  kidney and, 356
  newer insulins and, 353-354
  prevention of diabetes and, 347-349
  transplantation of pancreas and,
    349-350
Resistance, insulin, 100, 268
  hyperosmotic coma and, 258-259
  research and, 348-349
  type II diabetes and, 189-190
Retinitis, 271-272; *see also* Eye(s)
Retinol, 72*t*
Retinopathy, 272, *273*, *274*, 274-279; *see
    also* Eye(s)
  cesarean delivery and, 236
  photocoagulation laser and, 277-279
  pregnancy and, 223-224
  proliferative, 275
  research and, 355
Retrograde ejaculation, 288
Riboflavin, 72*t*
RNA, 6

Saccharin, 67-69, 67*t*
Saturated fat, 59, 389
Schedule of dosing, 169-170, *169*
School, 213
  insulin injection and, 210
Sclerosis of kidney, 283
Seasickness, 340, 342
Secondary diabetes, 19
Seizure, 360
Self-monitoring of blood glucose, 139-146,
    140*t*, 141-143*t*, 144-145*t*, 150-153,
    355
  child and, 205-207
  Diabetes Control and Complications
    Trial and, 355
  intensive insulin therapy and, 175-176
  older patient and, 244
Semilente, 113
Semi-synthetic insulin, 116
Sensory neuropathy, 285-289
Septra; *see* Sulfamethoxazole
Sexual function
  male, 332-335
    impotence and, 27, 286-287

retrograde ejaculation and, 288
  oral contraceptive and, 326
Ship travel, 340-342
Shoes, 296, 298
Sick day(s), 359-361
  insulin requirement and, 262-264
  prevention of illness and, 365
  pump and, 186
Skin, 26, 300-301
  foot and, 294-296
Sleeping pill, 325
Slow sugar, 55
SMBG; *see* Self-monitoring of blood
    glucose
Smoking, 323-324
Sodium, 76
Soluble fiber, 56-57
Somatostatin
  hormone and, 23
  pancreas and, 5-6
Somogyi effect, 250
Sorbitol, 65, 66-67
Spice list, 387-388
Split-mix insulin program, 170
  child and, 202-203
Spontaneous abortion, 232
Sports, 332
Starch list, 373-379
Stasis, urine, *281*
Stillbirth, 233
Sting of insect, 331-332
Storage, 119-120
Strength training, 84-85; *see also* Exercise
Stress, 24-25
Stress test, fetal, 232
Strip-reading meter, 139-140, 140*t*,
    141-143*t*
Stroke, 290
Subconjunctival hemorrhage, 272
  immediate treatment of, 362
Subcutaneous insulin infusion, 182-186
Sucrose, 65-66; *see also* Glucose
Sugar; *see* Glucose
Sulfamethoxazole, 342
Sulfonylurea, 94-106, 320
  availability of, 100-102
  function of, 97-100
  side effects of, 102-103
  type II diabetes and, 17-18, 191-194
  University Group Diabetes Program
    Report and, 104-105
Sunburn, 331
Surgery, 327-328
Sweetener, 65-69
Synthetic insulin, 116
  human, 353
Syringe, insulin, 120-121, 121*t*
  pump and, 184

Tape and infusion set, 184-185
Test strip, 148*t*
Tes-Tape, 148*t*
Testing; *see* Monitoring of blood glucose;
 Urine
Thiamin, 72*t*
Time zones, 339-340, *341*, 342
Tingling, 285-289
Tocopherol, 73*t*
Tolazamide, *98*, 392
Tolbutamide, *98*, 392
"Tourista," 342
Toxemia, 233
Toxicity, 103
Tracer, 143*t*
Training; *see* Exercise
Tranquilizer, 325
Transoceanic crossing, 340-342
Transplantation
 islet cell, 350
 of pancreas, 349-350
 renal, 282-284
Trauma, 25
 immediate treatment of, 362, 365
Travel, 335-344
 time zones and, 339-340, *341*, 342
Trends Lancet, 145*t*
Trendsmeter, 143*t*
TrendStrip, 140*t*
Triglyceride, 58-61
Trimethoprim, 342
Twenty-four hour urine test, 147-148
Type II diabetes; *see* Non-insulin-
 dependent diabetes mellitus

UGDP; *see* University Group Diabetes
 Program
Ultralente insulin, 113
 algorithm for, *177*
 intensive therapy and, 170, *171*
Ultrasound test, 231
Unconsciousness, 360
 hypoglycemia and, 257-262
Unilet Lancet, 145*t*

University Group Diabetes Program,
 104-105
Urinary tract, 280-284, *281*
 infection and, 227, 232-233
Urine
 acetone in, 148-149, 150*t*, 361
 glucose in, 29-30, 149*t*, 361-362
 home testing and, 134
 immediate treatment for, 361-362
 testing for, 146-149, 147*t*, 148*t*
 ketones and, 231
 pregnancy and, 227, 231
 stasis of, *281*

Vacation pump, 187-188
Vaccine, 292
Vaginal infection, 268
Valve, polster, 287
Vegetable list, 369-370
Vegetarian diet, 78-79
Vibramycin; *see* Doxycycline hyclate
Virus, 21-22
Visidex H, 140*t*
Vision; *see also* Eye(s); Retinopathy
 blurred, 27-28, 265-266
 immediate treatment of, 362
 double, 286
Vitajet, 393
Vitamin, 70-75, 72-73*t*
Vitrectomy, 279-280
Vitreous hemorrhage, 275

Wasp sting, 331-332
Weight
 loss of, 76-78
 type II diabetes and, 190
 pregnancy and, 234
White clasification of pregnancy, 223, 365
Wine, 320-322, 321*t*

Xanthoma, 26
Xenon-arc photocoagulator, 278

Yellow jacket sting, 332